BUSINESS/SCIENCE/TECHNOLOGY DIVISION
CHICAGO PUBLIC LIBRARY
400 SOUTH STATE STREET
CHICAGO, IL 60605

JM   HWLCSC

REF
RL
803
.C76
2004

Chicago Public Library

R0406475647

The poisoned weed : plants toxic to skin

D0205421

Chicago Public Library

REFERENCE

Form 178 rev.. 11-00

THE POISONED WEED

DONALD G. CROSBY

THE POISONED WEED

PLANTS TOXIC TO SKIN

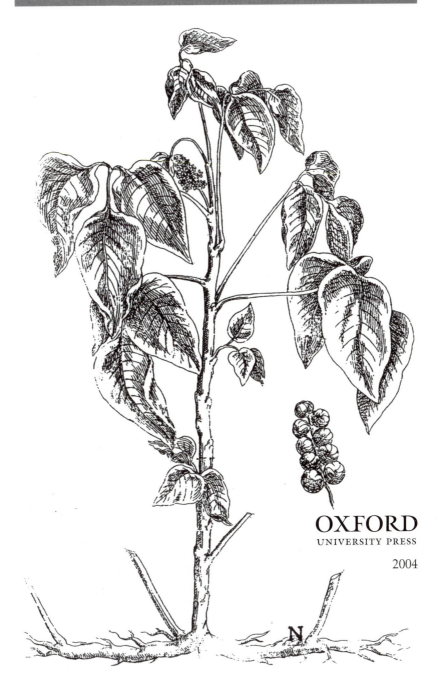

OXFORD
UNIVERSITY PRESS

2004

OXFORD
UNIVERSITY PRESS

Oxford New York
Auckland Bangkok Buenos Aires Cape Town Chennai
Dar es Salaam Delhi Hong Kong Istanbul Karachi Kolkata
Kuala Lumpur Madrid Melbourne Mexico City Mumbai Nairobi
São Paulo Shanghai Taipei Tokyo Toronto

Copyright © 2004 by Oxford University Press

Published by Oxford University Press, Inc.,
198 Madison Avenue, New York, New York 10016

www.oup.com

Oxford is a registered trademark of Oxford University Press

All rights reserved. No part of this publication may be reproduced,
stored in a retrieval system, or transmitted, in any form or by any means,
electronic, mechanical, photocopying, recording, or otherwise,
without the prior permission of Oxford University Press.

Library of Congress Cataloging-in-Publication Data
Crosby, Donald G.
The Poisoned Weed: Plants toxic to skin /
Donald G. Crosby.
p. cm.
Includes bibliographical references and index.
ISBN 0-19-515548-3
1. Dermatotoxicology. 2. Poisonous plants. 3. Plant toxins. I. Title.
RL803.C76 2003
616.5'07—dc21   2003046272

9 8 7 6 5 4 3 2 1
Printed in the United States of America
on acid-free paper

R0406475647

BUSINESS/SCIENCE/TECHNOLOGY DIVISION
CHICAGO PUBLIC LIBRARY
400 SOUTH STATE STREET
CHICAGO, IL 60605

To Nancy, whose struggles with T. diversilobum, T. radicans,

M. indica, S. terebinthefolius, E. maculata, U. dioica,

and sundry other plants inspired this book.

PREFACE

Human dermatitis from plants is almost universal. In the United States alone, more than two-thirds of the population reacts to poison oak, poison ivy, and their relatives—more than 160 million people, including me. Many familiar plants in our homes, fields, and gardens produce substances toxic to skin, and allergenic and irritant species are found on every continent except Antarctica. Considering the misery they cause, I was surprised at how few guides to them were available.

The idea for this project developed over a period of years as I watched my wife, Nancy, react to a series of toxic plants until, at age 60, I too became sensitized to poison oak. Then, in preparing a classroom lecture in the late 1980s, I discovered that the only existing book on poison oak and poison ivy (by James B. McNair) had been published in 1923—before the toxic constituents were identified, before a mechanism was proposed for their toxic action, and before the name *Toxicodendron* was established for their genus—even before I was born. An update seemed long overdue, but as reference material accumulated, so many other species with similar allergens and effects emerged that the scope had to expand.

As plans proceeded, I became aware of several recent books on poison oak and poison ivy for the lay reader, in particular those by Edward Frankel (1991) and Susan Hauser (1996). However, none was sufficiently technical for my purposes, and the classic *Botanical Dermatology* by John Mitchell and Arthur Rook (1979) and *Dermatologic Botany* edited by Javier Avalos and Howard Maibach (2000) were too detailed. Unfortunately, I did not discover the especially helpful 1986 *Clinics in Dermatology* volume on plant dermatitis, edited by Jere Guin and John Beaman, until my manuscript was almost complete. My sincere appreciation for the efforts of all these writers. Other key references are listed in appendix G.

The present book reviews the history, occurrence, classification, toxic constituents, and health aspects of allergenic and irritant plants that people contact in everyday life. Because the reaction of human skin to the poison ivy (cashew) family is especially severe and widespread, those species receive the most attention, but other familiar weeds, crop plants, ornamentals, and wild species are discussed also. Coverage is not intended to be encyclopedic, and references are provided for further exploration. Because chemistry defines a plant's dermatotoxic activity, species whose active constituents are still unidentified generally have been excluded.

The writing is intended to inform a broad cross section of chemical, medical, and biological scientists and students about common plant species and products that are toxic to human skin. However, parts of this book also may interest people involved with forestry, firefighting, utilities, parks, gardening, agriculture, outdoor recreation, and anyone else who has frequent contact with plants. The reaction of an individual's skin to any particular plant is unpredictable and recognizes no geographical boundary, so the coverage is international.

Almost all previous books on the subject have been written or edited by dermatologists, so one of my aims is to provide the viewpoint of a chemist and toxicologist. Consequently, the contents are heavily slanted toward the toxic species, their constituents, and people's exposure to them, and many biological and medical aspects are left to others more knowledgable. Because the information cuts across so many fields of activity, a glossary has been provided.

The choice of illustrations was difficult. Given the limited number agreed upon with the publisher, I chose those I thought would be especially interesting and representative of my own experience. Also, I wanted plants that were widely accessible, so most of the photos were taken near my home in Davis, California. Except where noted, the photographs and line drawings are my own, but I acknowledge, with thanks, permission to publish others, as indicated in their captions.

I am indebted to many friends and colleagues for their help. John Hylin, Howard Maibach, Bob McCandliss, Bob Rice, Warren Roberts, and Ellen Zagory provided helpful reviews of the various sections; Rick Crosby, Jere Guin, and Sandy Ogletree assisted with some of the photos, and I appreciate the help and advice of Senior Editor Kirk Jensen and Production Editor Lisa Stallings; any errors are mine, not theirs. I am especially grateful to my wife, Nancy, for her continued input, encouragement, and knowledge of plants.

CONTENTS

THE POISONED WEED

ONE

"The poysoned weede is much in shape like our
English Ivie, but being but touched, causeth rednesse,
itchinge, and lastly blysters, the which howsoever
after a while they passe away of themselves without
further harme..."
—Captain John Smith, 1609

Captain Smith's "Ivie" was well known to his Powhatan Indian neighbors. For centuries, they and other Native Americans had used it for medicine. Navajos made arrow poison from this native plant, and California's Miwoks made the Western version, *it-tum* in their language, into black dye for baskets (Balls, 1962). They were very aware of its harmful character—in Mexico, it was called *mala mujer*, the wicked woman—but to unwary European settlers, the attractive weeds became familiar as "poison ivy" and "poison oak."

With the latter blanketing the Pacific Coast and the former growing rampant over much of the rest of the continent, the two species were to become our nation's best-known toxic plants. Contrary to popular belief, Native Americans were just as susceptible to the poisons, and as fearful of them, as those whose skins were white or brown. The lingering notion that blacks and Asians also were immune proved equally incorrect, and at least two-thirds of our country's inhabitants, regardless of race or color, remain sensitive today to "the poysoned weede."

Of course, poison ivy and poison oak are not the only offenders. Literally thousands of other plant species or their products are known to damage human skin, and the most important and frequently encountered of them are the subject of this book.

1.1 History

From Captain Smith's account, we know that early settlers of our East Coast were quickly introduced to poison ivy. Similarly, missionaries, soldiers, and frontiersmen could hardly have avoided the plants as they explored westward across North America. One account tells of members of Mexican Governor Valverde's 1719 expedition into what is now New Mexico. Unaware as they were of poison ivy's toxic effects, they soon encountered it to their sorrow.

Although its description had been recorded in sixth century China, the common English name "poison ivy" was coined by Captain Smith (of Pocahontas fame) at the Virginia Colony in 1608–09, and he offered the first glimpse of its effect on his fellow colonists (Smith, 1624). Like the Captain, the seventeenth century Dutch physician J. P. Cornut (1635) considered it a form of English ivy and named it *Edera trifolia canadensis* (three-leafed Canadian ivy). Although he never set foot in North America, Cornut's 1635 drawing (fig. 1.1) shows us a plant identical to poison ivy, either *Toxicodendron radicans* or *T. rydbergii,* which we know and avoid today. The early history has been reviewed in detail by Barkley and Barkley (1938).

Poison ivy was probably the *hiedra maligna,* or "evil ivy," mentioned by the Spanish explorer Clavigero in his 1789 book, *Historia de la California*

Figure 1.1 The first likeness of "*Edera trifolia canadensis*" (poison ivy, *Toxicodendron radicans*) of Cornut (1635). From Barkley and Barkley (1938), by permission of the *American Midland Naturalist.*

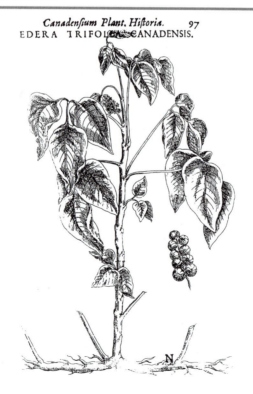

Canadenſium Plant. Hiſtoria.   97
EDERA TRIFOLIA CANADENSIS.

(Standley, 1923), written when California's area was much larger than it is today. The great Swedish botanist Linnaeus already had classified a North American specimen as *Toxicodendron triphyllum glabrum* in 1736, but he later renamed it *Rhus toxicodendron*, or "toxic sumac." *Rhus radicans*, already well known at that time, eventually was shown to be identical to *R. toxicodendron*, and although poison ivy's present scientific name, *Toxicodendron radicans*, is a compromise, many authors still refer to the plant as *Rhus*. Chapter 2 provides a more detailed description.

Western poison oak did not receive its name until much later. Botanist David Douglas (of the Douglas fir) discovered it during an 1825–27 visit to Fort Vancouver on the Columbia River, only 20 years after the explorations of Lewis and Clark (Wilks, 1914). Captain F. W. Beechey, of *HMS Blossom*, saw it at about the same time at the barren California seaport of Yerba Buena, now called San Francisco (Hooker and Arnott, 1832). As the ship's botanist, Hooker named his find *Rhus lobata*, but with that name already claimed for a nontoxic relative, botanists John Torrey and Asa Gray reclassified the new species in 1840 as *Rhus diversiloba*. A 1930s reorganization that put all the toxic *Rhus* species into one genus, *Toxicodendron*, finally provided today's official name: *Toxicodendron diversilobum* (Torrey and A. Gray, 1840). Gillis (1971a) offers a detailed history.

Although dermatitis from exposure to North American poison ivy has been recorded for almost 400 years, human reaction to some of the world's other allergenic and irritant plants can be traced back much further. The Chinese reported the caustic effects of croton (*Codiaeum* species) as early as 2700 B.C., and dermatitis from *Bhavachee* (scurf pea) was recorded in India before 1400 B.C. Egyptians of Moses' time, 3000 years ago, knew that bishop's weed (*Ammi visnaga*) and sunlight acted in concert on human skin.

By that time, a toxic black finish made from sap of the lacquer tree, *T. vernicifluum*, was being applied to oriental bowls like that seen in plate 1 (Casal, 1961; Toyama, 1918). In the Western Hemisphere, explorer Ovidio y Valdes observed in 1535 that dermatitis from poison ivy relatives known today as *Comocladia* and *Metopium* severely afflicted his soldiers when they were in the area that is now Chile (Mitchell and Rook, 1979).

However, plant dermatitis surely must have been recognized long before written records. For example, although not classified botanically until 1750, the corrosive rengas trees (*Gluta rengas*) of Southeast Asia would have brought grief to the earliest permanent residents, more than three millenia ago, and even to their primitive Protomalaysian (Hoabinhian) forebears who followed the glaciers 7000 years before that. Present-day poison oak and poison ivy originated over 30 million years ago in eastern Asia (Gillis, 1971a)—far predating our own species—and they may have reached North America via migrating land birds long ago (section 2.5).

Because even the earliest humans presumably would have been as susceptible to them as are we today, it is clear that plant dermatitis has been around for a long time.

I assume that readers have at least heard of dermatotoxic plants—plants toxic to skin—and the misery they bring. This chapter provides background for the rest of the book and for dealing with such species, the poisons and our exposure to them, and the dire consequences of carelessness.

1.2 The Plants

The allergenic and irritant plants are many and varied (table 1.1). They range in size from tiny liverworts to huge red cedars, and they are found on every continent except Antarctica (where probably no one has looked yet). Several plant families claim more than their fair share of dermatotoxic species: the Anacardiaceae, the family of mango, poison oak, and poison ivy; the Asteraceae (Compositae) or daisy family; and the Apiaceae (Umbelliferae) or carrot family. Irritant plants fall largely within the Euphorbiaceae (spurge family), Brassicaceae (mustard family), and Alliaceae (onion family), although anyone who has ever been "stung" by a nettle would add Urticaceae to the list. Fortunately, only a few such plants are truly dangerous for most people (table 1.1).

Table 1.1 Dangerously Dermatotoxic Plants of the United States

Common name	Species	Family	Toxic Part	Action[a]
Brazilian pepper[b]	*Schinus terebinthifolius*	Anacardiaceae	Leaf, fruit	A
Buttercup	*Ranunculus* spp.	Ranunculaceae	Sap	I
Candelabra cactus	*Euphorbia lactea*	Euphorbiaceae	Latex	I
Chili pepper	*Capsicum annuum*	Solanaceae	Seed, oil	I
Fig	*Ficus carica*	Moraceae	Latex	P
German primrose	*Primula obconica*	Primulaceae	Trichome	A
Hogweed	*Heracleum* spp.	Apiaceae	Sap	P
Persian lime	*Citrus aurantifolia*	Rutaceae	Peel, oil	P
Manchineel	*Hippomane mancinella*	Euphorbiaceae	Latex	I
Pencil bush	*Euphorbia tirucalli*	Euphorbiaceae	Latex (stem)	I
Poison ivy relatives[c]	*Toxicodendron* spp.	Anacardiaceae	All parts	A
Poison wood	*Metopium toxiferum*	Anacardiaceae	Latex	A
Stinging nettle	*Urtica* spp.	Urticaceae	Spine	I
Wood nettle	*Laportea* spp.	Urticaceae	Spine	I
Wild feverfew[d]	*Parthenium hysterophorus*	Asteraceae	Sap	A

[a]A = allergenic, I = irritant, P = phototoxic. [b]Also called Christmasberry and Florida holly. [c]Includes poison oak, poison sumac, and various lac trees (see table 2.1). [d]Congress grass.

Anacardiaceae

The Anacardiaceae, a particular focus of this book, includes some 70 genera and 600 species found in tropical and temperate climates throughout much of the world (Mitchell and Mori, 1987). Members of this family vary from desert shrubs to large trees of the rain forest, and most are harmless. Although some do indeed cause a serious skin rash in humans, even those may provide widely enjoyed foods and ornamentals such as mangoes, cashew nuts, and pepper trees. Summaries of the botany and toxicity of poisonous Anacardiaceae have been provided by Kligman (1958), Guin and Beaman (1986), Guin et al. (2000), and the next chapter of this book.

Asteraceae

Another family important to our subject, the Asteraceae, represents more than 10% of the world's known plant species. Unlike the Anacardiaceae, many of them have been used in human medicine for centuries, and early physicians including Dioscorides, Pliny, and Galen described their applications. The seventeenth century medicinal plant book, or herbal, by Culpeper (1653) details remedies from over 20 such species, and although the author makes his selection seem to fit almost any ailment, many claim to reduce inflammation. Daisies, for example, "applied to the privities, or to any other parts that are swollen and hot, doth dissolve and temper the heat," and because dermatotoxic substances often do regulate inflammation (chapter 9), the daisy's purported curative powers may be based on fact. Plants of this family indeed are used in folk medicines throughout much of the world—Mexico and Central America (Robles et al., 2000), for instance—and tincture of Arnica remains a common liniment in our own country.

Skin reactions to members of the Asteraceae generally are much milder than to those of the Anacardiaceae, but this family's wider distribution makes it a significant threat. For example, a serious 1956 outbreak of dermatitis in India was caused by an accidental introduction of seeds of congress grass (wild feverfew, *Parthenium hysterophorus*), already known to cause "weed dermatitis" in our Southeast states, in a humanitarian shipment of grain; thousands of the subcontinent's people were afflicted, some died, and the plants gained a reputation as "the scourge of India" (Towers and Mitchell, 1983; Paulsen, 1992).

Euphorbiaceae

The Euphorbiaceae, or spurge, family is another large one, many species of which invoke human dermatitis. Besides well-known weeds such as spotted spurge, prominent euphorbs also include ornamental poinsettias and crotons and the economically important Para rubber tree, castor bean, and tapioca (cassava). Where our reaction to poison ivy or chrysanthemums is delayed, Euphorbiaceae species "causeth reddness, itchyng, and ... blysters" immediately and corrosively; they are prime examples of irritant plants. Early explorers of the Caribbean reported that an almost legendary tree-size euphorb called manchineel, beach apple, or manzanilla (*Hippomane mancinella*) caused extreme dermatitis from even the runoff of dew from the leaves. Skin lesions finally became so prevalent among that region's U.S. military personnel in the 1900s that the Army had to train its troops to avoid the tree and conduct extensive (and only partly successful) efforts to eradicate it.

Other Species

Plants very different from the Anacardiaceae can contain poisons that are chemically and toxicologically similar to those of poison ivy, including wheat (family Poaceae), ginkgo (Ginkgoaceae), and even the familiar philodendron (Araceae). Hardwoods such as rosewood (Fabaceae) contain allergenic quinones, and many other species produce so-called essential oils (extractives with a pleasant odor or essence) that are used widely for flavoring and for fragrances in cosmetics, soaps, and other products. Citrus peel oils become toxic when skin exposed to them encounters sunlight, and the mustard oils from cole crops are highly irritant. Rash-producing constituents are present in such garden favorites as Peruvian lilies (family Alstroemeriaceae), English ivy and schefflera (Araliaceae), tulips and daffodils (Liliaceae), and even primitive plants such as liverworts (Hepaticaceae) growing on trees and garden walls. Chapters 3 and 4 show that dermatitis from plants or plant products may now be inescapable.

Conveyance

The poison must somehow make its way from plant to victim, but the process has received relatively little scientific attention. One mode is for toxic sap to be released directly onto the skin surface. *Toxicodendron, Euphorbia,* and many other species can accomplish this only by rupture of a resin duct at the leaf surface or in an injured stem—not necessarily a simple matter. The sap often forms a latex, that is, an emulsion of minute droplets of poison suspended in a liquid medium, like in cow's milk. If the toxicant is water-soluble, as is the case with tulips and buttercups, it is delivered in clear, watery juice when ducts are disrupted, or it may be formed in the rigid cells of a heartwood such as teak and released only upon cutting.

In other instances, a tiny volume of toxic fluid is contained in a glandular surface hair (called a trichome) that releases it when crushed or dislodged. An extreme example of this is a nettle; the nettle's trichomes take the form of quartz needles whose tips break off on contact and inject the contents under pressure into the skin. Airborne transport of toxic particles or vapor has long been controversial but now seems firmly established. And, of course, if stable enough, the offending substance may be transferred easily from hands, tools, or dog hair to bare skin (chapter 8).

1.3 The Poisons

Captain Smith's description of his contact with poison ivy (Smith, 1624), quoted in the epilogue of this chapter, is readily appreciated by anyone who is sensitive to the plant. The rash is caused by chemical constituents long a subject of considerable interest. Those from the various toxicodendrons are similar or identical to one another, irrespective of species, and are referred to as urushiol or laccol, depending on chemical structure. The first name is derived from *urushi*, the Japanese word for the sap that first afforded the toxic agents in 1909, whereas the second refers to the Japanese lac tree (*Toxicodendron vernicifluum*), the botanical source of *urushi*.

Poison ivy dermatitis was once thought to be caused by an "invisible, colorless vapor" released from the plants and inhaled by the victim (McNair, 1923). At the time, many diseases were believed to be spread this way, as suggested by the word *malaria* (from the Italian *mala aria*, bad air). Early attempts (1787–1800) to define the poison chemically were often abandoned because of the effect on the experimenters, and the toxic-gas theory proved long lived. For example, J. B. Van Mons (1797) collected the gaseous emanations of a *Rhus radicans* (poison ivy) specimen in a jar in daylight and exposed the hand of his highly sensitive brother to it. When no adverse effect was detected, Van Mons repeated the experiment with a darkened jar and noted an immediate burning sensation (in the brother's hand) followed by the typical rash, and he mistakenly concluded that the poison was a gaseous hydrocarbon released only at night.

Others claimed that dermatitis could be produced in people many meters away from a poison ivy plant, or even in those entering a room where experiments with the plant were in progress. The toxic principle was variously described as a hydrocarbon, an alkaloid, and a volatile acid ("toxicodendric acid"), although an aqueous distillate of the plants never produced the expected symptoms. Several writers commented in passing that poisoning seemed to follow the rubbing of *Rhus* (*Toxicodendron*) sap on the skin, or even the victim shaking hands with an experimenter, and a notion arose that the disease was caused by a bacterium that, even without isolation, was given the name *Mycobacterium toxicatus*.

By 1897, however, physician Franz Pfaff had decided that the poison must not be volatile, and he extracted an extremely toxic oil from *Rhus toxicodendron*—yet another name for poison ivy—that he termed "toxicodendrol." Some extractions required as much as 100 pounds of leaves and berries at a time, and one can only imagine what must have been experienced by the individuals actually doing the work. However, after Pfaff, experimentation lapsed for almost a century. An interesting history of these early chemical adventures has been provided by James B. McNair (1923).

In his book, McNair describes his own extraction experiments on western poison oak (termed *Rhus diversiloba* at the time). He was able to isolate "a clear, amber-red, oily, nonvolatile, viscous poisonous liquid," which he named "lobinol" and which proved very similar to the urushiol isolated from the Japanese lac tree (*Toxicodendron verniciflluum*) by R. Majima (1915). Lobinol would later be shown to be a complex mixture containing laccol (3-heptadecylcatechol) as the main toxic ingredient, a substance closely related to the 3-pentadecylcatechols accepted by that time as the poisons in urushiol. Surprisingly, the precise composition and structure of the poison oak allergens were not established until relatively recently (Corbett and Billets, 1975).

The powerful response of skin to these chemicals is based on their unusual physical and chemical properties, properties now known to be shared by toxic constituents from many other plant species. Fat solubility is especially significant, because it determines both the chemical's ability to be absorbed by skin and its tendency to move through the environment. An aversion to water (hydrophobicity) also leads to low solubility and suggests that evaporation of allergens from a wet leaf might explain how the plants could affect sensitive people without ever being touched.

Urushiol's allergenicity also requires the chemical's ability to react with skin proteins. This explains why even very different substances, from completely unrelated kinds of plants, can cause the same toxic response when high fat solubility is combined with this reactivity; any substance related to urushiols chemically and immunologically will be referred to here as a *urushioid*. Most urushioids are unable to combine with protein directly and are thought to be converted to a more reactive form, such as a quinone. Many other plants already contain or can form toxic, fat-soluble quinones, as discussed in section 6.2.

Allergenic asters and their relatives do not contain urushioids but, instead, a different type of reactive hydrophobic chemicals classified as sesquiterpene lactones. At least 95% of the 450 plant species reported to produce these substances belong to the Asteraceae (Herz, 1977) and include dahlias, marigolds, chrysanthemums, artichokes, and lettuce (chapter 3). Lactones are cyclic esters that, like quinones, react with skin proteins but generally differ from urushioids in other ways. In fact, a common theme among most allergenic and irritant chemicals is that they must be able to combine chemically with skin components (chapter 5).

In some cases, the original substance has to undergo a chemical conversion to provide the actual toxicant. Terpenes, the simple compounds responsible for the scent of roses or the taste of an orange, must be oxidized by air before they can become toxic. On the other hand, the extent to which a substance is broken further into nontoxic fragments by natural forces determines its mobility, skin penetration, effects on organisms, and persistence in the body or in nature.

The physical properties may be equally significant, as they affect a chemical's fate and availability. The most important factors are volatility, solubility in water, and solubility in fat (lipophilicity); although there is a surprising lack of physical data for dermatotoxic plant constituents, they are important (table 1.2). For instance, volatility—the rate at which a chemical vaporizes into the surrounding air—is related to the vapor pressure, P_v, measured in mm of mercury, or torr. A value of P_v greater than 1 torr suggests a very high volatility and less than 0.01 torr a low one. The simple terpene geraniol has a moderate vapor pressure of about 0.03 torr at 25°C, and thus can give roses the characteristic fragrance our noses detect.

As table 1.2 shows, data on water solubility range from freely soluble (helenalin) to almost insoluble (urushiol); on partitioning, from limited movement from water into fat (toluquinone) to extensive (limonene); and on volatility, from almost nonvolatile (helenalin) to highly so (limonene,

Table 1.2 Physical Properties of Dermatotoxic Plant Products

Chemical (Type)	Mol. Wt.	WS (mg/L)[a]	log K_{ow}	P_v (torr)[a]
Alantolactone (lactone)	232.32	38.4	3.38	3.16×10^{-5}
Benzyl benzoate (ester)	212.25	15.4	3.97	2.24×10^{-10}
Cinnamaldehyde (aldehyde)	132.16	1,400	1.90	0.025
Geraniol (terpene)	154.25	100	3.47	0.030
Helenalin (lactone)	262.30	11,800	0.87	4.69×10^{-9}
d-Limonene (terpene)	136.23	13.8	4.83	1.98
Linalool (terpene)	154.25	1,590	2.97	0.16
Methyl isothiocyanate (organosulfur)	73.12	7,600	0.73	3.54
Psoralen (furocoumarin)	186.16	1,930	1.67	2.24×10^{-5}
Toluquinone (quinone)	122.12	19,900	0.72	0.034
Urushiol I (catechol)	320.51	3×10^{-4b}	9.27	$<1 \times 10^{-10b}$
Vanillin (aldehyde)	152.15	1,100	1.21	1.18×10^{-4}

Data from Howard and Meylan (1997). [a]WS = water solubility and P_v = vapor pressure, both at 25°C. [b]Calculated.

methyl isothiocyanate). A combination of such chemical and physical information allows a degree of prediction of the relative dermatotoxicity of any particular chemical.

1.4 Skin

Many, many types of plant constituents cause dermatitis: acetylenes in English Ivy, irritant esters in euphorbs, and aldehydes in cinnamon, to name only a few. However, no matter what the chemical, skin is *always* the key element. The largest of the organs—up to 10% of a person's body weight—the skin provides a continuous, flexible envelope that holds and protects the internal organs, presents a barrier between them and the outside world, helps regulate water loss and internal temperature, affords sensory perception, and often represents the body's first contact with and defense against toxic chemicals.

Skin Structure

The skin surface is coated with a water-repellent called sebum. This layer, only about one micron (1 μm or 0.0001 cm) thick, consists largely of steroid relatives that include the $C_{30}H_{50}$ hydrocarbon, squalene. Sebum protects the outermost layer of cells, the thin stratum corneum (SC or "horny layer") that is dead, densely packed, and composed mostly of the same protein (keratin) as horn, hair, and bird feathers (fig. 1.2). Voids between SC cells are filled with "fat," more precisely a mixture containing 35% of C_{16}-C_{24} amides (ceramides or sphingolipids), fatty acids (25%), cholesterol and relatives (25%), and other lipids (Elias, 1992). As the SC wears away during everyday use, it is replaced from an underlying epidermis consisting of a thin granular layer (stratum granulosum), squamous cells (stratum spinosum) just below that, and finally a basal (germinative) layer in which

Figure 1.2 The structure of human skin

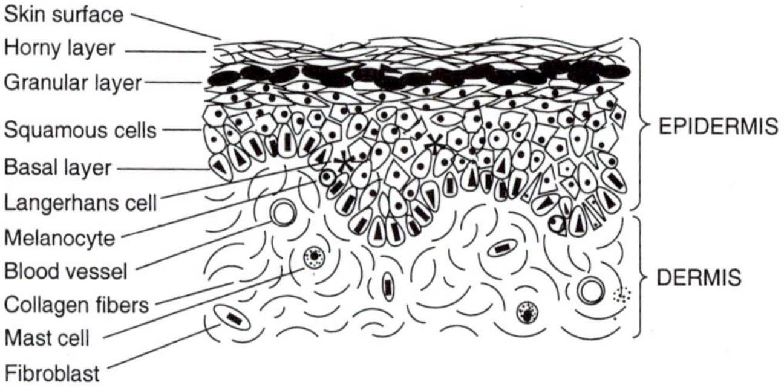

Skin surface
Horny layer
Granular layer
Squamous cells
Basal layer — EPIDERMIS
Langerhans cell
Melanocyte
Blood vessel
Collagen fibers — DERMIS
Mast cell
Fibroblast

new skin cells (keratinocytes) continually form and start their migration to the surface. Basal cells give rise to all the others.

Generally less than a millimeter thick, the *living* epidermis (excluding the SC) contains hair follicles, glands that secrete sweat or sebum, and, wandering through it, the oddly shaped Langerhans cells (LC) that extend numerous dendritic "arms" to form a monitoring network to detect the entry of any foreign substance (Schuler, 1991). Its keratinocytes are responsible for the initial breakdown ("metabolism") of absorbed chemicals, as discussed below, and the basal layer contains melanocytes that give skin its color. The entire epidermis is replaced monthly.

Beneath the epidermis lies a 3–5 mm layer of dermis made up mostly of bundles of cartilage (collagen) synthesized by fibroblasts (fig. 1.2). It contains the nerves required for pain and touch, the muscles we feel when our skin "crawls," fat bodies, and capillaries that carry blood or lymph. Near the blood vessels are granule-filled mast cells that release the so-called mediators responsible for the symptoms of allergy and irritation. In three dimensions, the rounded extensions of dermis into the epidermis (fig. 1.2) are actually protuberances (papillae) reminiscent of an egg crate (Milne, 1972). The significance of these cells and tissues is explored in chapter 9.

Absorption of Chemicals

The skin absorbs chemicals primarily according to their surface concentration and a partition coefficient (K_p) that measures their tendency to seek fat rather than water. An artificial but convenient surrogate for K_p is the *octanol-water* partition coefficient, K_{ow}, for which the fat is replaced by a fat-like, 8-carbon alcohol (1-octanol). A long list of K_{ow} values is available (Hansch et al., 1995), and table 1.2 gives a few examples, mostly from dermatotoxic plant constituents. Fat-soluble (lipophilic) chemicals whose K_{ow} exceeds 1000 can penetrate skin very readily, and the degree of uptake is directly proportional to the K_{ow} (Potts et al., 1992).

Although often thinner than a human hair, the SC provides the rate-limiting barrier to an absorption that depends on the skin's age, thickness, and physiological state as well as its resistance and bodily location. Movement of chemicals occurs by simple diffusion, largely through the fat-filled spaces between SC cells, and so is much faster through the relatively thin scrotum than through forehead, scalp, back, forearm, or palm, in that order. Liquids make better surface contact with the sebum than do solids and so are more readily absorbed. Urushiols and laccols penetrate rapidly.

Scraped knees and elbows reveal blood-filled capillaries, part of our circulatory system that lie just below the skin's surface. However, few people are aware that a comparable system transports a colorless fluid called lymph and also extends throughout the body, returning excess tissue fluid to the bloodstream. Because the heart pumps only blood, lymph is forced along, one way, by the skeletal muscles. Lymph occupies a key place in our internal defenses by transporting microorganisms, chemicals, and even occasional debris such as soil particles into collection and filtration units (lymph nodes) for final disposal.

Biotransformations

From the very onset of absorption, a foreign chemical (xenobiotic) is subject to the biochemical breakdown known as biotransformation or metabolism. The chief purposes of this process are to reduce the chemical's reactivity, increase its water solubility, decrease its K_{ow} and cause it to be more easily eliminated. In the first step (Phase I), the body oxidizes, reduces, hydrolyzes, or dechlorinates the entering compound, which in the second step (Phase II) is deactivated (conjugated), if necessary, in preparation for its removal via the urine. Breakdown products, referred to as metabolites, usually are much less toxic than the parent chemical, so the process is considered to be *detoxication*.

Most, and perhaps all, living cells are capable of some sort of biotransformation, and skin cells are no exception. Although it exhibits as little as 2% of the detoxifying ability of the most active organ, the liver, skin still is able to perform all the principal types of chemical change (Mukhtar, 1992). The reactions are largely enzyme-catalyzed (table 1.3), and oxidation is especially prevalent. For example, when a poison oak branch is cut, metabolic oxidation of the laccols quickly turns the ends black, which is similar to what happens in a cut slice of apple, providing a reliable test of whether the unrecognized plant may be dermatotoxic. This is the "black spot test" (section 5.3).

Table 1.3   Some Biotransformation Reactions in Skin

Reaction Type	Enzymes	Typical Substrates
Oxidation	Cytochrome P450	Parathion
	Arylhydrocarbon hydroxylase (AHH)	PAH[a]
N-Dealkylation	Monoamine oxidase (MAO)	Norepinephrine
Reduction	Cortisone reductase	Cortisone
Hydrolysis	Esterase	Paraoxon
Conjugation		
Mercapturation	Glutathione-S-transferase	Dinitrochlorobenzene
Glucuronylation	UDP-Glucuronyl transferase	p-Nitrophenol
Methylation	Catechol O-methyltransferase	Norepinephrine

See Kao and Carver (1991); Mukhtar (1992). [a]Polycyclic aromatic hydrocarbons.

Biotransformations in the skin are the body's second line of defense (after the SC), and although the epidermis is the most active, even the "dead" stratum corneum contains degradative enzymes. As a chemical penetrates the skin, part of it becomes bound to skin proteins or is degraded, and what remains enters the bloodstream to be acted on eventually by the liver and excreted in the urine. However, the high incidence of rash among humans exposed to poison ivy or other dermatotoxic plant suggests that detoxication often is too slow to offer complete protection.

1.5 Exposure

If skin is the gateway for plant dermatitis, exposure is the latch. Despite early recognition in China, Japan, and eventually most of North America, toxicodendron dermatitis long remained virtually unknown in Europe simply because people there were never exposed to the plants. However, the species are now a major factor in occupational illness for many places: In California, for example, poison oak exposure rates as one of the main lost-time accidents among farmers, foresters, telephone linemen, firefighters, and others who work out-of-doors. Hikers, campers, gardeners, and millions of other people worldwide have to miss work and suffer from exposure to toxicodendrons or other dermatotoxic plants during recreation. Mango, philodendron, and celery are more likely to exhibit their toxicity in the home, whereas lactone-bearing weeds and garden plants are most likely to affect commercial horticulturists, florists, farmers, and gardeners. Woodworkers and woodsmen are exposed to forest products, and children may become victims anywhere.

Exposure can be either direct or indirect. A run-in with poison oak on a mountain trail qualifies as direct exposure—that is, contact with the plant itself—whereas exposure via contaminated hands, pets, doorknobs, or garden tools is considered indirect (chapter 8). The "florist's finger" caused by handling cut flowers is direct, but very similar symptoms can occur indirectly just from unlacing one's shoes after a hike through poison ivy country. To correctly diagnose plant dermatitis, a dermatologist must examine *all* of a patient's recent activities; a "housecall and garden walk" by the physician is recommended in determining the source of a stubborn rash (Mitchell and Maibach, 2000). A single exposure is said to be *acute* and that of long duration *chronic*.

Opportunities for exposure, then, are almost unlimited and arise not only from the type of plant but also from the duration and frequency of contact, time of year, temperature, and even the victim's state of health. There is more about exposure and how to control it in chapter 8.

1.6 Adverse Effects

Toxic means poisonous. The dictionary defines a poison as "a substance that through its chemical action kills, injures, or impairs an organism," and that certainly describes urushioids, lactones, and the rest. Exposure via eyes (ocular), lungs (respiratory), and mouth (oral) are all possible—most toxicity values are for the oral route—but exposure via the skin (dermal) undoubtedly is the most prevalent.

Fat-soluble poisons are absorbed, enter the bloodstream, and then are carried throughout the body via the circulatory system to affect some key enzyme or process. The resulting effects often are increased by metabolic activation or decreased by detoxication. Toxic substances normally exert their effects by interference with some basic biochemical process—inhibition of nerve impulses by phosphate insecticides or of respiration by arsenic, for example—and the result is proportional to the amount of poison present. According to the old saying, "the dose makes the poison." However, dermatotoxic poisons don't work that way.

Toxicity

Although many plant constituents are highly toxic by mouth, few of the dermatotoxic ones are. The acute oral toxicity of dermatotoxic plant constituents is generally low (table 9.2), although the effect of some of them on the mouth and gastrointestinal tract is so violent that they can only be tested by injection. Urushioids are not highly poisonous in this sense—they do not seriously interfere with any vital process, and their toxicity is only vaguely related to dose. Rather than a barrier, the skin becomes an active and essential partner in the toxic action.

Effects on the Skin

The interaction of skin and chemical can produce any of several results (table 1.4). Irritation is the most common, but plants seldom cause chemical burns where skin is actually eaten away. *Irritant contact dermatitis* (ICD) is a surface inflammation like that from your grandmother's mustard plaster (Lammintausta and Maibach, 1990), whereas *contact urticaria* (Lahti, 1986) is similar but immediate and brief (a nettle sting, for example). *Phytophotodermatitis* refers to reddening and blisters caused by certain plant constituents in the presence of sunlight (Pathak, 1974).

Such maladies often are difficult for the lay person to distinguish from one another (see chapter 9). However, *allergic contact dermatitis* (ACD) is of particular interest to victims of toxicodendrons and other urushioid-bearing plants, and when ICD and ACD occur together, the result can be spectacularly bad. Allergic reactions will be discussed first.

Table 1.4   Skin Responses to Chemicals

Classification (Type)	Sensitization	Lag Time	Duration	Typical Elicitors
ICD[a]	no	minutes–hours	hours–days	euphorbs, mustard oil
Contact urticaria				
Nonimmunologic (I)	no	seconds–minutes	minutes–hours	nettles, cinnamon oil
Immunologic (IV)	yes	minutes–1 hour	hours–1 day	tulips, rubber latex
ACD[b] (IV)	yes	24–48 hours	4–10 days	poison oak, mayweed
Photo-ACD (IV)	yes	hours[c]	8–10 days	drugs, perfumes
Phototoxicity (I)	no	>8–48 hours[c]	days–years	lime peel, fig latex

[a]Irritant contact dermatitis. [b]Allergic contact dermatitis. [c]Requires exposure to ultraviolet radiation (sunlight).

Allergy

Since early in Earth's history, single-celled organisms such as amoebas have fought enemies by either engulfing them or poisoning them. We vertebrates continue this primitive trait through various types of defensive cells that can inactivate foreign objects and so confer protection ("immunity"). The cells, known as *leucocytes* or white cells, are of three main types: *phagocytes* (monocytes and macrophages) that engulf and digest invaders; *granulocytes* (basophils and mast cells) that release a toxic mediator, often via proteins called immunoglobulins; and T- and B-*lymphocytes* that interact with the others through chemical signals (lymphokines). Together, they form the protective skin immune system of Bos and Kapsenberg (1986).

The immune system is turned on by the presence of a foreign agent, such as a bacterium, that carries *antigens* (characteristic protein molecules) on its surface. The antigens stimulate phagocytes to engulf and digest the intruder, and B-cells to form defensive *antibodies*—antigen-specific proteins (immunoglobulins) designated IgM and IgG—to aid in its destruction. Furthermore, some long-lived memory cells persist, and the next visit of that particular antigen, be it days, months, or even years later, quickly triggers a new and specific defense.

However, in highly sensitive (hypersensitive) individuals, some antigens cause B cells to generate IgE, an antibody that sticks to granulocytes such as mast cells. No outward symptoms appear at the time, but the individual is now *sensitized*. A future appearance of the same antigen, called elicitation, triggers the granulocytes to release mediators that include heparin to prevent blood clotting and histamine to dilate blood vessels and cause them to leak. The result, documented by Captain Smith, is the inflammation ("reddness"), pruritus ("itchyng"), and eruptions ("blysters") that constitutes *allergy*. Where nature had intended protection, there is instead a mistaken and sometimes violent allergic reaction.

The same reaction also can be initiated by skin contact with small molecules to produce contact allergy. Of five types, only two—immediate (Type I) and delayed (Type IV) hypersensitivity—are caused by plants (table 1.4). Type I reactions come on quickly, as in those treated with an old-fashioned mustard plaster or its modern equivalent, whereas the Type IV reactions typical of poison oak may be delayed several days. As an antigen must be a relatively large molecule of at least 10,000 molecular weight, anything smaller, termed a hapten, has to combine with lymphocyte protein to form the *allergen*. The term *allergen* signifies here any substance that causes an allergic reaction, be it a hapten or a protein antigen. Substances such as urushiols that must be converted to a protein-reactive form are termed *pro-allergens* (allergen generators), whereas those that react directly with skin proteins are *direct allergens*.

Allergic Contact Dermatitis

Type IV reactions are especially complex, slow to start, and long lasting (Kalish, 1995). During sensitization, the hapten becomes attached to the surface of an epidermal cell, often a Langerhans cell, and the resulting allergen moves to a lymph node, where it is transferred to a specific T-cell. The next encounter with the allergen, even weeks or months later, induces memory T-cells to proliferate and release lymphokines (messengers, not antibodies) that eventually lead to mediator release and symptoms like those of Type I allergies. The actual process is much more complex than this (see section 9.5) and may require several weeks of itching, reddened skin, swelling, and perhaps oozing blisters to run its course. ACD is not a pretty sight.

Although the liquid in the blisters is harmless, contact with the affected area can spread surface allergen to other parts of the body, most often the face and genitals. Although a few victims end up in the hospital, breathing urushiol-containing smoke can end in the morgue (McNair, 1923). Once the immune response is set in motion, nothing can be done to stop it; although some individuals appear more resistent than others, perhaps because of age, frequent exposure, or simply lack of previous sensitization, probably *no one* is completely exempt.

ACD is more common than most people realize. At least 3000 chemicals are potential haptens, among them benzocaine in sunburn lotion, the over-the-counter antibiotic Neomycin, the silvery nickel in coinage and jewelry, and the rosin in varnish, ink, and paper. Plus, of course, the allergens of poison oak and ivy, prime offenders in this country. Primrose (*Primula*) allergens lead in Europe, "rhus" allergens hold that place in Australia, and those in asters and their relatives are found worldwide. Thus, another plant may be related to poison oak and ivy less by botany than by the physical and chemical properties of its allergenic constituents (chapter 5).

Irritation

A thorn's prick is unmistakably a mechanical irritation, whereas the painful sting of a nettle (*Urtica* spp.) is an instant chemical irritation, appropriately called *urticaria*. The unpleasant reaction of our skin to a decorative crown of thorns cactus (*Euphorbia millii*) in the parlor, varigated croton (*Codiaeum variegatum*) in the garden, or a backyard buttercup (*Ranunculus* spp.) is a similar chemically induced *irritant contact dermatitis*. Although the exact mechanism often is unclear (section 9.5), the rapid onset of inflammation, rash, and blisters obviously suggests a kinship with the final stages of ACD, and sensitization is indeed involved in ICU or immunological contact urticaria (table 1.4).

Some plants, such as the common fig, produce dermatitis (actually phytophotodermatitis) only after the irritant-bearing skin is exposed to sunlight. Light energy may be perceived as waves whose crest-to-crest distance (wavelength) is measured in nanometers (nm)—a billionth of a meter. The shortest, most energetic solar radiation reaching Earth's surface is classified as ultraviolet (UV, 280–400 nm); that visible to our eyes is seen as violet below 440 nm, yellow near 550 nm, and red above 620 nm; and infrared waves (heat) are even longer. This energy may be absorbed by some substances to drive chemical reactions.

It's no news to most people that sunlight penetrates human skin far enough to cause sunburn and eventual tanning, both a result of photochemical processes. The combination of sunlight, chemicals, and skin also can lead to *phototoxicity* (sections 4.1 and 9.4), in which reddening and blisters appear quickly and do not involve the immune system, or to *photoallergic contact dermatitis*, that is, a delayed immune response to certain light-absorbing synthetic chemicals but few plant constituents (Epstein, 1991).

1.7 Prevention and Treatment

Not surprisingly, people throughout history have tried to find relief from the symptoms of plant dermatitis. Some traditional treatments for "rhus dermatitis" seem harmless, such as 1790s remedies consisting of a mixture of soot and milk, a salt solution, or "sweet oil." More questionable were poultices made from ashes of the offending plant or leaves of the highly toxic jimsonweed. Still others now seem rather terrifying: *aqua regia*, the nitric-sulfuric acid mixture used to dissolve gold; liquid bromine mixed with oil; or an ointment made of copper sulfate, red mercury oxide, lard, and turpentine. McNair (1923) lists many others, including his own recommendation, bathing the entire body in a solution of iron chloride! Chapter 10 reviews these "cures" and others, although of course nothing stops the immune process.

Unfortunately, haptens such as urushiols and laccols are absorbed so rapidly that most traditional remedies are hopeless unless applied immediately. Even the old standby, strong soap and water, often removes only the poison remaining on the surface, and the damage already is under way by the time washing begins. Rinsing with alcohol has been recommended, but this may only spread the oily poisons around and hasten absorption. Gloves and barrier lotions are effective, and some new treatments also are promising; they, too, are discussed in chapter 10. In the end, however, avoidance of dermatotoxic plants is the only certain way to keep from "getting poison oak" or one of its unpleasant equivalents.

The modern way to detect an allergy is by a patch test or its equivalent (section 10.2). A standard allergen, a dilute extract of a suspect plant, or even a leaf or stem of the suspect plant is placed on the bare upper back or forearm and covered; this "patch" is removed after 48–96 hours, and any resulting skin reaction is noted and graded. No change may be visible in an unsensitized person, but erythema (reddening) or even blisters will be seen in one already sensitized. Several potential allergens can be tested at the same time, bringing multiple allergies or cross-reactions to light; in a cross-reaction, a substance of similar structure substitutes for the original or primary allergen. However, accidental sensitization of a previously nonallergic person always is possible.

1.8 Conclusions

Dermatotoxic plants existed long before people, and they are found almost everywhere. Probably anyone can develop some form of contact dermatitis from these plants, although a few people are either resistant or just never became sensitized. The allergy or irritation usually is short-lived but may recur with renewed contact. Most victims are exposed to the plants directly, although indirect exposure can occur via contaminated objects or persons. Although barriers such as gloves and lotions may help, the best way to avoid harm is to become familiar with your local plants and steer clear of the dangerous kinds.

Hundreds and perhaps thousands of plant species are toxic to skin, but they are not equally harmful. A large number of factors control just how severe a person's reaction will be—from mild, as with carrots, to strong, as with pencil bush—so how does one know what to avoid? Mostly, experience must show what is tolerated and what isn't, but a few common species so widely dangerous as *always* to require caution are listed in table 1.1.

Why do plants produce such frightful substances? Some, such as irritants, may actually help the plant's defense against insects and fungi. A toxicodendron's latex quickly hardens over a wounded leaf, but because insects, deer, and goats seem immune to the allergens, this must represent a healing mechanism like the clotting of our own blood. Also, the fault does not lie entirely with the plant: The human immune system is set up to recognize and deal with particular kinds of foreign proteins (antigens), and even when they are formed inadvertently by contact with a plant, the body has no choice but to go on the defensive. Deflating as this may seem to a sensitive human ego sure that such plants are acting out of spite, the victims usually have only their own carelessness and peculiar immune system to blame.

TWO

"Toxicodendron species are numerous, but
conservative botanists agree to three, viz. T. radicans,
T. querquifolium, *and* T. diversilobum, *while some*
add several varieties. ... Inevitably, however,
dermatologists will adhere to the vague and
botanically reprehensible common names, using
'poison ivy' for the climbers and 'poison oak' for
the shrubs, expecting the latter to have a more
oak-shaped leaf."
—Etain Cronin, 1980

2.1 Family Ties: The Anacardiaceae

To best understand and appreciate plants, one must relate them in some logical order. This is the function of taxonomy (table 2.1). For example, poison oak, poison ivy, and poison sumac all belong to the same large group or family of plants related to mango and cashew: the Anacardiaceae. Members of this family, some 70 genera representing 600 species (Mitchell and Mori, 1987), occur in tropical and temperate areas of the world except for New Zealand and the deserts of Asia, Africa, and Australia (Mitchell, 1990). Some of the familiar ornamental and economic species are discussed in chapter 3.

However, a major problem with some species of this family cannot be overlooked: They are seriously toxic to human skin. Although other plant families and genera may claim equally dangerous members, the present chapter will focus on the uniformly dermatotoxic genus *Toxicodendron* (Greek for "poison tree"), the major cause of plant-derived dermatitis among the peoples of the world. An informal introduction to the toxicodendrons has been provided by Frankel (1991).

2.2 Toxicodendrons

How do toxicodendrons relate to the rest of the Anacardiaceae? Botanists divide the family into five "tribes" based on form: Anacardieae such as

Table 2.1 Taxonomy of the Genus *Toxicodendron*

Taxonomy		Common Name (Location)[a]
Kingdom:	Planta	
Phylum:	Spermatophyta	
Class:	Angiospermae	
Subclass:	Dicotyledonae	
Order:	Sapindales	
Family:	Anacardiaceae	
Tribe:	Rhoeae	
Genus:	***Toxicodendron***	
Section:	Simplicifolia	
	T. borneense Stapf	(Borneo)
Section:	Venenata	
Species:	*T. striatum* (Ruiz & Pavón) Kuntze	Manzanillo de Cerro (C & S America)
	T. succedaneum (L.) Kuntze	Arkhol (India), rhus (Australia)
	T. trichocarpum (Miq.) Kuntze[b]	(China, Korea, Japan)
	T. vernicifluum (Stokes) Barkley	Japanese lac tree (Japan, China)
	T. vernix (L.) Kuntze	Poison sumac (E & SE US)
Section:	Toxicodendron	
	T. diversilobum (T. & G.) Greene	Western poison oak (W US)
Subspecies:	*pubescens* (P. Miller)[c]	Eastern poison oak (E/SE US)
	T. nodosum Blume	Jahor (Malaysia)
	T. rydbergii (Small ex Rydberg) Greene	Rydberg's poison ivy (N US, S Can)
Species:	*T. radicans* (L.) Kuntze	
Subspecies:	*barkleyi* Gillis	Aquiscle (Veracruz, Mexico)[d]
	divaricatum Greene	Yedra venenosa (Baja CA, Mexico)
	eximium Greene	Lambrisco (Coahuila, Mexico)
	hispidum Engler	Taiwan tsuta-urushi (Japan)
	negundo (Greene) Gillis	(C US)
	orientale Greene	Tsutsa-urushi (Japan)
	pubens Englem. ex Watson	(Mississippi Valley US)
	radicans (L.) Kunze	Poison ivy (E US, Can, Bahamas)
	verrucosum Scheele	(Texas)

[a] C = Central, Can = Canada, Carib = Caribbean, E = eastern, N = northern, S = south, SE = southeast, W = west. [b] Possibly identical to *T. vernicifluum*. [c] Also called *T. quercifolium* (Michx.) Greene, *T. toxicarium* (Michx.) Greene, or *T. pubescens* (Miller). [d] For other local names of Mexican subspecies, see Martínez (1979).

Anacardium (cashew); Rhoeae, whose type genus is *Rhus* (lemonade berry); Semecarpeae (type genus *Semecarpus*, the marking nut tree); and the lesser-known Spondiadeae (type genus *Spondias*, or hog-plum) and Dobineae (type genus the rather obscure *Dobinia*) (Mitchell and Mori, 1987). Dermatotoxicity may be found in any tribe, but it defines the Roeae's genus *Toxicodendron*.

Accepted taxonomic relations within the genus are shown in table 2.1. One expert says it may contain as many as 30 species, whereas another states there are only six (we will define nine, four of them native to North America). This difference of opinion arises from an inherent variability of form, a tendency to interbreed, and the multitude of botanical authorities who have studied the plants over the past three centuries. The scientific name originated before 1700, considerably predating Linnaeus' 1753 classification of the plants into the genus *Rhus*, but it apparently fell out of botanical favor for centuries and was not reinstated until the 1930s.

The structural differences between *Toxicodendron* and present-day *Rhus* seem clear enough. Among other traits, flower stalks (peduncles) of the former are *axillary* (in the axil or angle formed by leaf and stem), whereas those of the latter are *terminal* (occur at the end of the branch). Other *Toxicodendron* characteristics not seen in *Rhus* include poisonous resin, drooping clusters of small cream-colored to tan fruit, and minute (<32 μm) pollen grains (Gillis, 1971a). However, the nomenclature may never be settled because toxicodendrons often are referred to as *Rhus* even in the current scientific literature, and *Toxicodendron* poisoning still is called "rhus dermatitis."

Most of the species have had to endure frequent name changes—*T. diversilobum* (poison oak) at least 14 times, and *T. radicans* (poison ivy) over 50—and disagreement still remains over some current names. For example, most authors refer to eastern poison oak as *T. quercifolium*, but prominent poison ivy expert W. T. Gillis (1971c) calls it *T. toxicarium*, with *T. quercifolium* as an alternate. A recent poisonous plant book (Burrows and Tyrl, 2001) refers to it as *T. pubescens*, but current authority (Jones et al., 1997) considers it to be just a form of western poison oak.

Another cause of confusion is the ease with which the species interbreed. Although the poison oak found west of the town of Hood River in northern Oregon is clearly *T. diversilobum*, and the poison ivy east of the John Day River 40 miles to the east is readily identified as *T. rydbergii*, the plants in between represent hybrids between the two (Gillis, 1971d). There now appear to be only four accepted North American species: *T. radicans* (poison ivy), *T. diversilobum* (poison oak), *T. rydbergii* (Rydberg's poison ivy), and *T. vernix* (poison sumac). The worldwide total is probably no more than 10 (table 2.1).

However, poison ivy occurs as nine widely distributed subspecies (table 2.1), as indicated by the abbreviation subspp. or ssp., or simply by adding a third term to the name or epithet: *T. radicans* ssp. *orientale* or *T. radicans orientale*. Botanists usually include the name of the first authority who gave the plant its epithet (often L. for Linnaeus), so the correct full name of eastern poison oak should be *Toxicodendron diversilobum* (Torrey & A. Gray) E. Greene ssp. *pubescens* (P. Miller). As is increasingly common, this book usually will not include such attributions.

Advances in analytical chemistry often have provided a "chemical taxonomy" by which species are differentiated and classified according to the presence or absence of one or more chemical constituents. Surprisingly, this apparently has not yet been applied to *Toxicodendron* species or other Anacardiaceae, although limited analysis as well as the uniformity of poisoning symptoms suggest that the toxic agents—urushiols and laccols—surely provide a common chemical link not seen outside the genus (chapter 5).

The Plants

All members of the Anacardiaceae share certain basic features, including loosely branched clusters (panicles) of numerous, small, five-petaled flowers. However, beyond that, each genus and species claims its own particular character, as illustated by the toxicodendrons. Most species of *Toxicodendron* form small trees, or shrubs that can become vines bearing conspicuous aerial roots; their leaves are opposite and either ternate (in three parts) or compound with 7–13 leaflets; and they generally are dioecious (separate males and females), with the flowers in panicles axillary (in the leaf axils) and on stalks (pedicels). Fruits are clustered, small, spherical, and cream-colored to brown.

The genus *Toxicodendron* is divided into three sections: Simplicifolia, Venenata, and Toxicodendron (table 2.1). Section Simplicifolia contains only a single species, *T. borneense*, described in detail by Gillis (1971b) but so far seen only in the tropical forests of Borneo (Beaman, 1986). As the name suggests, its leaves are simple (single) rather than compound (of multiple leaflets), elliptical, and fairly large—up to 3 × 6 inches (8 × 15 cm); in fact, the entire tree is large.

Poison Sumac and Relatives

The second section Venenata is composed entirely of tree-like forms, of which only poison sumac (*T. vernix*, plate 2) is native to the United States. It is fast-growing, short-lived, and usually forms either a small tree or a multibranched woody shrub less than 15 feet (5 m) high, although some specimens may reach 40–50 feet (12–16 m; J. D. Guin, personal communication). Unlike the other North American toxicodendrons, its leaves are pinnately compound, that is, composed of 7–13 smooth-edged oval leaflets attached opposite each other, like barbs of a feather, along a central stem or rachis; the pale fruit provides winter food for quail, pheasant, turkey, and songbirds. The plants prefer the marshy places throughout much of the eastern United States. Although often similar to *T. vernix* in appearance, nonpoisonous sumacs can be recognized by their toothed leaf margins, erect stalks of red berries, and aversion to wet places.

Toxicodendron striatum, locally called *Manzanillo de Cerra* (little apple tree of the mountains), is much like *T. vernix* but is native from southern Mexico southward. Also, it generally tends to be taller and less shrub-like than its exclusively northern neighbor, and its 11–15 leaflets are oblong and acuminate (tapered with a sharp tip) rather than oval.

Known in Australia as "rhus," *T. succedaneum* was once restricted to the Himalayas but now grows widely throughout India, China, and Japan. Its spead is reflected in local names used across the Indian subcontinent (Chopra et al., 1965): *Kakar-sing* (Hindi), *Karkata-sringi* (Sanskrit), *Krakkadaga-chingi* (Tamil), *Ranivalai* (Nepalese), and *Arkhol* (Punjabi). This 15–25 foot (5–8 m) jungle-dweller, now sold as an ornamental in many warmer parts of the world, apparently was imported into Australia as an ornamental years ago and became established there.

In form, it exhibits a grayish-brown trunk and bright green, pinnately compound leaves that turn scarlet in autumn. Creamy white to yellow flowers form drooping panicles at branch tips in the spring and are followed by clusters of yellowish-brown fruit that remains over the next winter. This seemingly desirable addition to any garden causes a distinctly undesirable dermatitis even after the leaves fall, and it constitutes a real hazard for leaf-rakers. Thankfully, this tree has not yet found its way into American gardens.

A similar tree, the Japanese lac (*T. vernicifluum*), has been cultivated in Japan for centuries, both as an ornamental and as the source of black lacquer used to coat wooden utensils. The largest representative of the toxicodendrons (50–60 feet or 15–18 m tall), it has 10–20-inch (25–50-cm) compound leaves of 7–13 shiny, 6-inch (15-cm) elongated oval leaflets, and its pale yellow flowers form loose, pendulous panicles up to 8 inches (20 cm) long. However, like the other species, its sap is highly dermatotoxic and a hazard both to workers who produce and apply the lacquer (see section 8.7) and customers who buy poorly cured objects. The rarely seen *T. trichocarpa* from China, Korea, and Japan, described by Sargent (1916) as a "large bush or less commonly a slender tree from 6 to 8 m tall" with "brilliant tints in autumn" (vol. 2, p. 180) is closely allied with *T. vernicifluum* and probably is identical to it.

The third section, Toxicodendron, provides most of the plants in the genus. Although its species, and even individual plants, can differ markedly from one another, they obviously share certain traits: They are deciduous, woody vines or shrubs with slender, erect branches, and all of them contain the same allergenic urushiols and laccols (chapter 5). Unlike the pinnately compound leaves of members of section Venenata, these tend to have just three (or rarely five) rather broad leaflets that branch from the same base (palmately trifoliate) as typified by poison oaks.

Poison Oaks

Western poison oak (*Toxicodendron diversilobum*) is familiar to most North Americans on the West Coast. In full sun, it forms a multistemmed shrub whose leaves comprise three small, shiny leaflets often less than one inch (2.5 cm) long (plate 3, fig. 2.1). Shaded, it becomes upright and more delicate-looking, with terminal leaflets up to 5 inches (13 cm) long (plate 4), or a vine whose stem diameter may exceed 8 inches (15 cm) at the base and which can climb more than 50 feet (15 m) into a nearby tree by means of numerous red-brown aerial roots. Individual plants generally are connected by underground rhizomes and can form dense thickets covering as much as an acre (0.4 ha). Birds enjoy eating the cream-colored berries (called drupes, plate 5).

The small (0.2 inch, 5 mm), pale-yellow flowers appear during April and May in clusters that emerge from the leaf axils. The plants are dioecious, and males are recognized by their five bright yellow anthers; the fragrance is powerful but apparently nontoxic and serves as a warning to unwary

Figure 2.1 Leaf form and geographic distribution: North American *Toxicodendron* species

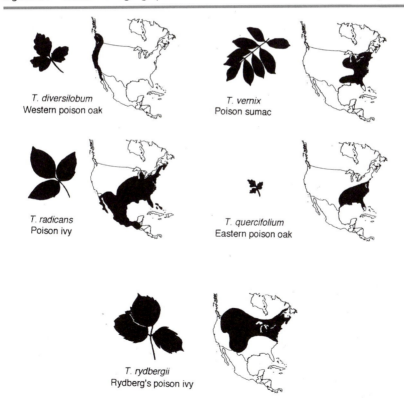

T. diversilobum
Western poison oak

T. vernix
Poison sumac

T. radicans
Poison ivy

T. quercifolium
Eastern poison oak

T. rydbergii
Rydberg's poison ivy

hikers. The striated fruit is somewhat smaller than a garden pea and under its tough exterior has a soft interior (mesocarp) containing a single, dark-colored seed. The autumn leaves are generally bright red (plate 6), although in dry, sunny locations, they tend to just dry up and turn brown.

The roots, stems, and leaves of all toxicodendrons, as well as the flowers and immature fruit, possess interconnected ducts, 5–10 μm in diameter, embedded in the plant's conductive tissue (phloem). These vessels are formed within clusters of specialized cells also located in the phloem, and the allergens are thought to originate there (McNair, 1923) as well as in the ducts (laticifers) themselves. When a duct breaks, the milky toxic sap (latex) squirts out under pressure and soon hardens to black plastic to seal the wound. Laticifers exist in addition to, and separate from, the plant's normal vascular system that carries mineral nutrients up from the roots and photosynthesis products down from the leaves.

The ducts between stem and leaf are sealed off just before the autumn leaf drop, and those leaves lose their toxicity as they dry. However, if the stems are cut when full of sap, as happens with herbarium specimens or when brush is removed in the spring or summer, the excised parts can remain toxic for years. Similar ducts are found even in species of Anacardiaceae whose sap is nontoxic, but *Toxicodendron* is distinguished by the powerful allergens of its latex that turn black when exposed to air (section 5.3). A more detailed description of the stems and laticifers is available from McNair (1923).

W. T. Gillis (1971c) provides a detailed description of so-called eastern poison oak, a plant he refers to as "the most misunderstood species in the poison ivy complex." As mentioned earlier, *T. quercifolium* (*T. toxicarium*, *T. pubescens*) recently has been demoted to just a variety of western poison oak, *T. diversilobum* ssp. *pubescens*. Unlike poison ivy and western poison oak, this 1–2-foot (30–60-cm) untidy shrub neither climbs nor has aerial roots, and its leaves and fruits are hairy (pubescent). The foliage can look even more oak-like than that of *T. diversilobum* (fig. 2.1), similar indeed to white oak (*Quercus alba*), but it is just as poisonous as its western cousin. However, the two poison oaks never grow near each other and are distinct except for their allergenic properties, and eastern poison oak seldom hybridizes with poison ivy because the two flower at different times (Guin et al., 1981).

Poison Ivy

Poison ivy actually comes in many forms, at least for botanists. The common *T. radicans* ssp. *radicans* actually looks a lot like poison oak, although its leaves sometimes do seem more ivy-like (plate 7, fig. 2.1). It occupies moist, shady areas throughout the Atlantic States and the Southeast, but it seldom grows west of the Mississippi River and never on the West Coast.

Like poison oak, it becomes a vigorous climber whose stem may flatten to a thick ribbon a foot wide as it ascends the trunk of a large tree.

The older climbing vines are characterized by thick mats of dark aerial roots, often arising from a narrow stem. Gillis (1971b) describes one place in New Jersey that exhibits "a roadside carpet [of poison ivy] for about 15 miles, covering every patch of ground not occupied by some protruding plant, house, or intersection, and [climbing] every tree on both sides of the road!" However, the subspecies *radicans* is joined by eight other distinct subspecies (fig. 2.2), and photos of the six that are native to the United States are displayed by Guin and Beaman (1986). *T. radicans negundo* is the common poison ivy of our Midwest, its range angling southwest from the Great Lakes across Iowa, Nebraska, and Kansas into Arkansas; the plants were first reported in 1853 from "Indian Territory" (Oklahoma).

Figure 2.2 Leaf form and geographic distribution: North American *Toxicodendron radicans* subspecies.

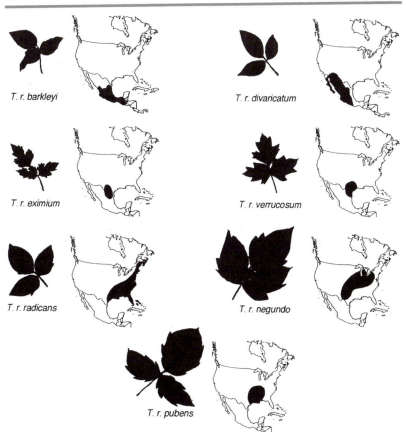

Subspecies *pubens* is found in the lower Mississippi Valley, whereas subspecies *eximium* and *verrucosum* occur near each other in Texas.

As might be expected, the subspecies are all very much alike. However, each has its own distinct range, the leaf shapes differ somewhat, and most have some other identifying characteristic as well (Table 2.2). For example, subspecies *negundo* might be difficult to distinguish from the coexisting *pubens* were it not for both its leaf surfaces being smooth and hairless (glabrous), whereas those of subspecies *pubens* tend to be rough (scabrous) on the upper side and hirsute (hairy) on the lower and, to quote Gillis (1971b),

Table 2.2 *Toxicodendron* Checklist

Locale[a]	Stature	Leaflets[b]	Classification
United States and Canada			
US, E of MS R	Tree/large shrub to <5 m	Pinnate, 7–13	*T. vernix*
US Pacific Coast, Baja–BC	Shrub/climber to 20 m, common	Oak-like, smaller in full sun, 3	*T. diversilobum*
N US, S Canada, UT–KS S to Mex	Shrub, never climbs	Spoon-like, ~3, rounded	*T. rydbergii*
US, E of MS R, S of Ohio R	Shrub/climber, aerial roots, common	Ivy-like, 3	*T. radicans* ssp. *radicans*
US Midwest to Plains	Low shrub	Ivy-like, Gl both sides	ssp. *negundo*
US, E TX, MS Valley, TX coast	Shrub/vine, aerial roots	Ivy-like, top rough, underside hairy	ssp. *pubens*
US, Rio Grande area	Low shrub/vine, rare	Deeply incised, pointed	ssp. *eximium*
US, N TX–OK	Shrub/vine, aerial roots	Gl Both sides, tips acute	ssp. *verrucosum*
SE US, TX, OK, LA	Small shrub, never climbs	Oak-like	ssp. *pubescens*
Mexico to South America			
E Mex, S to Guat, some on W Coast	Shrub/vine, aerial roots	Top Gl-velvety, hairy below	ssp. *barkleyi*
W Mex, Baja, N to AZ	Shrub or vine	Top Gl and darker, veins prominent	ssp. *diverticarum*
S Mex to Bolivia	Tree, to 12 m	Pinnate	*T. striatum*
Asia and Australia			
Japan, Kuriles	Shrub	Terminal leaf longer, 3	*T. r.* ssp. *orientale*
C China, Taiwan	Shrub	Tear-shaped, 3	ssp. *hispidum*
Austr, India, Orient	Tree, to 8 m	Pinnate, 9–15	*T. succedaneum*
Japan	Tree, 15–18 m	Pinnate	*T. vernicifluum*
Malaysia, Indonesia	Vine, to 16 m, rare	Pinnate, 5–7	*T. nodosum*
Malaysia (N Borneo)	Large tree, very rare	Large, simple	*T. borneense*

Most data from Gillis (1971a, b, c). [a]Abbreviations same as in table 2.1; also Austr = Australia, Guat = Guatamala, Mex = Mexico, R = River, US = United States. [b]Gl = glabrous (hairless).

"velvety to the touch." Indeed, these two do intergrade where they meet in Arkansas and Missouri, adding yet another difficulty in their identification.

Subspecies *eximium* and *verrucosum* also are very similar, occurring only in Texas and southernmost Oklahoma—subspecies *verrucosum* more to the north and the rare *eximium* nearer the Rio Grande. The term *verrucose* means wart-covered, an epithet mistakenly applied to leaves of an early specimen bitten by insects and thus covered with scabs of hardened sap. Actually, the main difference between the two, as between *verrucosum* and neighboring *pubens*, is that leaves of *verrucosum* actually are satiny on both sides, whereas those of the others are velvety (pubescent). The deeply cut and acutely pointed leaves of the south Texas *eximium* (fig. 2.2) also set it apart from all other *T. radicans* subspecies and make it look like an indoor ornamental ivy.

Subspecies *barkleyi* and *divaricatum* are almost exclusively Mexican (fig. 2.2). They overlap and intergrade across central Mexico, but the velvet-leaved *barkleyi* is thought to be derived from ssp. *pubens* of the Mississippi Valley rather than from the glabrous *divaricatum* (Gillis, 1971b). Another difference—one that limits an exchange of genes—is that *divaricatum* flowers mostly from April into May, whereas ssp. *barkleyi* flowers from June into July.

The two remaining subspecies are found only in Asia. The Japanese ssp. *orientale* probably was derived from the Chinese *hispidum*, and both are closely related to the North American ssp. *radicans*. A more subtle difference between the two is that fruits of *hispidum*, when viewed through a hand lens, are covered with 1 mm hairs (they are bristly or hispid), whereas those of *orientale* are either hairless or very short-haired. The reviews by Gillis (1971a,b,c,d) give further taxonomic details, maps, and photos of all nine subspecies.

Other "Poison Ivies"

There is yet another North American poison ivy. Rydberg's poison ivy, *T. rydbergii*, occurs across the northern tier of states, throughout most of southern Canada, and west into Washington and Oregon although not as far as the Pacific Coast (fig. 2.1). It looks somewhat different from either *T. diversilobum* or any of the *T. radicans* subspecies (plate 8): It lacks aerial roots (and does not climb), the mature plants are somewhat smaller, and younger leaflets tend to fold along the midrib to form a "spoon," as seen in the plate. Also, the trifoliate leaves occur at the tips of long (up to 25-cm or 10-inch), hairless stems (petioles), and their leaflets are somewhat rounded. It is often considered just another variant of *T. radicans*, a confusion due partly to the ease with which it hybridizes with nearby ssp. *radicans* or *T. diversilobum*.

Toxicodendron nodosum occurs on limestone soils along the Malay Peninsula and on the Indonesian islands of Sumatra, Java, Borneo, and Sulawesi (Celebes), but it is rare or at least inaccessible. This species forms a shrubby vine up to 50 feet (15 m) long, with slender red-brown branches and compound leaves of 5–7 long leaflets. It is the only vine among the toxicodendrons to bear pinnate leaves, and one is unlikely even to find it, much less mistake it for anything else. The so-called African poison ivy belongs to the genus *Smogingium*.

2.3   What to Look For

Plant taxonomy is based largely on anatomical details, especially flower parts, often not readily apparent to nonbotanists. However, besides the frequently trifoliate leaves, a few obvious characteristics of toxicodendrons help establish their identity (table 2.2). The plant's location can be diagnostic: For example, *T. diversilobum* is found only on the Pacific Coast of the United States (and a bit of Canada and Mexico), so check locale first. Next, the size and form of the mature plants may be distinctive—poison sumac (*T. vernix*) is the only tree type of *Toxicodendron* found north of Mexico City and then only in marshy places. Where ranges overlap, leaf form can be useful, as is the case with the two *T. radicans* subspecies from northern Mexico described in previous paragraphs. Some plants are uncommon, such as *T. radicans eximium* and *T. nodosum*; *T. trichocarpum* and *T. borneense* are so rare that even tropical botanists may never see them.

However, leaves of North American toxicodendrons are notoriously variable (figs. 2.1 and 2.2). Most people are familiar with the saying about poison oak and ivy, "leaflets three, let it be; leaflets five, let it thrive," but although the 3-leaflet (palmately trifoliate) form is by far the most common, a few plants do have 5 or even 7 leaflets. And although they can show brilliant orange or red fall colors, some may remain green all winter in warm locations or else simply turn brown. Still, leaves provide a quick means of tentative identification (table 2.2), and it would be hard to mistake a pinnate-leafed Japanese lac tree for a ground-hugging, trifoliate poison ivy or to find a poison oak shrub in the wilds of southern Mexico. If still in doubt, one can apply the black spot test (section 5.3), and recall that skin contact with any plant of the genus is likely to result in an allergic reaction if you wait just a few hours!

Western poison oak and the poison ivies are responsible for most of the skin rash caused by North American wild plants. Exceptions and botanical niceties aside, what one must watch out for in shady locations is a low, herb-like plant or climbing vine bearing clusters of three smooth, medium-green, oak- or ivy-like leaflets. In full sun, the plants appear as dense shrubs with small, dark-green shiny leaflets, still in threes. Leaflets always are light green and tender in spring, often orange or bright red in autumn, and except in very warm locations, gone by winter to be replaced by dead-looking sticks that are hard to recognize but still very toxic (Guin and Beaman, 1986).

2.4 Habitats and Geographic Distribution

Despite their extreme variability of form—from tender, low-growing herbs to large trees—toxicodendrons generally occupy a well-defined habitat. They require plenty of moisture and do poorly in the desert, but neither will they grow under marshy conditions (except for *T. vernix*). They are not fussy about sunlight and tolerate full sun by reducing leaf size (plate 4), but they do best in filtered shade under high trees and seldom live in deep shade.

They grow well near sea level but generally not above about 5000 feet (1500 m) even in warm climates, although the *T. radicans* ssp. *divaricatum* of Mexico does extend to over 9000 feet (2700 m), according to Gillis (1971d). When leafless, they tolerate subfreezing temperatures, except probably for strictly tropical species like *T. striatum*, whose cold-hardiness has never been recorded. However, they do not extend beyond about latitude 50° north (central Canada, Kurile Islands) and 40° south (introduced into New Zealand).

Although a fossil *Toxicodendron* has been found in Germany (McNair, 1923), no present-day species are native (endemic) to either Europe, Australia, or Africa. The genus is thought to have arisen in central China and spread later to North and Central America, upper South America, and throughout East Asia (fig. 2.3). However, the United States presently is home to the widest assortment, including at least four *Toxicodendron* species and most *T. radicans* subspecies (Gillis, 1971c,d).

Western poison oak occurs exclusively along our Pacific Coast, from Baja California to southern British Columbia (fig. 2.1); it has not crossed the Cascades or the Sierra Nevada and is halted on the south by the Great Basin desert. Eastern poison oak (*T. diversilobum* ssp. *pubescens*, previously *T. quercifolia*) is found from Appalachia and the piney savannas of the Southeast west to just across the Mississippi River, but it does not appear to hybridize and prefers sandy soils too dry and poor even for poison ivy. Rydberg's poison ivy, *T. rydbergii*, crosses our northern states and southern Canada and extends down the Plains states almost to the Rio Grande (fig. 2.1), whereas poison sumac (*T. vernix*) grows along the eastern seaboard from Florida to Quebec and from the Carolina coast to just west of the Mississippi River.

The most widely distributed species is *T. radicans* (figs. 2.2 and 2.3). The familiar *T. radicans* ssp. *radicans* (*the* poison ivy to most Americans)

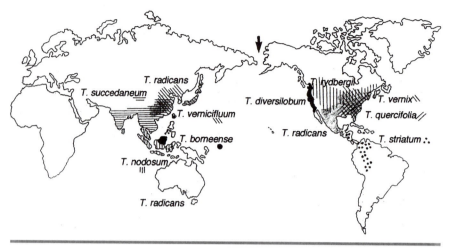

Figure 2.3 Worldwide distribution of the genus *Toxicodendron*. Arrow shows land bridge; *T. radicans* range in gray. Data from Gillis (1971a) and Mitchell (1990).

extends from Nova Scotia to the Florida Keys and Bahamas and west from the Atlantic Coast across Appalachia and the Southeastern United States as far as eastern Texas. It merges with *T. radicans* ssp. *negundo* in Michigan and across the Midwest, whereas *T. radicans* ssp. *pubens* runs down the Mississippi Valley and west into Oklahoma and central Texas to meet *T. radicans* ssp. *verrucosum*. An open strip of desert running south from central Idaho through Nevada and part of Arizona appears to be tox-icodendron-free, but the subspecies *eximium* and *divaricatum* reinstate the genus in Texas and northern Mexico and connect them to *T. radicans barkleyii* through southern Mexico and into Guatamala.

From Guatamala and Costa Rica, the arboreal *T. striatum* has moved into Venezuela (Blohm, 1962) and as far south as Bolivia (Mitchell, 1990; fig. 2.3). On the other side of the Pacific, *T. radicans* ssp. *hispidum* occurs in Taiwan and into central China but not in Japan and the Kurile Islands, home of *T. radicans* ssp. *orientale*. From China south, the wax tree, *T. succedaneum*, is widely established throughout Nepal, India, and Thailand (Chopra et al., 1965), whereas Japanese lac, *T. vernicifluum*, is found in northern China and Japan. The less common *T. nodosum* is seen in peninsular Malaysia, Indonesia, and southwestern Borneo (Sarawak), but North Borneo (Sabah, Sarawak, and Kalimantan) provides the only home for the rare *Toxicodendron borneense*. Somewhat surprisingly, *T. succedaneum* is the only toxicodendron species reported in Indochina, although others may once have lived there or simply still remain to be discovered.

Looking at a map of today's *Toxicodendron* locations (fig. 2.3), one can speculate about how such a distribution might have come to be. Two governing principles are that the plants tolerate neither extreme cold nor aridity, and that seed-eating birds (not seabirds) provide fairly rapid dispersal of the seeds. The parent genus, *Rhus*, is common throughout Asia and quite old, and what is now *Toxicodendron* probably diverged from it early in the Tertiary period, say, 45 million years ago; a rare Chinese plant, *Rhus paniculata*, may represent a common ancestor (Gillis, 1971a). Descendants of this primitive, pinnate-leaved species from section Venenata remained in Southern Asia, while a more advanced but now extinct trifoliate ancestor, *T. magnifolium*, moved east and north into Taiwan, Japan, and the Kamchatka peninsula—all of which were still joined to the mainland at the time. Two subspecies of *T. radicans* still grow there today.

During this epoch, a broad land bridge is thought to have connected Asia with North America (indicated by the arrow on fig. 2.3), across which these plants could migrate during periods of amenable climate. Later inundation of the bridge cut off access, but the bird-borne migration already had expanded south before the ice returned. *T. radicans* ssp. *radicans* of the East Coast bears a closer taxonomic resemblance to the Asian subspecies than to any other North American form, and 30-million-year-old fossils of *T. magnifolia* have been found in Northern California. The migration still has not progressed much beyond Central America, possibly because the present land bridge to South America was not in existence during most of the plant's New World history.

It is likely that *T. magnifolia* or its descendant, *T. radicans*, initially spread across much of what is now the continental United States. However, uplift of the Sierra Nevada and Cascades isolated the West Coast population, which evolved into *T. diversilobum* over the following 3 million years; uplift of other mountain ranges and development of the Western and Mexican deserts led to the separate evolution of other North American toxicodendrons into their present forms. An interesting review of such speculations is provided by Gillis (1971a).

The early Chinese species also spread south into what are now Malaysia and Indonesia, which at that time were continuous with the rest of Southeast Asia, but further expansion was blocked by rising sea levels and formation of the Himalayas and the Gobi Desert to the west. However, the migration logically should have continued into northern Australia before the sea returned and the genus may yet turn up in jungles of Queensland or the Northern Territories. However, Australia's isolation did not completely block establishment of toxicodendrons. Poison ivy (*T. radicans* ssp. *radicans* from the United States) was sold there as a garden ornamental especially coveted for its climbing habit and colorful fall foliage, and *T. succedaneum* was similarly imported (Parsons and Cuthbertson, 1992).

Poison ivy also has been imported into Holland to stabilize dikes, and it is said the same species reached England by ship within a few decades of the Pilgrims' arrival in Massachusetts; it certainly has been sold there in recent years for its dependable fall color (Huntington, 1998). The problem apparently has been averted temporarily in South Africa, where a single specimen introduced into a Capetown garden in the 1950s brought with it a case of dermatitis for its owner and resulted in the plant's destruction (Ross, 1959). Other countries, including Italy, Bulgaria, Poland, and Russia, have been slower to act and may be expected to suffer for it (Mitchell and Rook, 1979).

Because there is no reason to think that European and Australian birds relish poison ivy fruit any less than do their Asian and American kin, they and transoceanic human commerce provide an international distribution of "the poysoned weede" that nature could never have achieved on her own. The *T. radicans* and *T. succedaneum* introduced into South Australia and New South Wales have escaped their gardens and now spread across many acres of unoccupied land (Parsons and Cuthbertson, 1992), and the same probably happened to the poison ivy released in New Zealand (Connor, 1951). Our world map may soon show toxicodendrons almost everywhere.

2.5   Propagation

In addition to the sale of poison ivy and rhus as nursery stock in other countries, large quantities of western poison oak have been propagated in California. State law requires land developers and others who disturb natural vegetation to revegetate *with the same original species* whenever possible, and that includes *T. diversilobum*. Considering how much of it there is in the Golden State—it is said to be California's most abundant shrub—the plant is surprisingly tricky to grow intentionally. Mature seeds require a 2-month period of chilled after-ripening before they will germinate, although this can be shortened considerably by scarifying each seed or treating it with hot water followed by soaking for 24–48 hours. Seeds of *T. radicans radicans* achieved a germination rate as high as 80% in the greenhouse, and the subspecies *negundo* 60%, by simple chilling (Gillis, 1971d). However, the rate for other North American *Toxicodendron* species and subspecies did not exceed 3%.

Rhizome cuttings of *T. diversilobum* will regenerate in the greenhouse, but they are very prone to damping off, and only 3 out of 63 plants survived for even 3 months (Gillis, 1971d). Poison ivy, too, is rarely replanted successfully from rhizomes in the field, being influenced primarily by soil and light. Although tolerant of poor conditions, most toxicodendrons prefer rich, moist (but not wet) soil and plenty of sunlight. Adequate calcium is especially important (Gillis, 1971d), and poor success often may be attributed to inattention to the necessary cultural conditions. Athough aware of these difficulties, those of us who battle poison oak year after year are still shocked to enter a successful commercial greenhouse and see flat after neat flat filled with little poison oak plants.

Out in nature, each fruit contains a single 3–4 mm seed or "stone," which frequently is consumed by a bird or small mammal, carried off-site, and deposited in the droppings. There is evidence that these seeds germinate more readily than do those that fall on the soil directly, suggesting that the tough seed coat may be softened in passage. Birds are the principal reason for the wide distribution of *Toxicodendron* and its frequent occurrence near trees and under fence lines where birds perch (Kingsbury, 1964). McNair (1923) lists 38 species of California birds in whose innards the fruits and seed of *T. diversilobum* have been found, principally in October and November when the otherwise toxic drupes become ripe and nontoxic.

Seeds of poison oak or poison ivy germinate naturally in the spring to form a single, delicate, vertical stem whose basal nodes produce rhizomes during the first year. After a winter of dormancy, each rhizome sprouts secondary vertical shoots, together with adventitious roots at each stem junction, and each new stem in turn produces additional rhizomes. It is easy to see how dense stands of the plants could develop if given a little time.

In the summer of the second year, that year's stems produce flower buds on pedicels emerging from the leaf axils, but they overwinter and remain closed until the new leaves are fully expanded about May of the next year. Flowers of *T. diversilobum* have a sweet fragrance that attracts bees, and no doubt much of the resulting (nontoxic) wild honey makes its way into shops—a fact that never seems to be advertised. Fruit matures late in the summer but may stay attached to the stem until the following spring, so a complete life cycle can require three years.

2.6 Conclusions

As trees, shrubs, and vines of the family Anacardiaceae, the highly variable genus *Toxicodendron* now is found across much of the temperate and tropical world. Its spread is accomplished primarily by seed-eating birds, but in addition to natural radiation outward from its origin in China, it has also entered the international nursery trade and accidentally escaped.

For whatever reasons, the poison oaks, Rydberg's poison ivy, and the nine poison ivy subspecies are most common in North America. They are characterized by clusters of three (and rarely five) medium-green leaflets that emerge, palm-like, from a central point. The tree-like species—all of them except poison sumac from outside the United States—bear pinnately compound leaves of 5–13 pointed leaflets alternating along a central stem. All toxicodendrons are deciduous, become brightly colored in the fall, and are uniformly toxic. Largely because of their ornamental attributes, expansion of the toxicodendrons' range can be expected to continue worldwide.

THREE

*"Semecarpus laxiflora [Anacardiaceae] is the most
feared plant in the Bismarck Archipelago, as its
corrosive sap destroys skin and inflicts painful wounds
upon even the slightest contact."*
—P. G. Peekel, 1984

3.1   Dermatotoxic Plants

Rhus dermatitis can be due to many kinds of plants besides toxicodendrons
(Mitchell and Rook, 1979; Benezra et al., 1985). Numerous species produce
urushioids, including grasses (rice and wheat), vines (philodendron), and
large trees such as mango (table 3.1), whereas others contain dermatotoxic
quinones, lactones, or terpenes (table 3.2). This chapter deals with both
types of plants. Plants whose dermatotoxicity requires sunlight (phototoxicity), or which contain irritants whose poison ivy-like symptoms do
not involve the immune system, are reviewed in the next chapter.

3.2   More Anacardiaceae

Obviously, *Toxicodendron* is not the only dermatotoxic genus in the Anacardiaceae. Although a majestic rengas tree of the tropical jungle may seem
very different from a poison oak vine or a shrubby thicket of Hawaiian
Christmasberry, all these plants belong to the same family and produce
similar allergens and toxic effects. Although poison ivy and its relatives
are the particular focus of this book, other allergenic members of the
Anacardiaceae occur in, and even dominate, large areas of the tropical and
temperate world (table 3.3). Because everyday human contact with these
species is increasing, this is a good place to discuss some of the most dangerous and accessible among them.

Although table 3.1 lists a few of the well-known Anacardiaceae species
responsible for ACD throughout the world, table 3.3 suggests how many
there really are and how widely they are distributed. Not surprisingly, their

Table 3.1 Diverse Sources of Urushioid Allergens

Common Name	Species	Family	Occurrence[a]
Brazilian pepper[bc]	*Schinus terebinthifolius*	Anacardiaceae	CA, FL, HI, S Amer
Cashew[c]	*Anacardium occidentale*	Anacardiaceae	India, Trop S America
El Litre[c]	*Lithrea caustica*	Anacardiaceae	S Amer
Mango[c]	*Mangifera indica*	Anacardiaceae	Trop WW
Philodendron[d]	*Philodendron scandens*	Araceae	WW; Trop native
Poison oak	*Toxicodendron diversilobum*	Anacardiaceae	CA, OR, WA, SE US
Poisonwood[c]	*Metopium toxiferum*	Anacardiaceae	FL, Central Amer
Rice[e]	*Oryza sativa*	Poaceae	Trop/subtrop WW
Silky oak[c]	*Grevillea robusta*	Proteaceae	Australia, S US
Wheat[f]	*Triticum vulagare*	Poaceae	Almost WW

[a]Amer = America, Trop = tropical, US = United States, WW = worldwide. [b]Christmasberry (Hawaii), Florida holly (Florida, Bahamas). [c]See 0Avalos and Maibach (2000). [d]Knight (1991). [e]Suzuki et al. (1996). [f]Kozubek (1984).

allergens bear a striking chemical and clinical resemblance to the urushiols and laccols of poison oak and poison ivy, although the plants include common ornamentals, crop plants, utilitarian species, and even wild trees of the tropical jungle. Familiar as some of them may be, they all demand respect from anyone sensitive to toxicodendrons.

Table 3.2 Other Common Allergenic Plants

Common Name	Species	Family	Typical Allergen[a]
Artichoke (B)[b]	*Cynara scolymus*	Asteraceae	Cynaropicrin[c]
Chamomile (C)	*Chamaemelum (Anthemis) nobile*	Asteraceae	Nobilin[c]
Chrysanthemum (A)	*Chrysanthemum morifolium*	Asteraceae	Arteglasin A[c]
Cinnamon (A)	*Cinnamomum cassia[d]*	Lauraceae	Cinnamaldehyde
Dandelion (D)	*Taraxacum officinale*	Asteraceae	Taraxin acid[c]
English ivy (D)	*Hedera helix*	Aralaceae	Falcarinol
Lettuce (D)	*Lactuca sativa*	Asteraceae	Lactucopicrin[c]
Peruvian lily (B)	*Alstroemeria aurantiaca*	Liliaceae	Tulipalin A[c]
Prairie sage (D)	*Artemesia ludoviciana*	Asteraceae	Ludovicins[c]
Sunflower	*Helianthus annuus*	Asteraceae	Niveusin A[c]
Tulip (A)	*Tulipa* sp.	Liliaceae	Tulipalin A[c]
Vanilla (D)	*Vanilla planifolia*	Orchidaceae	Vanillin
Western ragweed (D)	*Ambrosia psilostachya*	Asteraceae	Isabelin[c]
Wild feverfew (A)	*Parthenium hysterophorus*	Asteraceae	Parthenin[c]

[a]Structures in figures 6.3, 6.5, and display 6.5. [b]Sensitizing power: A (strong)-D (weak), based on Gebhardt et al. (2000). [c]Indicates a lactone. [d]Also *C. zeylanicum*.

Table 3.3 Toxic Genera of Anacardiaceae

Genus	Species	Occurrence[a]
Anacardium	10	India, Central & S Amer
Astronium	10	S Mexico–Argentina
Blepharocarya	2	N Australia
Campnosperma	10	Trop WW
Comocladia	15	Mexico, Central Amer, Caribbean
Gluta[b]	~18	Trop Asia to New Guinea, Madagascar
Holigarna	8	India to Indochina
Lithrea	4	S. Amer
Loxopterygium	5	S. Amer
Mangifera	35	Trop WW, especially India to Melanesia
Mauria	8	El Salvador to Bolivia
Melanochyla	17	Malaysia, Indonesia
Metopium	3	S FL, Caribbean, S Mexico to Central Amer
Parishia	5	Myanmar (Burma) to Borneo and Philippines
Pentaspadon	6	SE Asia to Melanesia
Pseudosmodingium	7	S Mexico
Schinopsis	7	Peru, Brazil, Argentina
Schinus	24	Central S Amer, now Trop WW
Semecarpus	60	Indopacific and Austr
Smodingium	1	S Africa
Swintonia	12	SE Asia
Toxicodendron	~16	N Amer to Bolivia, E Asia to New Guinea
Trichoscypha	75	Trop Africa

Based on Mitchell (1990). [a]Abbreviations same as table 3.1; FL = Florida. [b]Includes Melanorrhoea (see Corner, 1952).

Cultivated Species

Perhaps the most familiar for many people is the mango (*Mangifera indica*), a tree that bears a delicious tropical fruit now sold in many local markets. Mangoes probably originated in sub-Himalyan Asia, and Neal (1965) recounts a Burmese legend of two brothers whose raft rose during the Great Flood until it reached heaven, where they saw a mango tree. The older brother plucked fruit to give to the world, but the younger selfishly climbed the tree to eat more; the water subsided, and he was left hanging there, "where he may be to this day." Over 500 mango varieties are found in India, some 40 of which now grow in Hawaii.

There are two races of mango: Indian and Philippine (Manila). Our Indian clones (Cornell University, 1976) are grown commercially in Florida, Hawaii, and frost-free locations in Texas and California. The handsome trees can reach 80 feet (24 m) in height, with glossy dark green foliage, numerous pinkish-white blossoms, and a heavy annual crop of red, oval 3–5-inch (8–12-cm) fruit. The taste is faintly like turpentine, and the odor of the crushed leaves is strongly so.

The juice and pulp of the fruit are safe, but biting into the peel can lead to lesions on the lips and mouth, and the clear sap causes allergic contact dermatitis in those who climb or cut the tree. According to Morton (1982), an individual may pick, peel, and eat the fruit for years and then one day be scratched accidentally by a mango branch and thereafter be unable to touch the fruit unless someone else peels it first. The fruit also must be washed well to remove any surface sap, and even the knife used to peel it should be washed before cutting the rest of the fruit.

For a sensitized person, no contact is safe. From a recent account of a young girl who had played in the fallen mangoes under a tree in Hawaii (Ferracane, 2001), "the relentless itching, which was bad from the start, intensified, and my rash grew redder and erupted into larger, oozing blisters that crusted over from head to toe. My facial features were so misshapen I hid indoors for the three weeks it took to subside, so hideous even my brother didn't tease me." In fact, mango is thought to be the principal cause of dermatitis in the state of Hawaii.

Cashew trees (*Anacardium occidentale*) support a multimillion-dollar industry. Cashews are grown widely in the tropics and subtropics, and their delicious nuts are familiar to most people. They come from untidy, 25-foot (8-m) trees grown on plantations primarily in India, and their small, fragrant blossoms produce 4-inch (10-cm) "apples" (swelled stems) that bear the husked fruit in which the nuts are embedded. The juice, husk, and a liquid found within the fruit shell (cashew nut shell liquid, CNSL) cause a persistent dermatitis among pickers and processors, and although well-roasted nuts are not allergenic, beware of the raw nuts often sold in health food stores.

The highly allergenic Brazilian pepper (*Schinus terebinthifolius*), once planted extensively as an ornamental in Southern California and Florida, is still available at nurseries today. However, this "Florida holly" eventually became a jungle that now covers thousands of acres in that state, threatens the Everglades, and will cost billions of dollars over the next 20 years to control. It also forms dense thickets in Hawaii (plate 9), where it was called *wilelaiki* (after Willie Lake, a politician who wore the berries on his hat) or *nani o hilo* (splendor of Hilo); people today call it Christmasberry—or worse. The shrub often is pruned (cautiously) into a 25-foot (8-m) single- or multitrunked tree that bears medium-green compound leaves made up of 5–13 short leaflets.

Pale greenish flower clusters yield small, red winter fruits that also are toxic to skin, and contact is most often due to touching Christmas wreaths, pruning decorative plantings, or clearing thickets for agriculture or development. Like poison oak and poison ivy, the allergens can be picked up from contaminated objects and pets (my wife had a run-in with a contaminated mailbox in Hawaii), and the common use of the dried berries as "pink peppercorns" can only lead to trouble, both internally and externally (Stahl et al., 1983). The popular California pepper tree (*Schinus molle*) is less dermatotoxic, and its berries have been used to adulterate commercial pepper.

Like the tropical tree forms of *Toxicodendron*, Burmese lac (*Melanorrhoea* spp.) produces a latex that provides the shiny black coating on Southeast Asian lacquerware. The tree's name is Greek for "black flow" and refers to the caustic sap that rapidly darkens in air. Without ever seeing one of the 150-foot (45-meter) giants, one may still contract ACD from poorly cured utensils (section 8.4), although lacquer is rapidly being replaced by less romantic (but less toxic) black plastic. Authorities sometimes place *Melanorrhoea* with the related genus *Gluta*, but we will consider the two to be separate.

Wild Species

Poisonwood (*Metopium toxiferum*) grows wild on the lime soils of South Florida and the Everglades, its seeds deposited there by tropical storms. It is native to Cuba and the Caribbean (Kingsbury, 1964; Rivero-Cruz et al., 1997), but the attractive shrub or small tree with compound leaves of 5–7 ovate leaflets is not commonly used as an ornamental. In the wild, it may reach 35 feet (10 m), and all of its parts are strongly allergenic. It is closely related to the equally toxic *M. brownei* that forms dense stands along Caribbean shores from Veracruz to Quintana Roo and whose beautiful wood makes it attractive for cabinetry despite the toxicity.

Semecarpus species are part of the poisonous rengas group that also includes *Gluta*, *Melanochyla*, *Melanorrhoea*, and *Swintonia* (Corner, 1952), and the dark sap affords a sure but risky means of identification of this group. They are among the largest trees of the tropical forest, and the red-brown heartwood is hard, durable, and strikingly marked but dangerous to handle. These woods seem never to lose their toxicity and cause agony or even death to foresters and timber dealers who try to harvest them. The trees also may be recognized by these characteristics: size, simple and spirally arranged leaves, panicles of pale flowers, tendency to grow near water, and dark blotches on the bark from sap; insects that feed on the juice are said to assume a lacquered appearance. The recurring tale that even rain-drip from the foliage causes skin lesions suggests that they should be admired from afar. The volumes by E. J. H. Corner (1952) provide extensive information.

The allergenicity of most other plants pales beside that of *Semecarpus*— its 40 species in Southeast Asia and the Pacific Islands are purported to be the most dermatotoxic of all the Anacardiaceae. Like the other *Semecarpus* species, the sap of *S. anacardium* (the bhilawa or "marking-nut tree") turns black when exposed to air and so is used as an ink and a fabric dye. However, once applied to cloth, the allergenic markings are permanent and can only be removed by cutting them out. The medium-size, deciduous trees are common across India and West Asia (Chopra et al., 1965), as shown by the local names *beladin* (Arabic), *biladur* (Persian), *bhelwa* (Hindi), *bhilawa* (Punjabi), and *bhalai* (Nepalese). The leaves are simple rather than compound, as much as 24 × 10 inches (60 × 25 cm), woolly underneath, and clustered at the branch tips. Yellow-green flowers form panicles, and each 1-inch (2.5-cm) black fruit is set in an orange cup! The nuts are the "golden acorn" of the early physicians Galen and Avicenna (King, 1957). *Semecarpus* is another tree most of us should avoid.

The 20 species of allergenic *Comocladia*, including the maiden plum (*C. dentata*), are shrubs or small trees (Oakes and Butcher, 1962). They bear pinnately compound spiny leaves, and are native to the Caribbean islands and southwestern coast of Mexico from Sinaloa to Oaxaca and into Guatamala (Lampe, 1986). To the south, *Lithrea caustica*, known locally as *el litre* or just *litre*, is abundant from central to southern Chile, and allergenic relatives *L. brasiliensis* and *L. molleoides* are native to Brazil. These unusually large and distinctive trees have a centuries-old reputation for severely afflicting anyone who rests in their shade (Hooker and Arnott, 1832; Hurtado, 1986), and yet its wood is used for lumber and firewood.

On the other side of the Pacific grows another 100-foot (30-m) giant of the jungle, *Campnosperma auriculata* (*terentang* or *serantang* in Malay). It has simple, glossy oval 3 × 8 inch (8 × 20 cm) leaves at maturity that may have been as large as 1 × 4 feet (30 × 120 cm) in the saplings (Corner, 1952). Although its allergenicity has been questioned, the fact that it contains a long-chain alkylphenol (Occolowitz, 1964) lends credance to the numerous reports of its dermatotoxicity (Beaman, 1986).

African poison ivy (*Smodingium argutum*), also called rainbow-leaf or tovana, can be a climbing vine, a woody shrub, or even a 20-foot (6-m) tree whose poison ivy-like trifoliate leaves turn bright scarlet in the fall. It comes from South Africa and has long been known to be poisonous

(Whiting, 1986). Despite causing symptoms similar to those of poison oak and poison ivy, it nonetheless is widely planted as an ornamental around schools and in parks and gardens (Findlay et al., 1974). The irritant *Pistacia vera*, source of the prized pistacio nuts, and the turpentine-producing *Pistacia terebinthus* are often mistaken for Anacardiaceae, but they are classified as Pistaciaceae.

Other Urushioid Species

A number of economically important cereal grains (family Poaceae) have been shown to contain dermatotoxic, long-chain alkylresorcinols identical to those of cashew and mango (Briggs, 1974; Kozubek, 1984; Suzuki et al., 1996). These species include rice (*Oryza sativa*), barley (*Hordium distichon*), rye (*Secale cereale*), and wheat (*Triticum aestivum*), and they differ from the broad-leafed plants already discussed in that they represent 3–4-foot (1–1.2 m) annual "grasses" (monocots) that bear flat narrow leaves, slim round stems, and heads of 0.15–0.3-inch (4–8-mm) seeds. The alkylresorcinols were found in seed extracts, except in rice where entire seedlings were extracted, and so they often present a hazard to millers and bakers—a factor in these professions that seems not to have been investigated adequately.

Philodendrons are well-known houseplants. Of more than 300 known species, *P. scandens* ssp. *oxycardum* (heart-leaf philodendron) has become the most popular indoor plant in North America (plate 10). This climbing vine can reach a height of 5 feet (1.5 m) indoors (but usually is much smaller), and its normally 4-inch (10-cm) leaves may be three times that size in older specimens. A much larger outdoor relative, *P. sellosum* (also called *P. bipinnatifidum*), is found in warm-climate gardens; the deeply notched, 18-inch (45-cm) dark green leaves are similar to those of its equally toxic relative called cutleaf philodendron (*Monstera deliciosa*).

The philodendrons (family Araceae) are well known for oral toxicity: *P. scandens* is eaten more often by small children than any other houseplant. This toxicity has been attributed to needle-like crystals of calcium oxalate that irritate the skin, mouth, and throat (section 4.2), but the ACD it causes generally has been overlooked (Knight, 1991). The dermatitis is like a moderate case of poison oak poisoning and is common among nurserymen, but housewives and office workers also are susceptible when pruning the vines. The allergens are long-chain alkylresorcinols similar to urushiols and laccols (table 5.2) but with the phenolic hydroxyls *meta* rather than *ortho*.

The maidenhair tree (*Ginkgo biloba*), commonly called ginkgo or *ginkyo* (its Japanese name), is used widely in landscaping because of its resistance to disease and insects and its bright yellow fall foliage. Originally from China, it is the last survivor of its genus, family, and order—more ancient and primitive even than the conifers—and it first appeared in Asia some 300 million years ago. Specimens can reach a height of almost 30 meters (100 ft) but are commonly less than half of that, and their bright green fan-shaped leaves are reminiscent of the maidenhair fern (*Adiantum* species). The trees are dioecious (separate males and females), but today's nursery stock is exclusively male; female trees drop copious purple fruit that give off an odor of rancid butter (butyric acid) when crushed, and children have contracted severe dermatitis from stepping on them (see Avalos and Maibach, 2000). The allergen is not this foul-smelling acid but a mixture of alkenylresorcinols like those of philodendrons. Although ginkgo leaves are not usually thought of as allergenic (Mitchell et al., 1981), they too contain 5-*n*-pentadecylresorcinol, which increases until about July and then declines until the leaves fall (Zarnowska et al., 2000).

Most of the numerous *Grevillea* species originated in Australia. Ranging from the 100-foot (30-m) silky oak, *G. robusta* (which is not an oak at all), to the low-growing hummingbird bush (*G. thelemanniana*), they have gained international recognition for their attractive foliage and spectacular yellow and red flowers (plate 11). With its pinnately compound, fern-like leaves, silky oak is used extensively as a street tree in warm regions and as a greenhouse specimen in other places. The strong and elastic wood, now imported mostly from East Africa, is valued for such diverse items as barrel staves, furniture, and telephone poles.

However, *Grevillea* sawdust produces severe dermatitis (May, 1960). Anyone who cuts the trees or branches is at risk, and telephone linemen are frequent poisoning victims in places like Honolulu and Los Angeles where the use of silky oak as large street trees is common. Cured lumber, necklaces, and bracelets remain toxic, as do the red or white blossoms of the related kahili (*G. banksii*) used in Hawaiian hat leis. The toxic agent is grevillol, yet another alkylresorcinol (table 5.2).

As pointed out previously, plants of the *Rhus* and *Toxicodendron* families do share such obvious features as compound leaves and brilliant fall color, but presumably not toxicity. However, the ornamental staghorn sumac (*Rhus typhina*) popular in Europe and along the eastern seaboard of the United States is reported to cause ACD in sensitive individuals (see Mitchell and Rook, 1979). The deciduous shrub, or up to a 15-foot (4.5-m) spreading tree, is valued for its brilliant red autumn foliage, red candle-like fruit, and fuzzy brown branches (hence its common name). Although its toxicity has been contested (Guin et al., 2000), the plants do contain low levels of some of the same allergenic 3-alkylphenols (cardols) found in cashew (Bestman et al., 1988) and probably should be handled with due caution.

3.3 Quinone-Containing Plants

Hundreds and probably thousands of plant species produce quinones (Thompson, 1971, 1987). Although the allergenicity of urushioids also has been attributed to quinones (section 1.3), even those that are structurally related do not appear to cross-react with their urushioid counterparts and so must be considered separately.

Ornamental Species

No members of the Anacardiaceae are native to Europe, where the main cause of plant-derived ACD is the primrose (*Primula* spp; Fisher and Mitchell, 1986). Many of the 400 *Primula* species, and the varieties developed from them, are available through nurseries and even in major chain stores in the United States and elsewhere. They are low-growing perennials (often planted as annuals) with showy umbels of flowers ranging in color from white and yellow through pink and red to deep purple (plate 12), and cheery blooms at Christmas lead to their frequent use as houseplants. A recent Random House book (Tumer and Wasson, 1997) describes 32 of the most common *Primula* species, and its spectacular colored photos illustrate the wide diversity of *Primula* flower forms. Another entire book is devoted to *Primula* (Richards, 1993).

Primroses are found all over the world. About 80% of the species originated in eastern Asia, particularly in the Himalayas, although some are native to Europe and a few, like the familiar cowslip (*P. veris*), are North American wildflowers. The brightly colored *Primula × polyantha* hybrid, a low-toxicity form sold widely in nurseries, is derived from *P. vulgaris* (English primrose) and *P. veris*. The leaves, stems, and flower heads of many primulas are covered with stout hairs (called trichomes) over 1 mm long, but it is the very short (0.1–0.3 mm) ones that contain the toxic oil whose principal active constituent is called primin (see table 3.4).

Trichomes occur widely in the plant kingdom. They may be single- or multicelled, usually represent outgrowths of the plant's epidermis, and take a variety of forms: short "stingers" of nettle leaves (plate 20), downy hairs of African violets, and the long fibers of cotton bolls. Many plant species produce glandular trichomes that biosynthesize and store toxic substances such as terpenes, lactones, and in primroses, dermatotoxic quinones (Rodriguez et al., 1984), which are exuded when the structures are broken upon contact. In primroses, the dissolved primin is held just under the outer

Table 3.4 Primin-containing Primroses (*Primula* species)

Species[a]	Common Name	Species	Common Name
P. alpicola var. *alba*	Moonlight primrose	*P. muscarioides*	
P. appenina		*P. obconica*[b]	Poison primrose
P. denticulata[b]	Drumstick primrose	*P. praenitens*[b,c]	Chinese primrose
P. elatior ssp. *elatior*[b]	Oxlip	*P. rosea*	Pink primrose
P. hirsuta (*P. rubra*)		*P. spectabilis*	
P. latifolia		*P. veris* ssp. *veris*[b]	Cowslip
P. malacoides[b]	Fairy primrose	*P. minima*	
		P. vulgaris ssp.	
		vulgaris	English primrose

[a]Hausen (1978a); Mitchell and Rook (1979). [b]Markedly dermatotoxic. [c]Also called *P. sinensis*.

cuticle of the hair, and cell rupture releases it as small, sticky drops that remain mostly on the flowers and flower stalks (pedicels) and less on stems and leaves.

In most instances, such hairs are harmless, and even in the Primulaceae, allergen release is passive. When a trichome actually can inject poison into the skin, the term *stinging emergence* is often used instead, particularly when the cells are other than epidermal. Stinging emergences occur in at least four plant families—Euphorbiaceae, Hydrophyllaceae, Loasaceae, and Urticaceae—probably the best known being the nettle (*Urtica* spp., section 4.2).

Through screening, Hausen (1978a) determined that 16 of the 83 primula species he tested contained primin (table 3.4), and a good example is the German primrose known in Europe as poison primrose (*P. obconica* Hance). These plants have characteristic backward-turning, serrated leaves, and the 1-inch (2.5-cm) blossoms are pale lilac to purple (plate 12). They were introduced into England from China in 1879 and quickly spread across Europe; Christensen (2000) has reviewed their botanical and toxic properties. The quinones, or perhaps related hydroquinone precursors, are synthesized and stored in the trichomes (section 6.2).

North American desert wildflowers of the genus *Phacelia* (family Hydrophyllaceae) also have adapted to urban gardens. Most of the 200 or so species are annuals less than 10 inches (25 cm) high, often pubescent (hairy) with trichomes from which the allergens are released. Seeds of the violet-flowered scorpionweed (desert heliotrope, *Phacelia crenulata*) and the bright blue desert bluebell (*P. campanularia*, plate 13) often are available in nurseries for spring and summer gardens, but the genus is most notable for the spectacular April flower displays it provides in the Southwest deserts. Many desert *Phacelia* species are allergenic, although others are not (Aregullin and Rodriguez, 2000); the lesions are like those from toxicodendrons and often occur in gardeners or in nature lovers who simply like to stroll through the springtime desert. The allergens, a group of which are known as phaceloids, are alkenylhydroquinones (section 6.2).

Orchids, too, can be allergenic. The *Paphiopedilum* species called slipper orchids or lady slipper are tropical natives, originally from India and Southeast Asia but now widely sold in flower shops. Unlike the wild lady slipper, *Cypripedium* (see below), they are relatively easy to grow, and allergic reactions to them have occurred in unsuspecting florists, orchid enthusiasts, indoor gardeners, and even botanists. The allergenicity is caused by a quinone, cipripedin (fig. 6.1; Hausen, 1980), and allergenic quinones also are found in the popular *Cymbidium* hybrids with their long sprays of flowers (Hausen et al., 1984). Vanilla orchids (*Vanilla planifolia*) cause ACD via their principal flavor chemical, vanillin (section 6.5; Collins and Mitchell, 1975).

The yellow lady slipper (*Cypripedium calceolus*, Latin for "Venus' slipper") is typical of this 35-member wildflower genus. It and similar species grow in cool, damp forests of North America and Europe, but being difficult to propagate, they have been collected almost to extinction. However, the plants produce an ACD similar to that from poison ivy but generally not as severe (Mackoff and Dahl, 1951). The allergy, first reported by a botanist collecting wild orchids for a herbarium (McNair, 1923), is caused by a "purplish secretion" (likely quinones) formed in the trichomes that cover the stems and leaves.

Tree Species

Two very common ACD-producing tree species, incense cedar (*Calocedrus decurrens*, formerly *Libocedrus decurrens*) and western red cedar (*Thuja plicata*), grow as part of vast forests in the western United States and Canada and also as ornamental trees in parks and private gardens. Both belong to the family Cupressaceae. Incense cedar is narrowly conical and slowly reaches a height of 70 feet (20 m), whereas western red cedar grows to over 80 feet (25 m) and is broader than *C. decurrens*. The woods are valuable, incense cedar more for amenities such as fine flooring or pencils and red cedar for lumber and posts that are slow to deteriorate.

Although Mitchell et al. (1972) proposed that their allergenicity is due to lichens and liverworts on the bark (section 3.6), cases of ACD in workers laying kiln-dried flooring, carpenters contacting the sawdust, and teachers using cedar pencils show that the wood itself is to blame (Bleumink et al., 1973). Shingles and shredded garden mulch are commercial cedar products not yet implicated. Airborne allergy (asthma) caused by the red cedar's plicatic acid is common in the Pacific Northwest (Chan-Yeung, 1994), but the allergen from incense cedar remains unidentified. The Mexican cedar (*Cedrela mexicana*), also called cigar box cedar, is actually a member of the mahogany family (Meliaceae), and its allergenicity is due to the dimethoxybenzoquinone (DMB) also present in other mahoganies (Hausen, 1978b).

A number of instances of contact dermatitis have been traced to paper birch (*Betula papyrifera*), a tree widely distributed across North America, and to white birch (*Betula pendula*, also known as *B. alba* and *B. verrucosa*), which is native to Northern Europe (Hausen, 1981). These species are common in both public and private gardens on both continents. The skin lesions are not due to any normal birch constituents but rather to betulachrysoquinone, the metabolite of a fungus, *Phanerochaete chrysosporium*, that has invaded and decayed the wood (Chen et al., 1977).

Exotic Hardwoods

Allergenic hardwoods, mostly from wild tropical trees (table 3.5), deserve special mention. For one thing, they represent a major industry—often *the* major industry—in parts of the tropical world. The logs and lumber are used locally for construction and are in great demand for export to make fine furniture, flooring, and decorative panelling. Among the most familiar are the rosewoods (*Dalbergia* spp.), teak (*Tectona grandis*), mansonia (*Mansonia altissima*), and mahogany (*Swietenia* spp.).

The numerous dalbergias of the Fabaceae (legume family) include Brazil rosewood (*D. nigra*), East Indian rosewood (*D. latifolia*), Siam rosewood (*D. cocchinchinensis*), Madagascar rosewood (*D. baroni*), Honduras rosewood (*D. stevensonii*), and cocobolo (*D. retusa*); all of them are allergenic. The more unusual cases of ACD include a cross-shaped rash on a man's chest caused by a rosewood religious pendant and a rash on the neck of a violinist whose chin rest was made of East Indian rosewood. Several dalbergias are also known as "jacaranda," not to be confused with the nontoxic, blue-flowered *Jacaranda mimosifolia* of the Bignoniaceae (bignonia family). The workers who fell, transport, or mill exotic hardwoods are particularly prone to severe ACD (Benezra et al., 1985), and the sawdust is especially a problem. Hausen (1981) has reviewed over 130 kinds of commercial woods that are irritant, toxic, or sensitizing, and Woods and Calnan (1976) describe these and others.

Working with the wood of ornamental hardwoods has become a popular pastime in the United States and elsewhere, so much so that many localities now sustain businesses that deal only in exotic woods and tools to shape them. There are many woodworking clubs and trade shows, and the names of common allergenic woods are now familiar (table 3.5), but dealers report increasing problems with dermatitis among both employees and

Table 3.5 Principal Allergenic Hardwoods

Common Name	Scientiic Name	Family	Allergen[a]
African blackwood	*Dalbergia melanoxylon*	Fabaceae	DLB[b]
Australian blackwood	*Acacia melanoxylon*	Fabaceae	Acamelin, DMB[c]
Brazil rosewood	*Dahlbergia nigra*	Fabaceae	DLB
Cocobolo	*Dalbergia retusa*	Fabaceae	DLB, obtusaquinone
Cordia	*Cordia goeldiana*	Boraginaceae	Cordiachromes
East Indian rosewood	*Dalbergia latifolia*	Fabaceae	DLB
Gonçalo, Zebrawood	*Astronium fraxinifolium*	Anacardiaceae	Laccols?
Honduras mahogany	*Swietenia macrophylla*	Meliaceae	DMB
Iroko, Kambala	*Chlorophora excelsa*	Moraceae	Chloraphorin
Lapacho, Ipé preto	*Tabebuia avellanedae*	Bignoniaceae	Lapachols, lapachenol
Litre, Aroeira	*Lithrea caustica*	Anacardiaceae	Laccols, urushiols
Macassar ebony	*Diospyros celebica*	Ebenaceae	Macassar II
Mansonia	*Mansonia altissima*	Sterculiaceae	Mansonone A
Pao ferra	*Machaerium scleroxylon*	Fabaceae	DLB
Peroba do campos	*Paratecoma peroba*	Bignoniaceae	Lapachols
Prima vera	*Tabebuia donnell-smithii*	Bignoniaceae	Lapachols, lapachenol
Rengas[d]	*Gluta rengas*	Anacardiaceae	Laccols
Silky oak	*Grevillea robusta*	Proteaceae	Grevillols
Singapore mahogany[e]	*Melanorrhea usitata*	Anacardiaceae	Laccols?
Sucupira	*Bowdichia nitida*	Fabacae	DMB
Teak	*Tectona grandis*	Verbenaceae	Deoxylapachol

Benezra et al. (1985); Hausen (1981); Mitchell and Rook (1979). [a]Structures in figures 5.1 and 6.1. [b]Dalbergiones. [c]2,6-Dimethoxybenzoquinone. [d]Also applied to tree species of *Melanorrhoea*, *Melanochyla*, *Semecarpus*, and *Swintonia* (Corner,1952). [e]Burmese lac.

clientele. The materials come almost exclusively from the heartwood of large trees; as the tree ages, the cells at the center of the trunk become compressed, chemical constituents in the cytoplasm are oxidized and concentrated, and the cells die and become tough fibers. Oxidation of the plant phenols provides quinones, so exotic hardwoods usually are highly colored—yellow, red, brown, or black—and the compression makes them very dense, fine-grained, and literally hard.

3.4 Asteraceae (Compositae)

Although urushioid-producing species understandably are to blame for most serious cases of ACD, common asters or "daisies" produce another type of powerful allergen known as sesquiterpene lactones or STL (section 6.3). Hundreds of lactones exist, in over a dozen plant families, but they occur most often within the daisy family—the Asteraceae.

The Asteraceae is an ancient clan, thought to have arisen from the now-extinct family Calyceraceae during the lower Cretaceous Period about

130 million years ago. Species in this family first appeared in the western part of Gondwanaland that later became northwestern South America, but they already were widely dispersed before the climax of continental drift; their fossils appear in Europe, North America, Africa, and Australia (Turner, 1977). Until recently, this family was referred to as the Compositae.

Unlike in any other dicotyledon, each reproductive structure consists of a composite of hundreds of tiny flowers thought by some to represent the apex of flower evolution and efficiency. Often, the central group of disc flowers is surrounded by a ring or rings of elongated and generally sterile ray flowers: Picture a common daisy, with its fuzzy yellow center (discs) and white rays (plate 14). Rather than a corolla of conspicuous petals that surrounds the base of most other flowers, the composite flower head is supported by an involucre, a whorl of green, leaf-like bracts. The allergenic lactones generally are contained in trichomes (see section 3.3) that cover the stems and leaves of plants such as sunflowers, as clearly seen in plate 15.

The family represents more than 10% of all flowering plants. Familiar members include chrysanthemums, dandelions, lettuce, marigolds, sunflowers, and zinnias. Most are herbaceous, and tree forms are rare. This superfamily is subdivided into three subfamilies, 17 tribes, 1535 genera, and 23,000 species dispersed worldwide (table 3.6). However, most allergenic

Table 3.6 The Asteraceae (Compositae)

Tribe	Genera	Species	Lactones[a]	Examples
Anthemideae	109	1740	412	Sagebrush, chrysanthemum
Arctoteae	16	200	13	Thistles
Astereae	135–170	3000	7	Aster, goldenrod
Barnadesieae	9	92	—[b]	Barnadesia (S. America)
Calenduleae	7–8	110	1	Calendula
Cardueae (Cynareae)	83	2500	132	Artichoke
Eupatorieae	160–170	2400	186	Joe Pye weed, ageratum
Gnaphalieae	162–181	2000	—[b]	Everlasting
Helenieae[c]	110	800	0	Marigold, Gaillardia
Heliantheae	189	2500	892	Sunflower, dahlia, ragweed
Inuleae	38	480	114	Elecampane
Lactuceae (Chicorieae)	98	1550	30	Lettuce
Liabeae	14	160	16	Liabum (S. America)
Mutisieae	76	970	29	Gerbera
Plucheae	28	220	—[b]	Marsh fleabane
Senecioneae	100–120	3000	744	Groundsel, cineraria
Vernonieae	98	1300	216	Ironweed

See Bremer (1994). [a]Number of reported sesquiterpene lactones (Seaman, 1982). [b]Not included by Seaman (1982). [c]Includes Tageteae.

forms belong to the tribes Anthemideae (chamomile-like), Heliantheae (sunflower-like), or Senecioneae (groundsel-like), although many tribes claim at least a few allergenic members. Sesquiterpene lactones are used in a chemically based taxonomy (Seaman, 1982).

All together, at least 200 species of the Asteraceae are known to cause ACD (Rodriguez et al., 1976b). It would be impractical to list them all, but a few especially important ones are listed in tables 3.2 and 6.3; structures of the allergens appear in figure 6.3. As the family was well established long before mankind emerged, we can assume that people have been exposed to its allergens from the beginning.

Certain members of the Asteraceae are notorious for producing allergies other than ACD. The pollen of ragweed (*Ambrosia* spp.), goldenrod (*Solidago* spp.), and sneezeweeds (*Helenium* spp.) is responsible for the widespread sneezing, coughing, and congestion of hay fever and related respiratory maladies. Some of the pollen allergens are proteins, but sesquiterpene lactones have also been detected and are thought to play a substantial role in the resulting human misery (Pecequeiro and Brandâo, 1985). Lactones are discussed more fully in section 6.3.

Crop Species

Lactone-containing foods from the Asteraceae include lettuce (*Lactuca sativa*), endive (*Chicorium endivia*), chicory (*Chicorium intybus*), and artichoke (*Cynara scolymus*). The first two are familiar from the grocery store; the blue-flowered roadside chicory is less common but does provide a coffee substitute in the southern United States, and the thistle-like artichoke is increasingly popular. The latex of the leafy species contains the STLs lactucin and lactucopicrin (fig. 6.3), and artichoke sap contains cynaropicrin. ACD from each of these is common among pickers, grocers, and housewives; at one time an estimated 20% of all artichoke handlers suffered from ACD.

Perhaps the most economically important species of the Asteraceae is the sunflower, *Helianthus annuus* (plate 15). This annual is grown for its seed oil, which is overtaking olive oil in popularity and starting to be produced throughout the world. Sunflowers are large, rather rough plants (up to 10 feet or 3 m tall), and they bear yellow, daisy-like flowers as much as a foot (30 cm) across. The leaves have been recognized for centuries as dermatotoxic, and at least seven toxic niveusin A derivatives are stored in and released from the round, glandular trichomes evident in plate 15 (Hausen and Spring, 1989).

A familiar relative is the pyrethrum daisy (*C. cinerariaefolium*), a common ornamental and the commercial source of pyrethrum insecticide. Extracted from dried flowers now produced primarily in Kenya and Australia, the insecticidal component is a mixture of nonallergenic esters called pyrethrins. However, another constituent, the lactone pyrethrosin, causes allergy among pickers, processors, and users.

Ornamental Species

One of the most familiar lactone-bearing ornamentals is the florist's chrysanthemum, once called *Chrysanthemum × morifolium* but now reclassified as *Dendanthrema × grandiflorum* (plate 14). Its botanical classification actually has been controversial for a long time (Schmidt, 1985); Linnaeus originally gave the name *Chrysanthemum* to a small European annual called corn marigold (*C. segentum*), and when the genus was later divided, name and plant had to remain together. Most chrysanthemums have been reassigned into one of at least six other genera: For example, marguerites, previously *C. frutescens*, are now classified as *Argyranthemum frutescens*; the common daisy *C. leucanthemum* has become *Leucanthemum vulgare*; and the feverfew that once was called *C. parthenium* is now *Tanacetum parthenium*. However, for most nonbotanists, "chrysanthemums" probably will continue to go by that name.

Likewise, taxonomists have been unable to influence the toxic character of the flowers and leaves of these popular plants, which are still allergenic and a frequent cause of ACD among florists, horticulturists, and gardeners (Hausen and Schulz, 1976). Arteglasin A and alantolactone are confirmed constituents (see fig. 6.3), but several other lactones also have been identified (Osawa et al., 1971). Although allergic reactions to the dozens of wild and cultivated species of Asteraceae differ widely, they are still related primarily to the frequency of one's exposure: seasonal in gardeners, perennial in florists.

Allergenic lactones are not confined to the Asteraceae. Notable exceptions are Peruvian lilies (*Alstroemeria* spp.) and tulips (*Tulipa* spp.); despite attempts to place *Alstroemeria* into the Liliaceae, it now has its own family, the Alstroemeriaceae (Avalos and Maibach, 2000). As the common name indicates, these beautiful plants with orchid-like flowers (plate 16) are native to South America but have become popular in north-temperate gardens. The flowers and leaves are allergenic for many people, and the allergens are the same as those in tulips and dog-tooth violets (*Erythronia* spp.)—tulipalin A and its related tuliposides (section 6.3).

However, there is no doubt that tulips belong to the Liliaceae. Originally from Asia, they became important in European commerce in the sixteenth century and are now one of the world's principal flower crops. Although the genus has more than 100 species, most commercial cultivars are derived from *T. gesneriana*, itself from an ancient line originally named by Linneaus. ACD ("tulip finger") is caused by handling the bulbs (Verspyck

Mijnssen, 1969). Because the allergenic tuliposides and tulipalins are also natural fungicides used by the plant for its own protection, *all* tulip bulbs must be suspect (Mitchell and Rook, 1979). The same is true to a lesser extent of the bulbs, leaves, and flowers of *Narcissus* (narcissus, jonquils, and daffodils) that cause "lily rash" on fingers, hands, and faces (Hjorth and Wilkinson, 1968).

So far, the lactone-producing plants we have discussed are small and either lily-like or herbaceous. However, a few tree species also make lactones, notably the Grecian laurel, *Laurus nobilis* (Lauraceae), a leather-leaved ornamental 30–40 feet (9–12 m) in height. This is the classic laurel awarded as a wreath to heroes in ancient Greece but now used as a flavoring in soups and stews and as an aromatic in soap and hair oil. Its lactones, principally laurenobiolide (fig. 6.3), do not contribute to either taste or odor, but they do lead to ACD (Cheminat et al., 1984). One wonders about the outcome of placing fresh laurel leaves on the sweaty brow of a winning athlete.

"Weeds"

Weeds may be just "plants out of place," but their home often includes sidewalks, vacant lots, and probably your garden. They usually exhibit rampant reproduction, accommodation to humans, and a penchant for self-protection via toxicity, repellent odor, or unpleasant taste. A surprisingly large proportion belong to the Asteraceae, but weed allergy is highly individual and there is no generally accepted "worst" species. However, a survey of human reactions to 19 common weeds of the central United States (Menz and Winkelmann, 1987) revealed that nearly all of the people tested were allergic to Mayweed (dog fennel, *Anthemis cotula*), 70% to cocklebur (*Xanthium pennsylvanicum*), 36% to wild feverfew (*Parthenium hysterophorus*), and 14% to fleabane (*Erigeron strigosus*).

Sagebrush (*Artemisia tridentata*), sneezeweed (*Helenium autumnale*), ragweed (*Ambrosia trifida*), and yarrow (*Achillea millefolium*) each caused an allergic response in 11% of people tested. The results differ from those of a similar test 35 years earlier (Mackoff and Dahl, 1951), when ragweed, sneezeweed, and wild feverfew were the chief offenders, in that order. Thus, both agricultural and population dynamics may alter ranking but not the basic allergenicity, so a brief review of these obnoxious Asteraceae species seems in order (see USDA, 1970).

Mayweed (dog fennel) was introduced centuries ago from Europe and has spread across the entire United States. This multibranched annual grows 4–24-inches (10–60-cm) tall and bears divided leaves and a profusion of white 0.5–1-inch (1.2–2.5-cm) daisy-like flowers with protruding yellow centers. All parts of the plant have a rank odor, blister human skin and the mouths of grazing animals, and cause ACD primarily via a lactone called anthecotulide, but these drawbacks have not kept it from being used as an ornamental ground cover. One dermatology patient at the Mayo Clinic reportedly planted it around her swimming pool "for decorative purposes" (Menz and Winkelmann,1987).

Its close relative, *Anthemis nobilis* (Roman chamomile, now renamed *Chamaemelum nobile*) has been used in folk medicine since medieval times, but both poultices and tea made from chamomile (sometimes spelled camomile) cause ACD because of the lactone nobilin. *Matricaria* (*Chamomilla*) *recutita*, the German chamomile commonly grown in gardens, is similar and contains the lactone desacetylmatricarin and its acetate, matricarin (fig. 6.3).

Cocklebur (*Xanthium pennsylvanicum*, also classified as *X. strumarium*) likewise occurs all over the world but is especially abundant in the Southeast and Central Plains of the United States. It is a bushy, erect plant 8–36 inches (20–90 cm) high, with alternate heart-shaped leaves and clusters of tiny flowers that appear from July to September. Its most obvious feature is the 0.5–1-inch (1.2–2.5-cm) burrs with hooked spines that cluster in the leaf axils (crotches) after early September. ACD is due to the lactones xanthinin and xanthatin (Deuel and Geissman, 1957).

Wild feverfew (*Parthenium hysterophorus*) is so named to distinguish it from another feverfew, *Tanacetum parthenium*. It seems to be just about the perfect weed (from a plant's viewpoint)—a tough, aromatic shrub from the Caribbean adapted to, and even dependent on, humans and their agriculture. It starts flowering at the tender age of 4 weeks and produces its small, white daisies for the next 6–8 months, during which it releases a prodigious amount of lactone-bearing pollen and, subsequently, seeds. As a result, the plant has spread to most of the eastern states of the United States and to every continent except Antarctica (Towers and Mitchell, 1983).

Its seeds often contaminate commercial agricultural products. This is how they entered India, in a 1954 shipment of grain, and spread catastrophically across that country (section 1.2). "The weed has invaded every nook and cranny along the sidewalks, in gardens and in vacant lots, both in the city and its outskirts, and large areas of agricultural land are overgrown by it" (Towers and Mitchell, 1983). ACD from this so-called congress grass developed into a major public health issue, especially among farmers and their families. As with other Asteraceae, the allergens—parthenin, coronopilin, and several other lactones—occur primarily in the short trichomes on the stems and leaves (Rodriguez et al., 1976a), but also in the pollen (Mitchell, 1981a; Picman and Towers, 1982).

A close relative, feverfew (*Tanacetum parthenium*, formerly *Chrysanthemum parthenium*), is an aggressive, 1–3-foot (30–90-cm) ornamental and a major weed problem in Europe. Native to that continent's southeast and to Asia Minor, it has been used for centuries as an effective folk medicine against arthritis, fever, migraine, unwanted pregnancy, and even insects. The plant is widely recognized to be dermatotoxic and responsible for ulcers in the mouths of any who chew the rank-smelling leaves for relief. As is the case in so many members of the Asteracee, the principal toxicant is the STL parthenolide (Hausen, 1991).

Fleabane, only one of a large number of weeds in the genus *Erigeron*, occurs west of the Pacific mountain ranges and again through the plains states to all the Atlantic seaboard except Florida. The plants are 1–5 feet (30–150 cm) tall but do not branch until perhaps halfway up the erect stalk. Leaves are long and narrow, and the white to lavender 0.8-inch (2-cm) daisy-like flowers with yellow centers cluster at the ends of almost bare branches. The ancient common name describes the plant's strong odor, once thought to drive away fleas.

Some kind of ragweed (*Ambrosia* spp.) can be found almost anywhere in the United States. Common ragweed (*A. artemisiifolia*) is a large, multi-branched annual reaching 3.5 feet (1 m) tall and sometimes more; it bears both opposite and alternate, deeply divided leaves and narrow terminal spikes of tiny, greenish flowers. It occurs widely, but especially from the plains states eastward. Western ragweed (*A. psilostachya*) is similar but perennial, somewhat shorter and bushier, and occurs primarily west of the Mississippi River, from Mexico north into Canada.

Ragweeds bloom from early summer into autumn, when their copious pollen can be a major source of ACD via the lactones ambrosin, isabelin, and psilostachyin (fig. 6.3; Mitchell et al., 1971). Hay fever is caused by inhaling either the lactone or protein allergens. The lactone content of ambrosias can be quite variable; for example, giant ragweed (*A. trifida*), with its broad, three-lobed opposite leaves and height of over 10 feet (3 m), contains no detectable lactones (Herz, 1977).

Other serious offenders include the mountain tobacco (*Arnica montana*), hillside arnica (*A. fulgens*), and seep-spring arnica (*A. longifolia*) of the American West (Hausen et al., 1978). The plants are found in moist meadows or on rocky hillsides across Europe, Western Asia, and North America and usually reach 1–2 feet (30–60 cm) in height, with paired, aromatic leaves and cheery yellow composite flowers. Since ancient times, the roots and flowers have provided "tincture of arnica," a concoction applied directly to the skin as a counterirritant to bruises, cuts, abrasions, and sore muscles and the principal cause of Arnica sensitization.

Members of the genus *Thapsia* (Apiaceae), native to the southern Mediterranean, rapidly produce erythema, blisters, and intense itching on contact (Christensen et al., 1997). Its medicinal resin, *Radix Thapsiae* or

Resina Thapsiae, were noted by the early Greek physician Theophrastos in the third century B.C., and the thapsigargin and thapsigargisin they contain are potent histamine liberators and general stimulants of the human immune system (Ali et al., 1985). Mature plants stand about 2 feet (60 cm) tall, bear large rounded umbels of yellow flowers, and are common in Spain and the Mediterranean region. Three species, *T. garganica, T. maxima,* and *T. villosa,* have been of recent chemotaxonomic interest (see Smitt, 1995).

3.5 Other Flowering Plants

Hundreds—perhaps thousands—of higher plant species have been reported to cause ACD (see Mitchell and Rook, 1979; Avalos and Maibach, 2000), only a few more of which can be mentioned here. However, because of wide and increasing use, species of the family Aralaceae require particular mention. These are familiar ornamental houseplants that include English ivy (*Hedera helix* ssp. *helix*), Algerian ivy (*H. helix* ssp. *canariensis*), schefflera (principally *Schefflera arboricola*), and fatshedra (*Fatshedra lizei,* actually a hybrid of *F. japonica* and *H. helix*). All of them contain allergenic polyacetylenes such as falcarinol (see section 6.4). Also, with the current interest in herbal medicines, the dermatitis suffered by users of ginseng (*Panax ginseng*) is worth citing. See Boll and Hansen (1987) and Hausen (2000b).

Food and Flavor Plants

If, indeed, "you are what you eat," we are all in deep trouble. A previous section described mango and cashew as common sources of ACD in humans; it is not the edible part that causes problems, of course, but the sap of the mango and the cashew nut oil. Wheat (*Triticum vulgare*) and rye (*Secale cereale*) seeds contain urushioids (Kozubek, 1984) that carry over into flour and present a health hazard for bakers, and the pink peppercorns from the Brazilian pepper tree (*Schinus terebinthifolius*) were said to be the principal source of ACD in South Florida at one time (Catalano, 1984). Sesame (*Sesamum indica*), a common source of cooking oil and flavored seeds, is both allergenic and irritant (Neering et al., 1975).

ACD from asparagus also is common among pickers, packers, and housewives. What we use as a vegetable is the immature shoot of *Asparagus offinalis,* which is widely valued by florists. The plants are grown commercially in the rich, damp, highly organic soils favored by ferns, and the spears are harvested as they emerge. The allergen is a sulfur-containing organic acid (section 7.4), not the volatile methyl mercaptan whose odor is so apparent in the urine soon after one eats asparagus (Hausen and Wolf, 1996).

Several common flavoring agents are convertible into allergenic *o*-quinones. For example, vanilla orchids (*Vanilla planifolia*) produce a "bean" (pod) whose main flavor constituent is vanillin; oil of cloves (*Eugenia caryophyllata*, Myrtaceae) owes its characteristic flavor to eugenol; and the tang of ginger root (*Zingiber officinalis*, Zingiberaceae) is due to zingerone and gingerol (fig. 6.5). Each of these can be demethylated metabolically to a 4-substituted catechol (display 6.6).

However, many natural flavor and fragrance compounds that cannot form quinones still are allergenic. They combine into the hundreds of complex, odorous essential oils (that is, oils with an odor or essence) extracted from a wide variety of plants but whose exact composition often remains poorly defined (table 3.7; de Groot and Frosch, 1997). The Lamiaceae (Labiatae or mint family) and Rutaceae (rue family) are strongly represented. Essential oils are used widely to flavor such everyday items as toothpaste, cold remedies, baked goods, confections, and even chewing gum, but the ACD they cause is generally due to handling rather than to eating them. Out of 200 random dermatology patients, 17 reacted to at least one of 35 different oils (Rudzki et al., 1976). For more on essential oils, see section 6.5, and for their ACD, see Scheinman (1996).

The essential oils are described in a monumental, multivolume monograph (Guenther, 1975), and the toxic properties of many individual oils are discussed by Opdyke (1975b). Although there are far too many to detail here, three that are in wide and growing use are typical: citrus oils, oil of

Table 3.7 Common Allergenic Essential Oils

Essential Oil[a]	Source	Family	Principal Constituent[b]
Anise	*Pimpinella anisum*	Apiaceae	Anethol (80–90%)[c]
Bitter orange	*Citrus aurantium*	Rutaceae	*d*-Limonene (90%)
Chamomile (Roman)	*Chamaemelum nobile*	Asteraceae	Butyl angelate (<50%)
Citronella	*Cymbopogon nardus*	Poaceae	Geraniol (60%)
French marigold	*Tagetes* spp.	Asteraceae	Tagetone (>50%)
Jasmine	*Jasminum officinale*	Oleaceae	Benzyl acetate (65%)
Lavender	*Lavandula officinalis*	Lamiaceae	Linalyl acetate (>30%)
Lemongrass	*Cymbopogon citratus*	Poaceae	Citral (>75%)
Peppermint	*Mentha piperita*	Lamiaceae	Menthol and esters (50%)
Rose (Bulgarian)	*Rosa damascena*	Rosaceae	2-Phenylethanol (65%)
Sage	*Salvia officinalis*	Lamiaceae	α- and β-Thujone (50%)
Vetiver	*Vetiveria zizanioides*	Poaceae	Vetevenols (>45%)
Ylang ylang	*Cananga odorata*	Annonaceae	Benzyl benzoate (>30%), sesquiterpenes[d]

[a]de Groot and Frosch (1997). [b]Guenther (1975); Srinivas (1986). [c]Structures in figure 6.5.
[d]60–65% in the distilled oil, almost none in extracted oil.

cinnamon, and tea tree oil, whose chemical properties are discussed in section 6.5. The citrus oils come from the fruit of 20–30-foot (6–9-m) spiny evergreen trees—particularly orange (*Citrus sinensis*, Rutaceae) and lemon (*C. limon*)—and have a long history as flavorings in baked goods, candy, and soft drinks. They are pressed or steam-distilled from the peels left over from commercial juice production, and current popularity of citrus drinks assures a large and continuous supply. Lemon and orange oils are commonly used in flavorings, fragrances, cleaning agents, and polishes, and orange oil also is used in fire-starters for home barbeques. The annual world production of orange oil has grown to about 160 million pounds (73,000 metric tons), mostly from Brazil and Florida (IARC, 1993).

Many children, present and past, recall making "cinnamon sticks" by soaking toothpicks in oil of cinnamon, an item of commerce for over 1000 years. The oil is produced by steam distillation of the bark of several moderate-size, tropical trees of the genus *Cinnamomum* (Lauraceae): *C. zeylanicum* of Sri Lanka, India, and Mexico; *C. loureirii* from Southeast Asia; and *C. burmanii* from Indonesia. Of the bark oil, 67% comes from Sri Lanka, whereas 85% of the leaf oil is from Southeast Asia. An acre (0.4 ha) of trees now provides 150–200 pounds (70–90 kg) of a brown inner bark containing 0.1–0.2% of oil, in addition to an even larger weight of leaves, so the world's total annual oil production is approaching 200,000 pounds (90,000 kg). The main uses are in perfumes, soaps, cosmetics, and flavoring for candy, baked goods, and especially soft drinks such as Pepsi-Cola.

Tea tree oil, from *Melaleuca alternifolia* (Myrtaceae), is becoming popular as a cleanser and antiseptic. The source is a medium-size native tree of Australia, 20–30 feet (6–9 m) tall, with narrow leaves and clusters of white to purple bottle-brush–shaped blossoms (the name "bottle brush," however, is reserved for related *Callistemon* species). All parts of the plant contain the allergenic oil, as do other *Melaleuca* species including *M. leucadendra* (*M. quinquenervia* or cajeput, pronounced "kaj-a-put") used for centuries as a rubiefacient and medicinal agent.

The taste and odor of most spices come from their essential oils, but because there are over 60 now in commercial and home use, only a few could be included in table 3.7. Besides the clove, cinnamon, and vanilla already mentioned, others such as bay laurel (*Laurus nobilis*, Lauraceae), nutmeg (*Myristica fragrans*, Myristicaceae), and ginger (*Zingiber officinale*, Zingiberaceae) also contain allergenic oils (Schwartz et al., 1957). Although not usually considered a food, propolis ("bee glue") is widely sold in health food stores as a pleasantly flavored cure-all. This is the comb cement made by bees, largely from the sap of the poplar (*Populus* spp.), whose composition reflects that of balsam of Peru (primarily cinnamate and caffeate esters), and the two cross-react (Hausen et al., 1992). Propolis causes ACD in beekeepers but also in a growing number of natural food devotees who purchase it in health food stores.

Food allergies and their recognition is of growing importance. Food allergy is much more prevalent than was once supposed and afflicts millions of people worldwide, but this complex subject can receive only superficial mention here. The term is usually applied to the dermatitis and other allergic reactions suffered by those who cannot tolerate certain specific foods (Metcalfe et al., 1997), but it also describes the contact urticaria produced directly on the skin of grocers, cooks, and housewives by certain uncooked food items (Czarnetzki, 1986). The flesh of fish, lobsters, and chickens, and many raw fruits and vegetables such as potatoes, carrots, and apples may bring about a Type I allergic reaction (see table 1.4).

Few food allergens have been identified chemically, but those that have been characterized are proteins or glycoproteins (Lahti and Hunnuksela, 1978). However, as suggested by the ACD caused by eating lettuce, endive, wheat flour, mango, or parsley that contain small, fat-soluble allergens, the rapid onset of contact urticaria from food allergy may eventually be related to some of the nonprotein allergens discussed in this chapter.

Fragrant Plants

The sap of most plants possesses an odor, although it is not always agreeable. However, some species produce aromas that are very pleasant indeed, and these have been cultivated since ancient times for perfume. Like flavors, with which they are closely allied, fragrances arise from the plant's essential oils—complex mixtures of volatile chemicals. Note that most of those listed in table 3.7 are recognized for their odor rather than their taste, and that they come from a wide range of plant sources. Perhaps several other species should be added for their high economic value: acacia (*Acacia farnesiana*, Fabaceae), carnation (*Dianthus caryophyllus*, Caryophyllaceae), geranium (*Pelargonium odoratissimum*, Geraniaceae), rosemary (*Rosmarinus officinalis*, Lamiaceae), orange blossom (*Citrus sinensis*, Rutaceae), and violet (*Viola odorata*, Violaceae).

Most of the oils are extracted or distilled from blossoms or leaves, but a few come from the wood of trees such as sandalwood (*Santalum album*, Santalaceae) and cedar (*Juniperus virginiana*, Cupressaceae); see section 6.5. Recovery and export of fragrance materials has been a large and lucrative industry and remains so today in many parts of the world, including France (lavender), Sri Lanka (cinnamon), and Australia (tea tree). However, as the composition of the natural oils becomes more accurately known, fragrance chemicals are increasingly man-made (table 6.4; de Groot and

Frosch, 1997), even though a blend of synthetics still does not convey the odor-equivalent of the natural mixture from the plant.

In earlier times, the use of plant fragrances was restricted almost entirely to toiletries and perfumes, and they were rare and high priced. Now they are applied to most items in our everyday lives, from laundry detergent to lipstick to toilet paper. Originally obtained from wild species of the jungle—sandalwood was collected almost to extinction in the late 1800s—essential oils today are largely commercially produced on extensive plantations. For example, in southern France, one can travel for miles though a virtual sea of purple lavender (*Lavandula officinalis*).

Balsam Species

Balsams are the aromatic liquids or resinous sap released from injured trees, and most of them either irritate or sensitize human skin (Hjorth, 1982). They are used in flavors, perfumes, and medicinals, the most common being tolu balsam (from *Myroxylon toluiferum*), balsam Canada (from the balsam fir, *Abies balsamea*), and balsam styrax (from *Styrax tonkinensis*), also known as Siam benzoin or storax. Another storax comes from liquidambar trees, *Liquidambar orientalis* (Levant storax) and *L. styraciflua* (American storax), but the most widely used is balsam of Peru.

Balsam of Peru is obtained from a tropical tree, *Myroxylon balsamum* var. *pereirae*, by tapping the resinous sap as is done to collect rubber latex or maple sap. The fragrant liquid is used in flavors, cosmetics, toothpaste, perfumes, hair tonic, throat lozenges, cola drinks, and other consumer goods that assure wide dermal and oral exposure. Occupational exposures can occur among dentists, bakers, painters, and even violinists (from wood finishes). Peru balsam, too, is a complex mixture, but chemical analysis as well as patch testing has shown the principal allergens to be benzyl cinnamate and related esters (fig. 6.5), known collectively as cinnamein.

Balsam of pine comes primarily from forest conifers, including *Pinus pinaster* (cluster pine) and *P. sylvestris* (Scotch pine) in Europe and *P. palustris* (long-leaf pine), *P. pinea* (stone pine), *P. taeda* (loblolly pine), and *P. elliottii* (slash pine) in North America. Trees are tapped and the liquid resin collected and distilled to provide "oil of turpentine" and a semisolid residue called colophony or gum rosin (Fregert and Horsman, 1963). World production of gum rosin in 1988 was about 1.6 billion pounds (720,000 metric tons), mostly from the United States. Until the 1970s, turpentine was the principal solvent for paints and varnishes, and its dermatotoxic action was utilized medically in rubefacients (substances to redden the skin); the skin reactions are not due to terpene constituents themselves but to their oxidation products (section 6.5).

Colophony should not be confused with either tall oil rosin (a by-product of the paper industry) or various chemically modified rosins now on the market. It is still applied widely in coatings, adhesives, printing inks, soap, paper, and many other products; Rietschel and Fowler (2001) list over 100 uses. Its age-old application to the bows of stringed instruments and the slippers of dancers makes it a source of occupational dermatitis among both industrial workers and musical artists (Ducombs, 1978). Norway spruce (*Picea excelsa*) is a source of turpentine and rosin, too, and *Abies balsamea* (balsam fir) yields Canada balsam, a substance which is familiar to microscopists as mounting material for slides.

3.6   Lower Plants

Up to this point, we have been concerned with the allergenic higher plants and plant products likely to be encountered in daily life and travel. However, skin contact with certain "lower" (nonflowering) species also can lead to dermatitis (Schmidt, 1996). The minute scale-mosses (liverworts of the family Hepaticae) are common offenders. Growing on damp rocks or tree trunks, they bear flat, scaly "leaves" (phyllidia), separate "flowers" (archegonia) and male structures (antheridia), and eggs and motile sperm that require a wet environment. They form small reddish or greenish mats, fluffy when moist and flattened when dry, best seen under a lens.

For such unobtrusive creatures, liverworts cause a lot of human suffering (Mitchell et al., 1970). Species of *Frullania*, especially *F. dilatata*, *F. nisquallensis*, and *F. tamarisci*, cause "forester's itch," also called cedar poisoning in Canada and pine poisoning in the northwestern United States. This is an ACD that affects loggers—especially lumberjacks—and anyone else intimately exposed to tree bark (Mitchell, 1981b, 1986). Rangers, truckers, and sawmill workers also are susceptible, and because the toxic constituents (lactones called frullanolides) penetrate to the wood underneath, lumber dealers, carpenters, and cabinetmakers, too, are at risk (Schmidt, 1996). An infested understory may even harass hikers and gardeners with "strollers' eczema" (Quirce et al., 1994).

Symptoms appear within a day or two and are gone within a few weeks if there is no further contact; this is similar to ACD from poison oak. However, serious cases may even require a change of profession to avoid further exposure. The most common sources of ACD from liverworts are the conifer species on which the lower plants live, such as fir (*Abies*) and spruce (*Picea*), chestnuts (*Castanea*), oaks (*Quercus*), sycamores (*Platanus*), and poplars (*Populus*), although some of the dermatitis may also be due to lichens rather than to liverworts (Dahlquist and Fregert, 1980).

Lichens represent a symbiosis between an alga and a fungus, the alga providing nutrients from photosynthesis and its ascomycete partner offering both form and moisture. They survive drought, cold, and high altitude, and occur all over the globe as crusts on bare rock, strands hanging from tree branches (such as old man's beard), or soft outgrowths on bark, fences, and other surfaces. Lichens come in a striking variety of colors— yellow, orange, red, grey—largely derived from the complex, phenolic substances they contain (Culberson, 1969); see section 6.6.

With at least 20,000 species of lichens in existence, it is fortunate that the dermatotoxic ones are only weak sensitizers. However, they can also be irritating, and Rademacher's list of 40 species that are of "dermatological significance" includes *Cladonia, Evernia, Parmelia, Lecanora,* and *Usnea* (Rademacher, 2000). Although many lichens survive on bare rock, they often live on tree trunks and branches, and skin contact is prevalent among loggers, foresters, wood cutters, and homeowners with fireplaces. Patch tests show that atranorin and evernic acid (section 6.6) most often are responsible. Use of an *Evernia* extractive called oakmoss in perfumery causes allergy even in people far removed from forests (Gonçalo et al., 1988).

Algae, by themselves, have also been implicated in dermatitis (Camarasa, 2000), and irritant agents have been identified in extracts of the marine cyanobacterium (blue-green alga) *Lyngbya majuscula* (Stafford et al., 1992); see section 7.5. The green microalga *Apatococcus constipatus* contains long-chain 5-alkylresorcinols, the exact composition depending on the strain, but its degree of dermatotoxicity has not been reported (Zarnowski et al., 2000). These authors also cite three other algal species that contain 5-alkylresorcinols, the same allergens found in mango. Although many fungi cause dermatitis (Mitchell and Rook, 1979), no specific agent has been implicated; however, tetracycline antibiotics (such as those from *Streptomyces*) have long been recognized to be phototoxic (Klaassen et al., 1996).

3.7 Photoallergenic Plants

ACD can result from simultaneous exposure to certain plant constituents and sunlight. Sandalwood oil, lime peel, and ragweed oleoresin are common offenders, but the problem occurs most often after use of perfumes, sunscreens, and aftershave lotions containing purely synthetic ingredients. Psoralens like 8-MOP (section 7.2) have also been implicated (Lunggren, 1977). Although instances of human injury have been claimed, the syndrome is considered rare (Chew and Maibach, 2000). However, *phototoxicity* (photodynamic action, section 1.6) certainly is very real and will be considered in sections 4.1 and 9.4.

3.8 Conclusions

It is apparent that toxicodendrons are not the only plants that cause ACD. Many kinds of higher and lower plants are allergenic or provide allergenic products, including ordinary foods such as mango, lettuce, and cashew; garden ornamentals like Brazilian pepper, orchids, and tulips; and such everyday items as perfumes, scented paper, food flavorings, houseplants, and hardwoods. The most frequent offenders are chrysanthemums, followed by tulips, Peruvian lillies (*Alstroemeria*), primroses, and, of all things, Christmas trees such as balsam fir. Many common weeds form allergenic lactones that reach a sensitive person by touch or on the breeze. Lichens, liverworts, and algae represent dermatotoxic lower plants. Indeed, exposure to plant allergens has become all but inescapable in modern life.

FOUR
PHOTOTOXIC AND IRRITANT PLANTS

"Kapparis (Capparis spinosa): But ye Caper ... from the Red Sea and Arabia is extremely sharpe, raysing pustules in the mouth, and eating up ye gummes to the bare bone, wherefore it is unprofitable to be eaten."
—Dioscorides, ca. A.D. 60 [Translated by J. Goodyer in 1655 (Gunther, 1959)]

4.1 Phototoxic Plants

Although many plant constituents are allergenic, others require sunlight for dermatotoxic action and so are said to be *phototoxic* (or photodynamic if visible light and oxygen are involved). When such substances contact skin that later is exposed to sunlight, the result can be anything from mild sunburn to large, painful blisters. Some phototoxic agents are absorbed into the blood stream, so eating a plant such as celery can produce the same result as skin contact. Although the effects usually last only a few days, some lesions may persist for years (Benezra et al., 1985). The disease is termed *phytophotodermatitis* (dermatitis due to plants and light).

The most common phototoxic constituents, called furocoumarins (section 7.2), occur throughout the plant world but principally in the Apiaceae (Umbelliferae) and especially in citrus species of the Rutaceae (see table 4.1). The following story illustrates the effects of furocoumarins. A major pharmaceutical firm once planned to market xanthotoxin (8-methoxypsoralen or 8-MOP) as an "oral suntan agent" whereby one had only to swallow a pill and then go out into the sunlight or sit beneath a UV lamp to become tan (or rather, burned). However, additional tests showed that tanning would not stop until the skin had turned to leather, so the project was abandoned. An extensive review of the occurrence, chemistry, and biological activity of plant furocoumarins has been prepared by Murray et al. (1982), and furocoumarins in food plants were reviewed by the Steering Group on Chemical Aspects of Food Surveillance of the UK (SGCAFS,1996).

Table 4.1 Common Phototoxic Plants

Species	Common Name	Family	Toxic Agent(s)[a]
Ammi majus	Bishop's weed	Apiaceae[b]	3,8,10,11,12,13,21
Anethum graveolens	Dill	Apiaceae	3
Angelica archangelica	Angelica	Apiaceae	1,3,10,12,13,15,16,21
Apium graveolens	Celery	Apiaceae	3,12,13
Citrus aurantifolia	Lime	Rutaceae	2,3,4,7,10,12,13
Citrus bergamia	Bergamot orange	Rutaceae	2,3,4
Citrus limon	Lemon	Rutaceae	2,3,4,5,7
Citrus paradisi	Grapefruit	Rutaceae	2,3,4,5
Citrus sinensis	Sweet orange	Rutaceae	4
Dictamnus alba	Gas plant	Rutaceae	3,19,21, Dictamnine[c]
Echinops exaltus	Globe thistle	Asteraceae	Butenynyl-2,2'-dithienyl[c]
Fagopyrum esculentum	Buckwheat	Polygonaceae	Fagopyrin[c]
Ficus carica	Fig	Moraceae	3,19,21
Heracleum lanatum	Hogweed	Apiaceae	1,3,10,11,13,14,18,19,21
Heracleum mantegazzianum	Giant hogweed	Apiaceae	1,3,5,10,11,13,18,19,21
Hypericum perforatum	St. John's wort	Hypericaceae	Hypericin[c]
Pastinaca sativa	Parsnip	Apiaceae	3,10,11,13,18,21,22
Pimpinella anisum	Anise	Apiaceae	3
Psoralea corylifolia	Scurf pea	Fabaceae	1,19
Ruta graveolens	Common rue	Rutaceae	3,5,12,13,19,21
Tagetes patula	French marigold	Asteraceae	α-Terthienyl[c]

See Murray et al. (1982) and Pathak et al. (1962) for more complete lists. [a]Numbers correspond to furocoumarins; see table 7.1. [b]Previously called Umbelliferae. [c]See section 7.2.

Rutaceae (Rue Family)

The Rutaceae is a family of 150 genera and about 1600 species distributed widely in temperate and subtropical regions. They are perennial shrubs or trees characterized botanically by odorous oil glands on the leaves and the outer peel of the fruit (Scott and Baker, 1947) and chemically by the frequent occurrence of furocoumarins; for example, bergapten (5-MOP) has been found in over 20% of the Rutaceae species examined (Murray et al., 1982). They are particularly prominent in the peel oils of most citrus fruits (table 4.1): Oil of lime (from *Citrus aurantifolia*) contains as much as 3.0 g/kg of bergamottin and 3.3 g/kg of bergapten (SGCAFS, 1996). A friend doing research on the furocoumarins in grapefruit oil (from *C. paradisi*) unwittingly spilled a few drops of extract down his shirtfront, returned home to mow his sunny lawn shirtless, and suffered a row of painful blisters down his chest as a consequence.

In another instance, a New York physician treated several young women whose bellies and inner thighs were inflamed and blistered. It seems they had vacationed at a Caribbean resort, where a popular game had young men attempt to roll a Persian lime (*C. aurantifolia*) from a woman's neck to her knees using only his chin! The unpleasant results arose from contact of lime oil with bare skin and sunlight (Sams, 1941). However, such outcomes are highly variable: Persian limes (also called Tahitian or Bearss limes) obviously are phototoxic, as are West Indian limes (*C. medica*) and Bergamot orange (*C. bergamia*), whereas Key limes (also known as Mexican limes) and certain other citrus species apparently are not (Sams, 1941).

Contrary to Sams's report, oranges (*C. sinensis*) can indeed produce dermatitis, although how much of this is photodermatitis and how much is allergic contact dermatitis is uncertain. Orange oil is phototoxic, and Hjorth (1982) cites the report of a patient with severe eczema on his hands who patch-tested positive to balsam of Peru of similar composition. To test the diagnosis, he ate an entire jar of orange marmalade, and after the worst eczema attack of his life, avoided perfumes, soft drinks, throat lozenges, and other items containing orange oil constituents and was soon cured of his illness.

In this case, there was no mention of his exposure to light, but citrus oils generally produce little or no dermatitis in the dark (Pathak et al., 1962), and this includes the oil of sour orange (*C. aurantium*) often added to marmalade. The oil glands occur in the colored, outermost layer of peel, the flavedo (Scott and Baker, 1947), and this so-called zest—both homemade and prepackaged—has become popular in gourmet cooking. However, the oils are composed primarily of terpenes such as *d*-limonene (90%), citral, and linalool, all of which are considered dermatotoxic by themselves (Benezra et al., 1985).

Common rue (*Ruta graveolens*), a two-foot (60-cm) perennial shrub with deeply divided, 2–4-inch (5–10-cm) aromatic leaves and small yellow flowers, is strongly phototoxic (Heskel et al., 1983). Native to Eurasia, it came early to the United States via Europe, where it was used for centuries in medicine; it now grows wild in the eastern United States and Pacific Northwest as well as in gardens elsewhere. It contains half a dozen furocoumarins (Murray et al., 1982), but the oil still is used as a fragrance ingredient in soaps, lotions, and perfumes (Opdyke, 1975a).

Other wild species of the Rutaceae also are recognized to be phototoxic, although human exposure to them is uncommon. The hop tree, *Ptelea crenulata*, is a 7–16-foot (2–5-m) furocoumarin-containing native of the margins of California's Great Central Valley, whereas its close relative *P. trifoliata* or water ash, occurs in the eastern United States (Muenscher and Brown, 1944). *Phebalium* (blister bush) species are 3–7-foot (1–2-m) Australian shrubs or small trees that produce no immediate reaction on contact with skin, but erythema commences within three days and blisters within four, and dark pigmentation can last as long as 5 years (Cleland, 1914). Despite its increasing use as an ornamental and its provocative name, dermatitis from blister bush is not mentioned by Wrigley and Fagg (1988) in their book on Australian native plants. Mokihana (*Pelea anisata*), the island flower of Kauai, Hawaii, causes dermatitis when used as a lei (Arnold, 1968).

Phototoxic *Dictamnus albus* has many common names, including burning bush, dittany, gas plant, and fraxinella. It is a woody-stemmed perennial about 3 feet (1 m) tall with glossy, 1–3-inch (2–8-cm) aromatic leaves and star-shaped white blossoms. If a lighted match is brought near the leaves on a still summer day, vaporized oil can briefly and harmlessly burst into flames. The Bible describes how God spoke to Moses from a "burning bush," and because dittany is native to the Near East, some consider it a prime candidate to explain this "miracle."

Apiaceae (Umbelliferae, Carrot Family)

Many species within the Apiaceae contain phototoxic furocoumarins (Murray et al., 1982; Pathak et al., 1962). The family consists of about 250 genera and 2000 species, distributed almost worldwide and characterized by a flat- or convex-topped flower head (umbel) surmounting narrow flower stalks (pedicels) that arise from a common point like an umbrella (hence the older family name). Familiar plants belonging to the Apiaceae include the common vegetables carrot (*Daucus carota*) and celery (*Apium graveolens*), persistent weeds (hogweed, *Heracleum* spp.), and the dangerous poison hemlock (*Conium maculatum*).

Celery has long been known to cause dermatitis, not only by eating it but also by handling it. Field workers and packers are especially prone to celery-picker's disease, a severe dermatitis of the hands, arms, and face. The problem is increased by pink rot fungus, *Sclerotinia sclerotiorum*, which causes the plants to produce fungitoxic furocoumarins in self-defense (Scheel et al., 1963). Pickers, packers, and grocerymen inevitably get the juice on their hands and suffer photodermatitis when later exposed to sunlight. Furocoumarins are normal constituents of celery leaves and stalks (Diawara et al., 1995), but their levels rise sharply if stalks are damaged or stored too long in the refrigerator (Beier et al., 1983; Chaudhary et al., 1985); see section 7.2.

The foliage of wild carrot (Queen Anne's lace, *Daucus carota*) is similarly phototoxic, but the situation with domestic carrots is unclear. Vickers (1941) and Van Dijk and Berrens (1941) offer evidence of phototoxicity, but Ivie et al. (1982) did not detect furocoumarins in extracts of carrot roots or foliage. However, canners handling raw carrots indoors often complain of rashes on their fingers and hands and give positive patch tests

(Klauder and Kimmich, 1956), so their reactions might actually be due to nonphototoxic substances such as polyacetylenes (see section 6.4). A similar-looking phototoxic species, angelica (*Angelica archangelica*), is used to flavor candy and liqueurs and in perfume (Opdyke, 1975b).

Other phototoxic vegetables include dill (*Anethum graveolens*), fennel (*Foeniculum vulgare*), parsley (*Petroselinum sativum*), and parsnip (*Pastinaca sativa*), both wild and domesticated. All are rich sources of furocoumarins (Murray et al., 1982; Nielsen, 1971), but phototoxicity may not be the greatest danger they present. Many wild members of the Apiaceae look a lot like the relatively harmless vegetables but are fatally poisonous when eaten. Poison hemlock (*Conium maculatum*), fool's parsley (*Aethusa cynapium*), water hemlock (*Cicuta* species), water parsley (*Oenanthe* spp.), and water parsnip (*Sium suave*) are among the most dangerous.

The phototoxic genus *Heracleum*, originally from the Caucasus Mountains, has only a single native North American representative, *H. lanatum*, although many of the 60 other species grow here. The genus is named for Hercules (*Herakles*), perhaps for its size and robustness or because the hero is supposed to have used it as medicine. "Herbaceous" *H. mantegazzianum*, which has escaped Europe into the United States, can reach 6–17 feet (2–5 m) in height, with a stem up to 4 inches (10 cm) thick. The deeply indented leaves grow to be 10 feet (3 m) long, so it is known in Germany as *Kaukasischer Bärenklau* (Caucasian bear's claw) and in our less-romantic English, giant hogweed.

Our common *H. lanatum* (also called *H. sphondylium*, cow parsnip) is somewhat smaller but still grows to be 3–10 feet (1–3 m) high with 1-foot (30-cm) deeply incised leaves and broad umbels of white flowers (plate 17). The plants seek moist areas and are common along both the East and West Coasts of the United States. The sap produces large blisters called bullae (see fig. 9.6), as does that of the Tromsø palm (*H. laciniatum*) that grows wild on the coast of northern Norway, far above the Arctic Circle (the city of Tromsø is located at 69°50′ north). Although snow often covers the ground there until late May, by the end of June this phototoxic plant can reach a height of 10 feet (3 m) and form jungles on open land, according to Kavli et al. (1983).

Ammi majus (bishop's weed) and *A. visnaga* (toothpick Ammi) are similar phototoxic annual weeds that grow 3 feet (1 m) high, mostly along roadsides and in gardens, and bear lacy leaves and small umbels of whitish flowers. These plants are common throughout much of the world, and their ground seeds have been used since ancient times to darken skin bleached by vitiligo, a depigmentation of the skin. However, dosing is tricky and may result in serious injury (Benezra et al., 1985).

Moraceae (Mulberry Family)

The milky latex of the common fig (*Ficus carica*, Moraceae) has been recognized as phototoxic for thousands of years and, like *Ammi*, has been applied to the treatment of vitiligo. According to the Greek herbalist Dioscorides, as translated by Goodyer in 1655 (Gunther, 1959), "But ye vitiligines albae are cataplasmed [poulticed] with ye leaves or ye boughs of ye Black Figge." Fig latex photodermatitis still is common, and as usual, commercial fruit pickers are the hardest hit. In addition to potentially serious irritation and blisters, injured skin develops a bronze discoloration that may last for years (Benezra et al., 1985).

Obviously, the snake was not the only danger to Adam and Eve! Fig leaves contain up to 480 mg/kg of the furocoumarin bergapten, and the latex has as much as 620 mg/kg (SGCAFS, 1996). A deciduous tree, *F. carica* grows to be 30 feet (9 meters) tall and as wide, with 9-inch (21-cm), five-lobed leaves and edible fruit. The phototoxic latex drips out of broken branches, crushed or excised leaves, and unripe fruit. Other *Ficus* species are sold as houseplants, among them India rubber tree (*F. elastica*), weeping fig (*F. benjamina*), and fiddleleaf fig (*F. lyrata*), and although Alber and Alber (1993) state there is no evidence that these irritate skin, all of them produce latex and many contain the same toxic furocoumarins found in *F. carica* (Murray et al., 1982).

Other valuable members of the Moraceae include breadfruit (*Artocarpus communis*), mulberry (*Morus* spp.), and Osage orange (*Maclura pomifera*), but apparently they are not considered phototoxic (Mitchell and Rook, 1979).

Other Phototoxic Plants

The 10 genera and 400 species of the Hypericaceae (previously Clusiaceae, or mangosteen family) occur scattered throughout the temperate world; the genus *Hypericum* is found both in the wild and as garden plants popular for bright yellow flowers with showy stamens. Aaron's beard (*H. calycinum*), a 1-foot (30-cm) perennial with opposite leaves, is a familiar ornamental ground cover, but the Klamath weed (St. John's wort, *H. perforatum*) introduced onto California range lands in the early 1900s eventually infested more than 2 million acres over a period of 30 years. Grazing cattle, horses, and sheep were so afflicted by its phototoxicity that it was said to have caused "the heaviest financial losses ever found on pasture and range lands of California" (Samson and Parker, 1930). The toxicity is due to a dianthrone, hypericin, and its relatives (Nahrstedt and Butterweck, 1997).

Today, *H. perforatum* is largely controlled on the range by the imported herbivorous beetles *Chrysolina quadrigemina* and *C. hyperici* (Huffaker and Kennett, 1959). Poorly absorbed by the skin, hypericin is toxic only by ingestion. Although no one would eat the intensely bitter fresh leaves, St. John's wort extracts have become a popular herbal medicine (*Hyperici herba*) sold over the counter to treat depression. Most *Hypericum* species contain the poison (Brockmann, 1957) and can be expected to be photo-toxic, and closely related species such as *H. hirsutum*, *H. maculatum*, and *H. montanum* are used to adulterate the herbal medicines (Nahrstedt and Butterweck, 1997).

From a completely different family and genus, species of *Fagopyrum* (Polygonaceae or buckwheat family) contain fagopyrin, a phototoxic qui-none similar in structure to hypericin (section 7.2). The common buckwheat (*F. esculentum*) used in pancake flour and the greenish Japanese noodles called *Soba* bears no resemblance to wheat (Poaceae); the plant is a 3-foot (1-m) broadleaf that bears fragrant white blossoms and numerous pyramid-shaped seeds (achenes) from which a nutritious flour is milled. The flour is mildly allergenic in humans (Blumstein, 1935) and probably not phototoxic. Used as a cover crop and forage in the northern United States and Europe, the plant has caused serious phototoxicity in light-skinned domestic animals (Kingsbury, 1964). Blumstein (1935) mentions a phototoxic, "hypericin-like" pigment in the lecheguilla (*Agave lecheguilla*, Agavaceae) that has poisoned sheep and goats, but later work suggests that the pigment is more likely a porphyrin generated in the animals by liver damage from a steroidal sapogenin in its feed (Camp et al., 1988).

Marigolds (*Tagetes* spp., Asteraceae) are common both as wildflowers and as popular garden plants. The genus contains about 50 species and many commercial varieties, among the most common *T. erecta* (African mari-gold), *T. lemmonii* (mountain marigold), *T. lucida* (Mexican marigold), and *T. patula* (French marigold). These New World plants, originally from Mexico or Central America, now have spread around the world. Most grow to 1–2 feet (30–60 cm), although a few species may reach 5 feet (1.5 m); blossoms can be single or double, yellow to orange or brown, and the glossy leaves are pinnately dissected. Marigolds are phototoxic to many people, the effects having been discovered in laboratory workers extracting the plants (Kagan, 1991).

The wild marigold (*T. minuta*) is a 1–3-foot (30–90-cm) noxious weed native to Central America but now found everywhere. Its sap is phototoxic, vesicant, irritant, and malodorous. *Tagetes* leaves have oil glands that con-tain tagetone, making them strongly scented—another name for *T. minuta* is stinking Roger. However, the phototoxicity is due to thiophenes (Kagan, 1991; section 7.2), which may also be allergenic (Hausen and Helmke,

1995). Over 30 genera of the Asteraceae are known to contain phototoxic thiophenes (Kagan, 1991), including such familiar species as cornflower (*Centaurea*), globe thistle (*Echinops*), coneflower (*Rudbeckia*), blanket flower (*Gaillardia*), and creeping daisy (*Wedelia*).

Among the numerous less-common phototoxic species, those of the genus *Psoralea* warrant mention if only because they were the original source of psoralen, the most phototoxic of all plant furocoumarins (Musajo and Rodighiero, 1962). *Psoralea pinnata* (blue pea, Fabiaceae) is a garden ornamental bearing bright green, needle-like foliage and blue and white sweet pea–like blossoms. Seeds of *P. corylifolia* (bavachi, ku-tzü, scurf pea) have been used for over 3000 years in Asian and African folk medicine as a "cure" for the vitiligo (leucoderma) previously cited.

4.2 Irritant Plants

Many plants produce symptoms similar to those caused by toxicodendrons but that are immediate, short-lived, and mostly nonimmunologic (Klaassen et al., 1996). A large number of substances have been reported to irritate skin, and as far back as 1887, J. C. White (1887) mentioned several hundred and L. F. Weber's list exceeded 1000 (Weber, 1937). However, most irritant plants tend to occur within just a few families: the Euphorbiaceae, Brassicaceae, Alliaceae, Urticaceae, and Ranunculaceae. Although there is evidence of ACD from some species, they will be described here for their obviously irritant properties. Structures of common plant irritants are shown in figure 7.5.

Euphorbiaceae (Spurge Family)

Euphorbs are among the most seriously irritant plants. This family of 300 genera and 8000 species is found everywhere but in the polar regions, and they vary in form from prostrate annual weeds like your garden's spotted spurge (*Euphorbia maculata*), through perennial shrubs such as poinsettia (*E. pulcherrima*), to the 30-foot (9-m) cactus-like pencilbush (*E. tirucalli*) and 40-foot (12-m) deciduous Chinese tallow tree (*Sapium sebiferum*). One thing many of these diverse plants have in common is corrosive sap— often a latex—that can severely damage human skin and eyes. Only a few of the most potent are listed here (table 4.2), and chemical features of their irritant constituents (diterpene esters) are discussed in section 7.3.

One expert, Radcliffe-Smith (1986), refers to the Euphorbiaceae as "a taxonomic dustbin" into which have been dumped a collection of rather odd and disparate plants. Although at least a half-dozen taxonomic classifications have been proposed for the family, including the widely used system of Pax and Hoffman (1931), we will defer to a more recent

Table 4.2   Common Dermatotoxic Euphorbs

Genus	Typical Species	Common Name	Use
Aleurites	A. fordii	Tung tree	Tung oil
Chamaesyce	C. (E.) maculata	Spotted spurge	Weed
Codiaeum	C. variegatum	Varigated croton	Houseplant
Cnidoscolus (Jatropha)	C. stimulosus	Tread-softly	Weed
Euphorbia	E. characias wulfenii	Euphorbia wulfenii	Ornamental
	E. lactea	Candelabra cactus	Ornamental
	E. lathyris	Mole plant	Weed
	E. marginata	Snow-on-the-mountain	Ornamental
	E. milii	Crown-of-thorns	Ornamental
	E. peplus	Petty spurge	Weed
	E. tirucalli	Pencilbush	Ornamental
Hevea	H. brasiliensis	Pará rubber	Rubber
Hippomane	H. mancinella	Manchineel	Cabinetry
Hura	H. crepitans	Sandbox tree	Ornamental
Ricinus	R. communis	Castor bean	Castor oil
Sapium	S. sebiferum	Chinese tallow tree	Ornamental
Synadenium	S. grantii	African milkbush	Ornamental
Tragia	T. ramosa	Noseburn	Weed

classification by Webster (1975) as being especially applicable to dermatotoxicity. Webster groups most toxic members into three out of the five subfamilies: (1) Acalyphoidae, which includes those species with stinging hairs; (2) Crotonoideae, which includes species whose seed oils are toxic; and (3) Euphorbioideae, in which are found genera such as *Euphorbia* and *Hippomane* whose sap is poisonous. Euphorbs most often are characterized by a milky latex in which the vesicants are dissolved or suspended; those with stinging hairs are mentioned later in this section.

Despite any actual or suspected toxicity, several members of the Euphorbiaceae have economic importance. These tree-size species are tropical or subtropical and produce valuable seed oils and protein-rich animal feeds. *Aleurites moluccana* (Kukui or candlenut) is typical, a shapely 60-foot (18-m) tree with iridescent foliage and dark nuts that are made into jewelry and whose oil was burned at one time for illumination. Similarly, the seed oil of the Chinese tallow tree (*Sapium sebiferum*) is used for soap and cosmetics and still fuels lamps in China. The tung tree, *A. fordii*, now classified as *Venicia fordii*, produces seeds from which the important drying oil for coatings is extracted, and castor beans (from *Ricinus communis*) provide castor oil. Nuts of the 35-ft (10-m) *Jatropha curcas*, called physic nut or purge nut, likewise causes violent purging of the bowels and severe abdominal pain if the nuts are eaten raw.

Originally thought to be due to saponins, the potentially lethal toxic effects of swallowing any of these oils actually are due in part to irritation by diterpenes (section 7.3), although highly neurotoxic proteins in the remaining seed meal also are a serious hazard. Evidence for skin irritation by the oils was uncertain until an article by Seip et al. (1983) identified the irritant and tumor-promoting esters in *S. sebiferum*; the dermatotoxicity is now widely recognized. Such large euphorbs often grow only in a limited area; 75 species of *Hura*, *Hippomane*, and *Manihot* are confined to tropical America and 60 others to tropical Asia, whereas 50 more occur only in Africa, and 14 are native only to Australia (Pax and Hoffman, 1931; Good, 1953).

Chapter 1 introduced the manchineel tree (*Hippomane mancinella*), a native of Panama, the Caribbean, and southern Florida's Everglades. These broad, 50-foot (15-m) gray-barked trees are found mostly near the sea and bear 2-inch, yellow- to red-skinned fruit, hence the local name beach apple. All parts rapidly induce severe erythema and blistering of the skin, and eating the fruit affects the mouth and throat in same way (Morton, 1982).

A more widespread Caribbean hazard is the pencilbush (*E. tirucalli*), up to 30 feet (9 m) high and 15 feet (4.5 m) wide, whose ascending branches form a thicket of narrow, cylindrical pencil-like branches (plate 18). It produces a few small leaves and clusters of tiny white flowers. The African native now is grown in any warm climate, including parts of the United States, and is even sold as a novelty in garden stores and supermarkets. Just a scratch on a "pencil" produces a copious flow of corrosive milk that is responsible for severe dermatitis and even temporary blindness if it gets into one's eyes (Morton, 1982).

However, most euphorbs are low shrubs like croton (*Croton texensis*), a Texas species that produces immediate skin blisters as a result of the phorbol esters in the leaves, stems, and seeds. In earlier times, croton oil pressed from seeds of the Old World *C. tiglium* was used in medicine as a violent purgative, but this practice has been largely abandoned because only a few drops could kill the patient. Presently, there are about 45 *Croton* species in the United States, mostly dryland weeds (Burrows and Tyrl, 2001) that proliferate across prairie land because cattle do not willingly eat them. Although crotons once served as garden ornamentals, the common variegated croton (*Codiaeum variegatum*) actually is from a different genus, a familiar 1–2-foot (30–60-cm) houseplant or small garden shrub with colorful, glossy, oval leaves. The mild effect of its milky sap on skin is nothing like the powerful corrosive action of true crotons, and in fact Hausen and Schulz (1977) offer evidence that *Codiaeum* is allergenic rather than irritant.

Other popular euphorbs include the crown-of-thorns (*E. milii*), a succulent, spine-covered "cactus" that bears flat panicles of tiny yellow flowers arising from showy red bracts, and the candelabra cactus (*E. lactea*), a fleshy houseplant with flattened stems that carry vertical rows of spines along the edges. Both species leak toxic latex, and Morton (1982) provides chilling descriptions of their dermatotoxic effects. Fifty-three out of the 60 species of *Euphorbia* tested for inflammatory ability showed positive activity (Kinghorn and Evans, 1975), 12 of them at very low exposures (table 9.3), but only a few of the 12 were commonly available: caper spurge or mole plant (*E. lathyris*), Canary Island spurge (*E. canariensis*), *E. resinifera*, source of the folk medicine "Euphorbium," and *E. characias* ssp. *wulfenii*.

This last species, sometimes called simply *E. wulfenii*, is used widely as an ornamental (plate 19), even though it is highly dermatotoxic (plate 24). Originally from the Mediterranean area, this shrubby, evergreen perennial grows to 4 feet (1.2 m), with large clumps of bluish leaves and clusters of yellow flowers, but its old name—*E. venenata*—reveals its irritant character. At the other extreme, hazards from familiar Christmas poinsettias (*E. pulcherrima*) are still controversial. Although Morton (1982) presents a gruesome picture of its effects and D'Arcy (1974) reports severe contact dermatitis in humans, Alber and Alber (1993) review the lack of evidence for any toxicity at all. Experiments by Winek et al. (1978) concluded that poinsettias were neither orally nor dermally toxic to rats, although possibly phototoxic to albino rabbits. Kinghorn and Evans (1975) saw no primary skin irritation on mouse ears, and no diterpene esters have been detected by chemical analysis (Evans and Kinghorn, 1977).

The discrepancy may lie partly with whether rodents or humans are being considered and partly with the relative dose. Further, toxicity may vary with plant variety: The tall (up to 12 foot or 3.5 meter) outdoor kinds, such as 'Henrietta Ecke,' differ from the usual semi-dwarf indoor varieties that include 'Annette Hegg' (red), 'Lemon Drop' (yellow), and 'Rosea' (Pink), but variety was seldom specified in the tests. As Santucci et al. (1985) suggest, young poinsettias from the greenhouse may not be as toxic as the mature wild specimens. As a child, I had frequent skin contact with latex from the outdoor variety without noticable harm, but avoiding unnecessary exposure still seems prudent.

The African milkbush (*Synadenium grantii*) is yet another ornamental euphorb, originally from Africa but now found widely in nurseries in other warm climates. Outdoors in southern Florida, it may reach 8–12 feet (2.4–3.6 m), but its smaller indoor size and lance-shaped 6 × 4-inch (15 × 10-cm) fleshy leaves make it an attractive houseplant. Cubans call it *dinamita* for its profound effect on the skin, eyes, and respiratory system.

Mature castorbean plants (*Ricinus communis*) generally form 10–12-foot (3–4-m) trees with large, deeply cut leaves and spikes of spiny seed pods, although tropical conditions can lead to a height of 40 feet (13 m). The mottled, tan seeds contain a toxic protein, ricin, that is lethal to eat, the milky sap is irritant, and the castor oil pressed from the "beans" is accused of causing contact dermatitis (Brandle et al., 1983). However, the only diterpene to be reported from *Ricinus* so far is the hydrocarbon casbene (fig. 7.4; Robinson and West, 1970), and it was extracted from whole seedlings. The well-known purgative effects of castor oil are attributed to glyceryl esters of ricinoleic acid (12R-hydroxy-9Z-octadecanoic acid), which alter the walls of the intestinal tract to cause loss of water and electrolytes (Bruneton, 1999).

However, many and perhaps most other euphorbs are reported to cause dermatitis, and *any* species of the genus *Euphorbia*, especially, should be approached with caution. This even extends to two common little garden weeds: the prostrate spotted spurge (previously classified as *E. supina* or *Chamaesyce maculata* but now called *E. maculata*) and the 6–10-inch (15–25-cm), yellow-green petty spurge (*E. peplus*). Many gardeners root them out with bare hands, and a tell-tale sign of potential trouble is the "milk" that appears immediately at the ends of broken stems and that has been responsible for a lot of sore, red hands.

As members of the closely related family Thymelaeaceae, species of *Daphne* including *D. odora* (winter daphne) and *D. mezereum* (February daphne) produce a group of what are considered the most irritant of all plant chemicals. Most daphnes are evergreen shrubs 1–4 feet (30–120 cm) high that bear creamy, sweet-smelling flower clusters, although *D. mezereum* is deciduous. Since ancient times, they have been recognized as lethal to eat, but their dermatotoxicity has remained almost a footnote. A classic book about poisonous plants (Kingsbury, 1964) states that the plants are "intensely acrid, producing vesication when the leaves are rubbed on the skin" and that ingestion "produces a burning sensation in the mouth and corrosive lesions of the oral membranes." The book lists coumarin glycosides as the poisons, although such compounds are generaly nontoxic, but irritant diterpene esters closely similar to those of the euphorbs are well established in the family and genus and seem much more likely suspects (section 7.3).

Brassicaceae (Mustard Family)

The irritant properties of mustard, a classic medicinal plant, have been apparent since antiquity. Culpeper's *Complete Herbal* of 1653 (Culpeper, 1653), republished in 1869, prescribes

The outward application [of mustard] upon the pained place of the sciatica, discusses the humors, and eases the pains ... and is much and often used to ease the pains in the sides or loins, the shoulder, or other parts of the body, upon the plying thereof to raise blisters ... (p. 125)

Mustards—*Brassica* species belonging to the family Brassicaceae (previously called Cruciferae)—are typical of and indeed define the family; whatever their other properties, all crucifers release odorous oils (isothiocyanates) when crushed. Likewise, they exhibit pastel-colored or yellow, cross-shaped flowers of four equal rectangular petals and six stamens (four long and two short).

The Brassicaceae represent over 350 genera and 3500 species, and new ones continue to be introduced. They occur throughout temperate regions of the world, at least 90% from the Northern Hemisphere but relatively few from the tropics. They provide familiar foods, including cabbage, cauliflower, and radish, the flowering stock, candytuft, and sweet alyssum, and common weeds such as hoary cress, wild mustard, and shepherd's purse. Once ancient foods, they have remained popular because of their simple culture and the pungent taste and aroma of the mustard oils. Plants from other families produce the same oils (table 4.3), including capers (Capparaceae) and mignonettes (Resedaceae), papaya (Caricaceae), some spurges (Euphorbiaceae), nasturtiums (Tropaeolaceae), pokeweeds (Phytolaccaceae), and plantains (Plantaginaceae).

Table 4.3 Mustard Oil Plants

Genus[a]	Typical Species	Common Name	Use
Alyssum	*A. montanum*	Alyssum	Garden border
Arabis	*A. alpina*	Mountain rock cress	Rock gardens
Brassica	*B. nigra*	Black mustard	Condiment, weed
Brassica	*B. oleracea*	Cabbage	Vegetable
Carica (C)	*C. papaya*	Papaya	Tropical fruit
Erysimum[b]	*E. cheiri*	Wallflower	Flower gardens
Eutrema	*E. wasabi*	Japanese horseradish	Condiment (*wasabi*)
Iberis	*I. sempervirens*	Evergreen candytuft	Garden border
Mattiola	*M. incana*	Stock	Flower gardens
Nasturtium	*N. officinale*	Water cress	Salad vegetable
Raphanus	*R. sativus*	Radish	Vegetable
Reseda (R)	*R. odorata*	Mignonette	Flower gardens
Tropaeolum (T)	*T. majus*	Nasturtium	Flower gardens

For a more complete list, see Kjaer (1960). [a]All are Brassicaceae except for Caricaceae (C), Resedaceae (R), and Tropaeolaceae (T). [b]Also called *Cheiranthus*.

Mustard oils seldom occur as such in the plants but are generated from water-soluble glucosides (called glucosinolates) that occur in all parts, especially seeds (section 7.4; Kjaer, 1960; VanEtten et al., 1969). The oil-generating reaction is catalyzed by an enzyme, myrosinase, that is stored in the vacuoles of special myrosin cells, whereas the glucosinolates are biosynthesized and stored in surrounding tissue (Werker and Vaughn, 1976). Disruption of the cells by a chewing insect or human mixes enzyme and substrate, and the isothiocyanate is formed (display 7.5).

Early German chemists called the oils *Senföl* ("mustard oil"), sometimes erroneously translated as "senevol." They are the active ingredients of the mustard plasters once common for warming the skin and alleviating aches and pains (via a form of dermatitis). Crushed seeds of black mustard (*Brassica nigra*), the familiar 1–3-foot (30–90-cm), yellow-flowered annual weed, usually provide the main ingredient, although seeds of Indian mustard (*B. juncea*) and other *Brassica* species may be substituted. Horseradish (*Armoracea rusticana*) and pungent *wasabi* (Japanese horseradish, *Eutrema wasabi*) are especially potent, and anyone who inadvertently puts too much "Japanese mustard" on their sushi can appreciate what it might do to tender skin.

The Capparaceae, sometimes called the Capparidaceae, form a family of over 35 genera that is the tropical equivalent of the Brassicaceae. They are not as well known as their northern counterparts, and only a few species are at all familiar. One is the caper bush, *Capparis spinosa*, whose dried and pickled flowers provide the condiment called capers, and another is the attractive spider flower (*Cleome hasslerana*). All Capparaceae tested contain at least one glucosinolate, generally the methyl homologue, and the literature gives numerous accounts of their rubefacient (reddening) and vesicant (blistering) medicinal action on skin (Mitchell, 1974).

Alliaceae (Onion Family)

Another ancient group of medicinal plants are the alliums, members of the onion family that includes, among others, onion (*Allium cepa*), garlic (*A. sativum*), leek (*A. porrum*), and chives (*A. schoenoprasum*). The familial connection has long been in dispute—some authorities seeing lilies (Liliaceae) and others Amaryllis (Amaryllidaceae)—but the question may have been circumvented temporarily with the invention of a new family, the Alliaceae. *Allium* is its principal genus, and all 600 or more species share the characteristics of an underground bulb (occasionally more like a rhizome), an often-spherical umbel of flowers on a tube-like stalk (peduncle), and 1–5 basal leaves that commonly are narrow and grass-like.

They also share an onion-like odor: If it smells like an onion, it probably is an allium, although a few other kinds of plants, such as *Triteleia* (Brodiaea), have the same aroma. The source is an oily mixture of allyl sulfides generated from odorless amino acids in the sap by the action of the enzyme alliinase (section 7.4). The sulfides and related compounds are fat-soluble and mostly volatile, and so are detected in the breath and skin of people who have been exposed. The ramp (*A. tricoccum*), a wild delicacy of the Appalachian hills, is especially notorious for this, and local ramp festivals are not for the timid.

Similarly, these compounds are absorbed into the milk of dairy animals that consume alliums from their pasture or hay, and the resulting off-flavor makes the products unsalable. Human breast milk also picks up the odor and taste from the mother's diet (Mennella and Beauchamp, 1991), and the 140% increase in milk volume consumed by nurselings of garlic-eating mothers suggests that babies develop a taste for it early in life (Mennella and Beauchamp, 1993).

This not to say that all alliums are alike. Garlic is a relatively large plant, often exceeding 3 feet (1 m) in height, whose bulb is divided vertically into segments ("cloves") and whose flower heads are encased in a papery sheath or spathe. Conversely, the onion bulb is round and composed of concentric layers of tissue, and the flower stalk is a hollow cylinder. Leeks have almost no discernible bulb, but instead a thick solid stem on whose lower end is a cluster of thin roots. Chives form neat mounds of slim cylindrical leaves, under a foot (30 cm) tall and topped by puffballs of minute, pale purple flowers. Scallions are the usual *A. cepa* harvested before the bulb forms, whereas shallots represent a kind of *A. cepa* known as green bunching onions.

Besides being food plants, many *Allium* species are found in the flower garden. Giant allium (*A. giganteum*) reaches 6 feet (1.9 m) tall and is topped with a large ball of purple flowers, whereas bear garlic (*A. ursinum*) forms broad leaves topped with clusters of starry white flowers. Some alliums are serious weeds, especially wild garlic (*A. vineale*), which is everything a real weed must be: drought- and cold-hardy with a preference for heavy, poorly drained soils, malodorous, difficult to eradicate, and nearly ubiquitous (USDA, 1970).

Alliums are found throughout the Northern Hemisphere except the Arctic; a compendium of California native plants lists 67 wild species in that state alone (Hickman, 1993). They have been used in folk medicine for centuries (Koch and Lawson, 2000), especially to ward off disease (although the self-imposed isolation of garlic eaters may help), and they have long been known to cause occupational dermatitis (Burgess, 1952). Again, the effects may involve ACD rather than simple irritancy (Bleumink et al.,

1972), because the dermatitis appears to be due to the allyl sulfides (Papageorgiou et al., 1983). The well-known tears brought on by a sliced onion are caused by a volatile, enzyme-generated propylsulfine (Block and Revelle, 1980); see section 7.4.

Urticaceae (Nettles)

Stinging nettles (*Urtica* spp.) are common in moist woods and on stream banks throughout much of the temperate world, especially in North America and Europe (Avalos, 2000). The plants were known in ancient times; the name comes from the Latin *urere* meaning, aptly, "to burn." The principal U.S. species is *U. dioica*, whose subspecies, *gracilis* (American stinging nettle), classified earlier as *U. californica* or *U. lyallii*, is found along the West Coast (plate 20). The subspecies *holosericea* (creek nettle) grows throughout most of the continental United States and Canada into Alaska.

These 2–7-foot (0.6–2-m) medium-green perennials bear opposite, coarsely serrated, heart-shaped leaves, 2–6 inches (5–15 cm) long and covered with short (1–2 mm) stinging hairs on the underside and stem. The smaller (18-inch, 45-cm) but still painful annual, *Hesperocnide tenella* (literally, western nettle; Hickman, 1993), grows in inland California and Hawaii, but the similar round-leaved rock nettle (*Eucnide urens*, family Loasaceae) is found only in Southwestern deserts: California's Death Valley, western Arizona, and northern Mexico.

The brush of a bare arm or leg against a nettle is memorable. The immediate pain sets one's teeth on edge, and itching and redness (urticaria) quickly follow as the fragile bulbous tips of tiny quartz needles (fig. 4.1) break off under the skin and inject a mixture of bioactive amines (see sections 7.6 and 9.5; Thurston, 1974). Nettles were grown as a food and fiber crop in Europe at one time, and the tender new leaves still are cooked as spring greens. Boiling water removes the stinging hairs (trichomes), but caution obviously is required to harvest and handle the plants beforehand.

Leaves of the imported annual dwarf nettle (*Urtica urens*), are only 1–1.6 inches (2.5–4 cm) in length, shorter and more rounded than those of other urticas. This species grows to about 2 feet (60 cm) tall and has become established in gardens and orchards, especially in Southern California. Its "sting" is said to be the worst of any North American plant but is still mild compared to that of Australia's "stinging trees." These *Dendrocnide* species (family Urticaceae, classified also as *Laportea*), are natives of Queensland's rain forests and are cultivated in nurseries for their attractive foliage (Wrigley and Fagg, 1988).

The largest, *Dendrocnide excelsa* (*Laportea gigas*), the giant stinging tree, ascends 100 feet (35 m) and bears 8-inch (20-cm) heart-shaped leaves

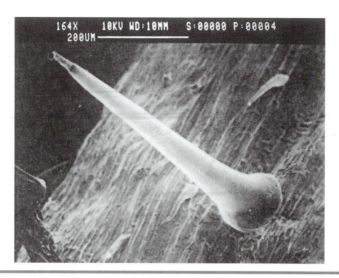

164X   10KV WD:10MM   S:00000 P:00004
200UM

Figure 4.1 Electron micrograph of a "stinging hair" (trichome), 0.6 mm long, of the nettle *Urtica dioica*. From Benezra et al. (1985), by permission of Mosby Publishers.

covered with stinging hairs. The pink fruit is said to be tasty, but even the slightest contact with the leaves causes intense pain that may last 3–4 *weeks*. However, *D. moroides*, or gympie bush, a popular houseplant "down under," is even worse. This species and its close relative, *Laportea canadensis* (wood nettle) of the eastern United States and Canada, can cause a person or an animal literally to go mad with pain. All together, there are at least 24 species of Urticaceae, Loasaceae, Euphorbiaceae, and Hydrophyllaceae that can sting (Evans and Schmidt, 1980).

Although they are in the Euphorbiaceae rather than the Urticaceae, plants of the 75-member genus *Cnidoscolus* inflict dangerously dermatotoxic wounds via nettle-like trichomes on their stems and leaves. The four North American representatives are warm-climate herbaceous weeds or small trees, for example, the bull nettle (*Cnidoscolus stimulosis*, or treadsoftly). This shrubby perennial bears ragged, 3–12-inch (8–30-cm) leaves, 3–5 lobed and studded with needles on both surfaces. It grows in sandy areas from Florida north into Virginia and west to Texas, and people have been known to faint from its sting. The very similar spurge nettle, *C. texanus*, also called bull nettle, is found from Arkansas south into Mexico, the larger and less common *C. angustidens* from Arizona into western Mexico, and *C. aconitifolius* from the U.S. border south into Panama. *Cnidoscolus* (pronounced "nid-os'-co-lus," Greek for pointed nettle) has been called "probably the most painful of all the stinging plants in Central America" (see Morton, 1982), and any plant of the genus *Jatropha* that bears stinging hairs has now been reclassified into this genus.

Perhaps the most bizarre type of sting is from euphorbs of the genus *Tragia* (commonly known as noseburn). Each hollow trichome contains a single needle of crystalline calcium oxalate (Thurston, 1976), which is ejected on contact, punctures a hole in the skin, and then is flooded by an irritant solution from the hair. The plants are found in warm climates worldwide, and our western species (*T. ramosa*) is a dryland shrub with narrow leaves and spiny stems.

Other Irritant Plants

A list of other common irritant plants is provided in table 4.4. Several are in the Ranunculaceae, whose irritant members include buttercup (*Ranunculus*), anemone or windflowers (*Anemone*), pasque-flower (*Pulsatilla*), old-man's beard (*Clematis vitalba*), and marsh marigold (*Caltha* spp.). Buttercups and anemones possess an acrid juice that contains a powerful vesicant called protoanemonin (display 6.3), and wild buttercups present a particular hazard to children and livestock—the former from picking wildflowers with their bare hands and the latter from eating the spring shoots that results in blistered lips and tongues. The most dangerous (Turner and Szczawinski, 1991) are the tall field buttercup (*Ranunculus acris*), bulbous buttercup (*R. bulbosus*), creeping buttercup (*R. repens*,

Table 4.4 Common Irritant Plants Other Than Euphorbs

Common Name	Species	Family	Typical Irritant[a]
Anemone	*Anemone* spp.	Ranunculaceae	Protoanemonin
Anthurium	*Anthurium andreanum*	Araceae	Ca oxalate
Bulbous buttercup	*Ranunculus bulbosa*	Ranunculaceae	Protoanemonin
Calla lily	*Zantedeschia aethiopica*	Araceae	Ca oxalate
Century plant	*Agave americana*	Agavaceae	Unknown
Chili pepper (fruit)	*Capsicum annuum*	Solanaceae	Capsaicin (in fruit)
Old man's beard[b]	*Clematis vitalba*	Ranunculaceae	Protoanemonin
Creeping buttercup	*Ranunculus repens*	Ranunculaceae	Protoanemonin
Creosote bush	*Larrea tridentata*	Zygophyllaceae	NDGA[c]
Daffodil, narcissus	*Narcissus* spp.	Amaryllidaceae	Ca oxalate (bulb)
Dumbcane	*Dieffenbachia picta*	Araceae	Ca oxalate
Marsh marigold	*Caltha palustris*	Ranunculaceae	Protoanemonin
Mayapple (mandrake)	*Podophyllum peltatum*	Podophyllaceae	Podophyllotoxin
Pasque-flower	*Pulsatilla vulgaris*	Ranunculaceae	Protoanemonin
Persian ranunculus	*Ranunculus asiaticus*	Ranunculaceae	Protoanemonin
White jasmine	*Jasminum officinale*	Oleaceae	Jasmone

[a]For structures, see figure 7.5. [b]Also called virgin's bower. [c]Nordihydroguaiaretic acid.

plate 21), and the cursed crowfoot (*R. sceleratus*). All of these are attractive, with cheerful, shiny yellow flowers in early spring and deeply incised leaves that lend the common name, crowfoot.

Chili peppers (*Capsicum annuum*, Solanaceae), common plants that bear irritant fruit, have been cultivated around the world as a vegetable and condiment since antiquity, but they are no longer found in the wild. The chili pepper is an 8–20-inch (20–50-cm) shrub with smooth, tapered fruit that may be yellow, orange, red, brown, or almost black. The principal irritant, capsaicin (section 7.5), is the basis of the Scoville scale, a measure of the pepper's perceived "heat" (that is, irritancy). With the limit of sensory detection defined as 1 unit, pure capsaicin represents 16 million Scoville units, the red habanero pepper 100,000–577,000 units, serrano pepper 5000–15,000, jalapeño pepper (*chipotle*) 2500–5000, and a yellow wax pepper 500–1000; bell peppers represent zero. The pungency is proportional to the level of capsaicin and its relatives (Krajewska and Powers, 1988), but these substances contribute nothing to the taste.

Capsaicinoid irritants are produced by glands on the fruit's placenta rather than in the flesh or seeds, but seeds occasionally do absorb them. I inadvertently allowed those of a tiny yellow jalapeño to touch my lower lip and was quickly rewarded with pain, swelling, and a blister. Pepper oil, Cayenne pepper, and the popular Tabasco sauce are all rich (up to 1%) in capsaicin, but although a little can enhance the flavor of scrambled eggs, none should *ever* be allowed to contact sensitive skin (Smith et al., 1970). Although one's first reaction is intense irritation, capsaicin also is allergenic (Benezra et al., 1985).

Mayapple (*Podophyllum peltatum*, Berberidaceae) is a highly poisonous plant that grows in moist woodlands of the eastern United States and southeast Canada. The 1-foot (30-cm) stem grows from a fleshy rhizome, and its deeply indented leaves cover the rest of the plant like an umbrella. The single 1–2-inch (3–5-cm) flower is white, waxy, and arises from the crotch of the two leaf stalks (petioles). Mayapple has been used in folk medicines for centuries, by Native Americans and settlers alike; alcohol extracts are extremely caustic to the skin and remain the treatment of choice for genital warts, although resin from a less common species, *P. emodi* of Tibet and Afghanistan, is even more corrosive (Rietschel and Fowler, 2001).

Beware of "swimmer's itch"! The blue-green alga that causes it, *Lyngbya majuscula* (a Cyanobacterium), lives in warm salt, brackish, and fresh waters of the Hawaiian islands and throughout the Pacific. It causes severe irritant dermatitis in bathers, among whom the effects are suffered widely—even if they seldom report it. The irritants lyngbyatoxin A, debromoaplysiatoxin, and aplysiatoxin are at least as potent as the diterpene ester, TPA, and like the esters, they activate protein kinase C, promote tumors (Fujiki et al., 1990), and compete with TPA for the phorbol ester receptor (see section 7.5).

Many other irritant species have been reported—Lewis and Elvin-Lewis (1977) list 29 *families* of irritant plants—but the ones reviewed here are among the most common and most dangerous. Some eventually will prove to be allergenic, certain *Brassica* species, for example (Mitchell and Jordan, 1974), but a number of allergens such as urushiol also will become more widely recognized as having irritant properties.

Mechanical Irritation

The action of irritant species discussed in this chapter has been to affect some specific biochemical process—that is, to cause a toxic response. However, some irritant plants damage the skin *mechanically*, by means of spines or other sharp objects. Although they do not meet the basic premise of this book, these plants deserve mention because this mechanical action sometimes has obscured a true biochemical toxicity, as was long the case with *Philodendron* (section 3.2). Needle-like calcium oxalate crystals (raphides) are the irritants often found in members of the Araceae such as dumbcane (*Dieffenbachia* spp.) and the bulbs of many Liliaceae (Khan, 1995). The sharp, 200-μm mineral slivers penetrate and disrupt mast cells in the skin, releasing the histamine responsible for the symptoms of dermatitis (section 9.5).

As an illustration, many *Agave* species (family Agavaceae) are reported to produce irritant contact dermatitis (ICD). Among them is the well-known *A. americana*, or century plant, and one victim developed severe dermatitis of the scalp after using *Agave* juice as a presumed hair restorer (Kerner et al., 1973). In another instance, hemorrhagic dermatitis appeared among workers soon after they were showered with agave juice while harvesting the leaves with a chain saw (Fuller and McClintock, 1986). A similar problem arises with workers in tequila distilleries (Salinas et al., 2001), where this Mexican industry consumed 1.3 billion pounds (610,000 metric tons) of *Agave tequilana* leaves in 1998 to produce 45 million gallons (170,000 m^3) of the liquor. *Agave* juice contains 4000–6000 calcium oxalate raphides per cubic centimeter—not something one wants to be around—but the distilled product presumably contains none. See sections 7.6 and 9.5 for more on calcium oxalate.

Another example is the genus *Dieffenbachia*, which consists of about 30 species of tropical members of the family Araceae that are among the most dangerous for small children. These popular ornamentals, usually varieties of *D. maculata* (*D. seguine*) known as dumbcane, bear broad, oval medium-green leaves with cream-colored blotches and are common around homes and offices. Their popular name arose because biting into the plant produces such swelling of the throat that one can neither speak nor breathe—hence the need to keep them out of little mouths. In their 1996 review, Krenzelok et al. (1996) reported that out of 912,534 cases of plant poisoning emergencies recorded by U.S. poison control centers between 1985 and 1994, 96,659 (10.6%) involved either *Philodendron* or *Dieffenbachia*, almost all (93%) in children under 6 years of age. The effects are due mostly to a release of calcium oxalate raphides into the mucous lining of the mouth and throat, although simply touching a leaf can discharge surface cells and cause dermatitis (Arditti and Rodriguez, 1982).

Calcium oxalate is a frequent constituent of other plants such as rhubarb, sorrel, and spinach, but ordinarily in harmless form. However, its toxicity is most often encountered in the Araceae, where it takes the form of raphides. Besides dieffenbachias, common offenders include caladium (*Caladium bicolor*), taro or elephant ear (*Colocasia esculenta*), philodendron (which also contains an allergenic resorcinol), and calla lilies (*Zantedeschia* spp.), all of which are used as houseplants.

4.3   Conclusions

In addition to the plethora of allergenic plants, many species produce non-allergenic skin irritants whose dermatotoxicity mimics ACD, at least superficially. Some, like buttercups, are common wildflowers, others are familiar houseplants such as variegated croton, and still others are table items, including mustard and garlic. Some require light to be active (phototoxic) and are dangerous partly because so many of them are associated with common foods—figs and celery, for example. Many ornamental euphorbs release caustic latex when injured and are especially dangerous to the eyes. Nettles are in a class by themselves for literally injecting histamine and other mediators directly into the skin. Similarly, ordinary houseplants such as dieffenbachia possess stinging cells that expel needles of crystalline calcium oxalate that irritate the skin mechanically. As is the case with allergens, exposure to irritant and phototoxic plants has become almost inescapable.

FIVE

*"The controversial nature of many recent publications
dealing with allergy to poison ivy may be attributed
in part to the lack of a standard allergenic substance,
and the experimentation in its stead with crude,
unstandardized, and unstable extracts of the
irritant plant."*
—Howard S. Mason, 1945

5.1 Urushioid Allergens

Literally thousands of plant constituents affect the skin in some way, from simple irritation to full-blown allergy. Most allergy sufferers are well acquainted with the effects of urushiols and laccols from poison oak, poison ivy, and their toxic relatives, so this chapter will focus on the underlying chemical characteristics of the substances and their occurrence in the plant world (table 5.1).

These powerful allergens are found in many members of the Anacardiaceae but apparently not outside that familly. However, allergens similar to them both chemically and immunologically do exist in other families, and we will refer to this entire class as *urushioids* (table 5.2). Some plant quinone and hydroquinone allergens bear a close structural resemblance to urushioids but differ from them immunologically in not cross-reacting. Another large group, called lactones, are not structurally related to either quinones or urushioids but appear to share a common mechanism of allergenic action with them. Quinones and lactones will be discussed in chapter 6.

5.2 Urushiols and Laccols

An understanding and appreciation of both human exposure to toxico-dendrons and the toxicity of the genus require some knowledge of the physical and chemical properties of urushioids, and more than a century of

Table 5.1 Urushiols and Laccols in *Toxicodendron*[a]

| | | | % of Purified Extractives | | | | | |
| | | | *T. diversilobum*[b] | *T. radicans* | *T. vernix* | *T. succedaneum*[c] | *T. striatum*[d] | *T. vernicifluum*[e] |
Form	R	Olefin						
Saturated	$C_{15}H_{31}$		22	0–6	15	5	7	4
	$C_{17}H_{35}$		2	0–0.2	0	—[f]	0	0
Monoolefin	$C_{15}H_{29}$	8	8	14–42	41	25	50	10–23
	$C_{17}H_{33}$	10	11	0.3–0.8	0	—	0	2
Diolefin	$C_{15}H_{27}$	8, 11	3	50–68	33	15	23	4
	$C_{17}H_{31}$	10, 13	19	0.7–3	0	—	0	2
Triolefin	$C_{15}H_{25}$	8, 11, 14	0	3–17	11	55	20	64–71
	$C_{17}H_{29}$	10, 13, 16	35	0–0.8	0	—	0	1

[a]See appendixes A and B for more detail. [b]*T. diversilobum*, poison oak; *T. radicans*, poison ivy; *T. vernix*, poison sumac (Gross et al., 1975). [c]*T. succedaneum*, Indochina lac (Du, 1990). [d]*T. striatum*, manzanillo (Nakano et al., 1970). [e]*T. vernicifluum*, Japanese lac (Du et al., 1984a). [f]Not reported.

serious investigation has gone into that subject. The following history reviews the sustained research effort that eventually provided our present understanding of urushiols and their allergenicity.

Because the symptoms of poisoning were so similar, it took people over 150 years to realize that the allergens of *Toxicodendron diversilobum* were not the same as those of *T. radicans*, and that those of other toxic Anacardiaceae species differed from both. With the idea laid to rest that the poison ivy allergen was a vapor (section 1.3), its true chemical features began to emerge. Yoshida (1883) was first to report urushic acid extracted from the latex of the Japanese Lac, but although it was similar to what we now know as urushiol, its composition ($C_{14}H_{18}O_2$) was not.

In 1897, Franz Pfaff (1897) reported that extraction of the leaves of poison ivy (then called *Rhus toxicodendron*) with alcohol eventually provided an oily black tar, which, after purification and the addition of lead acetate, gave a solid with the composition $C_{21}H_{30}O_4Pb$ whose subsequent workup provided a nonvolatile, toxic liquid he named toxicodendrol. Unfortunately, research was abandoned at this point.

It was two decades before James McNair continued Pfaff's work (McNair, 1916). Leaves, bark, and woody stems of western poison oak (*T. diversilobum*) yielded a viscous, yellowish allergenic liquid, which he named lobinol (McNair, 1921a). Its chemical reactions (such as acetylation,

Table 5.2 Urushioids in Genera Other Than *Toxicodendron*[a,b]

Plant Species	Urushioids
Anacardiaceae	
Anacardium occidentale L. (cashew)	Resorcinol, $5\text{-}C_{15}(0,1,2,3)$; $2\text{-}Me\text{-}5\text{-}C_{15}(0,1,2,3)$; $2\text{-}Me\text{-}5\text{-}C_{17}(0,1,2,3)$
	Phenol, $3\text{-}C_{15}(0)$
Campnosperma auriculata (Bl.) Hook	Phenol, $3\text{-}C_{19}(1)^c$
Gluta rengas L. (rengas)	Catechol, $3\text{-}C_{17}(2)$
Holigarna arnottiana Hook.	Catechol, $3\text{-}C_{17}(1)$
Lithrea brasiliensis March	Catechol, $3\text{-}C_{15}(0,1)$; $3\text{-}C_{17}(1,2)^m$
L. caustica (Mol.) (litre)	Catechol, $3\text{-}C_{15}(0,1)$; $3\text{-}C_{17}(1,2)^d$
L. molleoides (Vell.) Engler	Catechol, $3\text{-}C_{15}(0,1)$; $3\text{-}C_{17}(1,2)^m$
Mangifera indica L. (mango)	Resorcinol, $5\text{-}C_{17}(1)^e$
Melanorrhoea usitata Wall	Resorcinol, $5\text{-}(C_6H_5C_{12})$
(Burmese lac)	Catechol, $4\text{-}C_{17}(0)$; $3\text{-}C_{17}(1)$; $3\text{-}(C_6H_5C_{10})$, $3\text{-}(C_6H_5C_{12})^f$
Metopium brownei (Jacq.) Urb.	Catechol, $3\text{-}C_{15}(0,1,2)$; $3\text{-}C_{17}(0,1)^g$
M. toxiferum Krug & Urb. (poisonwood)	Catechol, $3\text{-}C_{15}(0,1,2,3)$; $3\text{-}C_{17}(1,3)$
Pentaspadon officinalis	Phenol, $3\text{-}C_{17}(1,2)^c$
Schinus terebinthifolius (Brazilionpepper Florida holly)	Phenol, $3\text{-}C_{15}(1)^n$
Semecarpus anacardium L. (marking nut)	Phenol, $3\text{-}C_{15}(2)$
S. heterophylla Bl.	Phenol, $3\text{-}C_{15}(1)$
S. travancorica Bed.	Phenol, $3\text{-}C_{17}(2)$
Smodingium argutum E. Mey (African poison ivy)	Phenol, $3\text{-}C_{15}(0,1)$; $3\text{-}C_{17}(0,1,2)$
Toxicodendron spp.	See appendixes A and B.
Araceae[i]	
Philodendron radiatum	Resorcinol, $5\text{-}C_{13}(0)$; $5\text{-}C_{15}(2,3)$; $5\text{-}C_{17}(1,2)$
P. erubescens	Resorcinol, $5\text{-}C_{15}(1)$; $5\text{-}C_{17}(1)$
P. scandens oxycardum Schott (philodendron)	Resorcinol, $5\text{-}C_{15}(0,1)$, $5\text{-}C_{17}(0,1,2,3)$
Ginkgoaceae[b]	
Ginkgo biloba L. (ginkgo)	Resorcinol, $5\text{-}C_{15}(0,1)$; $5\text{-}C_{17}(0,1)$
Poaceae	
Oryza sativa (rice)[i]	Resorcinol, $5\text{-}C_{13}(0)$; $5\text{-}C_{15}(0,1)$; $5\text{-}C_{17}(0,1)$
Hordeum distichon (barley)[j]	Resorcinol, $5\text{-}C_{19}(0)$; $5\text{-}C_{21}(0)$; $5\text{-}C_{23}(0)$; $5\text{-}C_{25}(0)$; $5\text{-}C_{27}(0)$
Secale cereale (rye)[k]	Resorcinol, $5\text{-}C_{11}(2)$; $5\text{-}C_{13}(1,2)$; $5\text{-}C_{15}(0,1,2)$; $5\text{-}C_{17}(0,1,2)$; $5\text{-}C_{19}(0,1,2)$; $5\text{-}C_{21}(0,1)$; $5\text{-}C_{23}(0,1)$; $5\text{-}C_{25}(0,1)$

(continued)

Table 5.2 (*Cont.*)

Plant Species	Urushioids
Triticum vulgare (wheat)[k]	Resorcinol, 5-C_{15}(1,2); 5-C_{17}(0,1,2); 5-C_{19}(0,1); 5-C_{21}(0,1); 5-C_{23}(0,1); 5-C_{25}(0)
Proteaceae[b]	
Cardwellia sublimis F. Muell.	Resorcinol, 5-C_{15}(0,1); 5-C_{17}(0,1), 5-C_{19}(2)
Grevillea banksii R. Br. (Kahili)	Resorcinol, 5-C_{11}(0); 5-C_{13}(0); 5-C_{15}(0,1)
Grevillea hilliana F. Muell.	Resorcinol, 5-C_{13}(0); 5-C_{15}(0,1); 5-C_{17}(0,1,1); 5-C_{19}(0,1)
Grevillea pteridifolia Knight	Resorcinol, 5-C_{13}(0); 5-C_{15}(01,1)
Grevillea pyramidalis	Resorcinol, 5-C_{13}(1); 5-C_{15}(1)[c]
Grevillea robusta A. Cunn. (silky oak)	Resorcinol, 5-C_{13}(0); 5-C_{15}(0,1,1)[l]
Hakea persiehana F. Muell.	Resorcinol, 5-C_{13}(0), 5-C_{15}(0); 5-C_{17}(0,1)
Opisthiolepis heterophylla Smith	Resorcinol, 5-C_{13}(0); 5-C_{15}(0); 5-C_{17}(0,1)
Persoonia eliptica R. Br.	Resorcinol, 5-C_{11}(0), 5-C_{11}(1); 5-C_{13}(1)
Persoonia linearis Andr.	Resorcinol, 5-C_{9}(0); 5-C_{11}(0,1)
Petrophila shirleyae Bail	Resorcinol, 5-C_{15}(1); 5-C_{17}(1)

[a]Code: 3-Pentadecadienylcatechol = catechol, 3-C_{15}(2). [b]See Evans and Schmidt (1980), except as noted. [c]Occolowitz (1964). [d]Gambaro et al. (1986). [e]Bandyopadhyay et al. (1985). [f]Du et al. (1986). [g]Rivero-Cruz et al. (1997). [h]Knight (1991). [i]Suzuki et al. (1996). [j]Briggs (1974). [k]Kozubek (1984). [l]Ritchie et al. (1965). Ridley et al. (1968). [m]Ale et al. (1997). [n]Stahl et al. (1983).

nitration, and methylation) classified lobinol as a phenol, whereas color tests, complexes with metals, and reducing properties suggested that it contained two phenolic hydroxyl groups adjacent to each other—a type of chemical called a catechol. Other tests indicated the presence of a multicarbon side chain, and McNair proposed (correctly) that lobinol was an alkylcatechol.

For centuries, the shiny black coating on Japanese bowls was produced by the action of moist air on the allergenic sap—called *ki-urushi* (kee oo-roo-she)—from the Japanese lac, *T. vernicifluum*. In an investigation extending from 1907 to 1922, R. Majima and his coworkers in Japan found the lacquer-forming monomer to be a mixture of phenols that they named urushiol (Majima, 1909) and which could be hydrogenated to a single product, hydrourushiol. This could be methylated and acetylated (Majima, 1912), and a 15-carbon side chain was proved by oxidation of hydrourushiol to hexadecanoic (palmitic) acid. The methylated hydrourushiol was thought to be 3,4-dimethoxy-*n*-pentadecylbenzene (Majima and Nakamura, 1913).

However, a laborious synthesis showed that this was not the right dimethylhydrourushiol (DHU) after all. Its 2,3-dimethoxy isomer did prove to be identical to the methylated natural urushiol (Majima, 1915; Majima and Tahara, 1915), and removal of the methyl groups indeed provided hydrourushiol. Ozonolysis showed that the original urushiol was in fact a mixture of hydrourushiol (structure 1) and several close relatives containing unsaturated side chains (Majima, 1922a) in which the diene **2** was later found to predominate (display 5.1).

1 (Urushiol I)   2 (Urushiol III)   5.1

Charles Dawson and his students at Columbia University fractionated methylated natural urushiol from Majima's Japanese lac into its constituents by careful distillation, column chromatography, and repeated rechromatography (Sunthankar and Dawson, 1954). The four resulting compounds proved to be 3-pentadecylveratrole (dimethylhydrourushiol, DHU) and three olefins easily hydrogenated to it.

Majima proposed structures for olefinic urushiols based on ozonolysis and permanganate oxidation of methylated extracts, but the complex mixture could not be resolved at the time. However, ozonolysis of Dawson's purified veratroles gave evidence of urushiol I (DHU), a monoene urushiol II, doubly unsaturated urushiol III, and triply unsaturated urushiol IV (table 5.1; See Symes and Dawson, 1954). Infrared spectra suggested that the double bonds were *cis* (or Z), but later work showed poison ivy urushiols to include partly *trans* (E) isomers (appendix A).

The close resemblance of poison ivy urushiol to that from Japanese lac (*T. vernicifluum*) had not escaped G. A. Hill at Wesleyan University, and he demonstrated that they both contained hydrourushiol and its unsaturated relatives (Hill et al., 1934). Dawson's group finally resolved poison ivy extract into the same components as those from *T. vernicifluum*: urushiols I (2%), II (10%), III (64%), and IV (23%) (Markiewitz and Dawson, 1965). In addition to Japanese lac, Majima (1922b) found urushiols in a number of other Anacardiaceae species.

The allergens of western poison oak remained unidentified. In 1975, Corbett and Billets (1975) showed by NMR and mass spectra that its allergens were very similar to those of poison ivy and Japanese lac but with side chains of 17 rather than 15 carbons (appendix B). Diolefin was again the most abundant congener and the saturated one the least, but the positions of the unsaturation remained undefined. Majima much earlier had reported "laccol" (3-heptadecylcatechol) in the resin of Indochina lac (*T. succedaneum*) and Formosa lac (*T. vernicifluum*) (Majima, 1922b), and

Gross et al. (1975) found that extracts of poison oak, poison ivy, and poison sumac all contained catechols representing *both* C_{15} and C_{17} side chains (table 5.1). Poisonwood (*Metopium toxiferum*) and the related *Metopium brownei* of Central America also contain both, as well as a new C_{15} congener in the latter (Rivero-Cruz et al., 1997).

Urushiols and laccols generally possess an *n*-alkyl sidechain containing an odd number of carbons (table 5.1). Besides the usual C_{15} and C_{17}, traces of C_{11}, C_{13}, and C_{19} homologs have been reported. However, in his 1934 book, Georges Brooks (1934) detailed the isolation and analysis of a laccol from *Rhus succedanea* (now *T. succedaneum*), which he claimed contained a 16-carbon side chain. Modern chromatography and mass spectrometry revealed that these urushioids actually were a C_{17} monoene and C_{15} triene and the corresponding alkylphenols (Du, 1990); there was no hexadecyl isomer. The carbon and hydrogen content of Brooks's laccol indeed is that of the proposed $C_{22}H_{38}O_2$, corresponding to a C_{16} side chain, but it also fits an equal mixture of C_{21} urushiol (C_{15} side chain) and C_{23} laccol (C_{17} side chain). Oxidation gave stearic acid, expected from a C_{23} laccol, so the odd-carbon rule remained intact.

Over the years, a number of "new" urushiols have been reported, but they always turn out to be just the ordinary ones. For example, the "bhilawanol" from *Semecarpus anacardium* (Mason, 1945b) proved to be a mixture of *cis*- and *trans*-isomers of a urushiol, and the "renghol" in *S. heterophylla* was found to be urushiol I. Although 4-substituted catechols and others with unusual side chains have been reported in Burmese lac (*Melanorrhea* spp.) in recent years (fig. 5.1), isolation of major new urushiols and laccols now seems unlikely.

5.3 Isolation, Identification, and Analysis

Isolation of the urushiols from *T. radicans* and *T. diversilobum* normally has been accomplished by solvent extraction of the macerated leaves and stems followed by vacuum distillation of the extract. Major losses to polymerizaton and thermal decomposition are reduced by prior methylation, but this requires later demethylation. Now, extracts are fractionated by some form of chromatography, a much more efficient and benign process. Mixtures are purified initially by column chromatography on aluminum oxide, and thin-layer chromatography (TLC) provides good separations of some congeners.

The polar nature of the catechol ring enables urushiols and laccols to dissolve in alcohols and in benzene, whereas the long hydrophobic side chain provides solubility in petroleum ether but not in water (see section 5.5). The side chain apparently also masks the reactivity of the phenolic

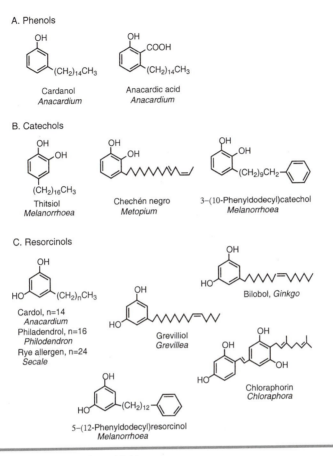

Figure 5.1 Unusual natural urushioids.

hydroxyls, and extractives are even insoluble in a dilute base and can be solvent-extracted out of alkaline slurries of plant materials, leaving other phenolics and acids behind. However, the ability of catechols to form colored complexes with metals is not impaired, and urushiols give positive color tests with ferric chloride and with Millon's reagent (mercuric nitrate in nitric acid).

Identifications originally were based on the separate chemical properties of the side chain and the catechol ring, as illustrated by the monounsaturated urushiol II (fig. 5.2). The ring is very reactive and can be nitrated to give a solid dinitro derivative of convenient melting point, but extensive oxidative degradation by the nitric acid makes prior protection of ring hydroxyls mandatory. The hydroxyls are easily acylated or benzoylated (Majima and Nakamura, 1913), and methylation, benzylation, or silylation forms the corresponding ethers (fig. 5.2).

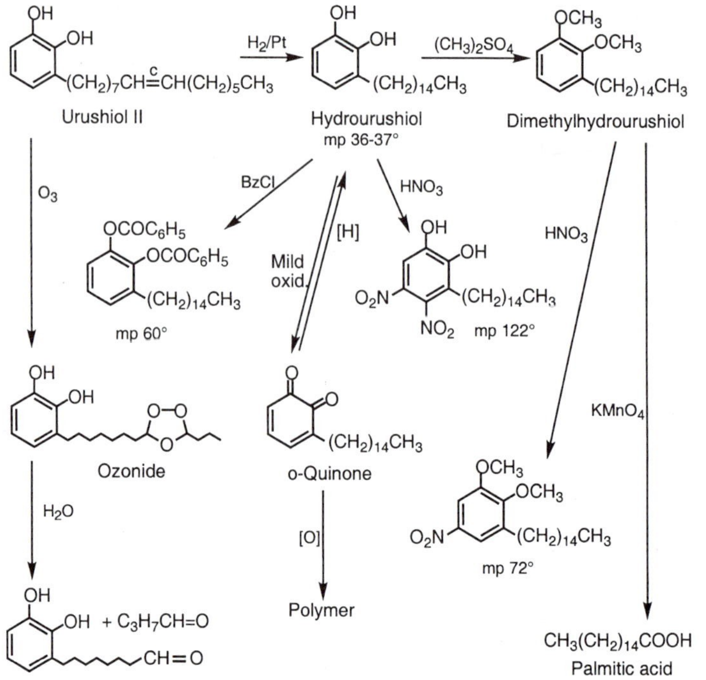

Figure 5.2 Chemical reactions of urushiols.

Polymerization

A saturated urushiol side chain is unreactive, but unsaturation permits normal catalytic hydrogenation, ozonolysis, Diels–Alder reactions, and polymerization. Indeed, it was polymerization that first drew attention to the urushiols. The coatings on oriental lacquerware, a product of the oxidative cross-linking of the side-chain double bonds, are possibly the toughest and most durable of all natural films (Kumanotani, 1983). With electron microscopy, the film is seen to be composed of densely packed cells or grains about 0.1 μm in diameter that contain polymerized urushiol inside a plant gum (polysaccharide) shell. Consistency and flowability depend on the proportions of C–O and C–C coupling, with molecular weights of the polymers ranging from 20,000 to 30,000 Daltons. The polymers become black in color, leading to shiny black bowls, black spots on damaged *Toxicodendron* leaves, and black marks on contaminated clothing and tools.

Oxidation

Urushiols and laccols can be oxidized under mild conditions (fig. 5.2). A dilute mixture of complexed copper and ammonium persulfate converts them quantitatively to the *ortho*-quinones, whose ultraviolet absorption maxima near 400 nm provide a means of colorimetric analysis (Quattrone, 1977). Silver oxide also oxidizes urushiols to quinones (Liberato et al., 1981), whereas more drastic oxidation with permanganate quickly destroys the catechol ring and converts urushiol I into palmitic (hexadecanoic) acid (Majima and Nakamura, 1913).

When a solution of urushiol I in ethanol or methanol was allowed to stand in air at room temperature, its ultraviolet (UV) spectrum immediately started to change and soon became that of the corresponding *ortho*-quinone (Balint et al., 1975; appendix C). Thin-layer chromatography (TLC) confirmed the oxidation and also revealed that the alcohol had added across a double bond in the quinone ring to return it to the catechol structure. This emphasizes the degree of care required when working with the catechols, and makes one wonder how earlier chemists were able to identify them at all.

More powerful oxidizing agents such as hydrogen peroxide or hypochlorite (bleach) cause oxidative polymerization of the quinone to black resin, as do oxidative enzymes or just plain air. Besides a black finish on bowls, the polymeriztion provides a simple test for urushioids. In the black spot test, a piece of leaf or stem of an unrecognized plant is cautiously crushed onto a piece of white paper and then removed; the rapid appearance of a brown spot that turns black within a few hours indicates a positive result (Guin, 1980).

In addition to the usual free-radical olefin polymerization, the reaction probably involves a series of intermediate polyphenyl ethers (display 5.2) generated by successive additions of phenolic hydroxyls across the quinoid double bond (Tyman and Mathews, 1982). This is followed by a reoxidation to form a new quinone of higher molecular weight, and the possibilities for cross-linking are almost endless. This type of Michael addition is discussed in section 5.6.

The results of classical chemical identification methods have been substantiated and extended by modern spectrometric techniques (appendix C). With the advent of high-resolution separations by capillary gas chromatography (GLC) and high-pressure liquid chromatography (HPLC), often with a mass spectrometer as detector (GCMS and LCMS), the laborious isolation of individual constituents of a urushioid mixture seldom is necessary for identification and quantitation.

Analysis

GLC and HPLC are now applied routinely to urushioid analysis. Colorimetric methods (Quattrone, 1977) may be useful for screening but lack sensitivity and specificity. GLC relies on the sensitivity of a flame ionization or mass spectrometric detector, either of which can readily measure nanogram $(10^{-9}\,\text{g})$ quantities of urushioids. A UV detector for HPLC achieves about the same sensitivity. A good capillary GLC method for underivatized urushioids (Du et al., 1984b) produced almost the same results as did reverse-phase HPLC (Du et al., 1984a). The most recent methods employ HPLC with a mass spectrometer detector (LCMS), which is sensitive, specific, and provides a lot of information (Shin et al., 1999).

Higher analytical sensitivity allows smaller samples, but more care is required to assure that they are representative. Table 5.1 shows the typical composition of urushioid mixtures from several *Toxicodendron* species; variations are due not only to species and individual plants but also to location, season, and other factors. For example, the ranges for poison ivy (*T. radicans*) represent three samples, from the same location (in Maryland), prepared in the same laboratory by the same procedure (Gross et al., 1975). In another example, the level of 8'Z,11'Z-urushiol III in Japanese lac from Ibaraki, Japan, was 3.2 times greater on July 5 (7.8%) than on September 30 (Du et al., 1984b). Even from a single *T. radicans* plant, leaves closest to the top (younger) contained 8–10 times more total urushiol than did those lower down, although the composition remained roughly the same (Baer et al., 1980).

In addition to the genus *Toxicodendron*, other members of the Anacardiaceae, Ginkgoaceae, Poaceae, and Proteaceae also contain long-chain catechols or 5-substituted resorcinols that induce ACD (table 5.2). The resorcinols may bear side chains of 9–27 carbons rather than the usual C_{15} and C_{17}, and some *Grevillea* species provide at least two different resorcinols with C_{19} side chains. All of these can be analyzed by methods similar to the ones used for urushiols (Tyman and Mathews, 1982; Du et al., 1984a; Kozubek et al., 1979), but many plants also contain corresponding anacardic acids and long-chain phenols (table 5.3) which generally must be methylated before analysis because the acids are so easily decarboxylated.

Extracts containing resorcinols and monophenols (and presumably catechols) can be analyzed directly by mass spectrometry to identify type,

Table 5.3 Allergenic Phenols and Phenolic Acids

Chemical Name[a]	Common Name	Source	Family
Salicylic acids[b]			
6-Pentadec-8-enyl-	Ginkgoic acid	*Ginkgo biloba*	Ginkgoaceae
6-Pentadecyl-	Anacardic acid	*Anacardium occidentale*	Anacardiaceae
6-Undecyl-	Anagigantic acid	*Anacardium giganteum*	Anacardiaceae
6-Heptadec-10-enyl	Pelandjauic acid	*Pentaspadon motleyi*	Anacardiaceae
6-Tridecyl-	Ginkgolinic acid	*Ginkgo biloba*	Ginkgoaceae
Phenols[b]			
3-Pentadecyl-	Hydroginkgol	*Ginkgo biloba*	Ginkgoaceae
3-Pentadec-8-enyl-[c]	Cardanol	*Anacardium occidentale*	Anacardiaceae
	Cardanol[d]	*Schinus terebinthifolius*	Anacardiaceae
	Ginkgol	*Ginkgo biloba*	Ginkgoaceae
3-Pentadecadienyl-	Cardanol diene	*Anacardium occidentale*	Anacardiaceae
3-Heptadecadienyl-[e]		*Melanorrhea usitata*	Anacardiaceae
3-Tridecyl-[f]		*Ginkgo biloba*	Ginkgoaceae

[a]Structures in figure 5.1. [b]See Tyman (1979). [c]Tyman et al. (1984). [d]Stahl et al. (1983). [e]Du et al. (1986). [f]Itokawa et al. (1987).

chain length, number of double bonds, and often their location, as well as to provide accurate quantitation (Occolowitz, 1964).

5.4 Physical and Environmental Properties

The physical and environmental properties of any chemical are closely linked. Aqueous solubility, volatility (and vapor pressure), distribution between water and fat, as estimated by Kow, and sorption onto surfaces control its environmental movement, whereas chemical reactivity such as transformations by sunlight and microorganisms (photodegradation and biodegradation) control its chemical form and toxicity.

Physical Properties

Key physical properties of urushiol I, urushiol III, and laccol III are summarized in table 5.4. They determine each chemical's mobility in water, its evaporation into the atmosphere, and its penetration into the skin. The melting point of urushiol I is surprisingly high (59°C) and reflects the polar nature of the catechol part of the molecule, whereas unsaturation in the other two causes them to be liquid at room temperature.

Although there are no data, calculations by the method of Lyman et al. (1990) indicate that the normal boiling points of urushiols and laccols

Table 5.4 Physical Properties of Urushiols and Laccols

	Urushiol I	Urushiol III	Laccol III
Side chain	15:0	15:2	17:2
Formula	$C_{21}H_{36}O_2$	$C_{21}H_{32}O_2$	$C_{23}H_{36}O_2$
Molecular weight	320.50	316.47	344.50
Melting point, °C	58–59°	liquid	liquid
Boiling point, °C	470°[a]	439°[a]	461°[a]
	190–200° (0.3 torr)		
Vapor pressure, torr[a]	$<1 \times 10^{-10}$ (25°C)	1×10^{-7} (25°)	5×10^{-8} (25°C)
Water solubility, µg/L[a]	0.3 (25°C)	3.2 (25°C)	0.2 (25°C)
Henry's constant, H'[a]	$<7 \times 10^{-6}$	6×10^{-4}	5×10^{-3}
log K_{ow}	9.27 (9.08)[b]	7.25[c]	8.57[c] (10.16)[b]

[a]Calculated (Lyman et al., 1990). [b]Roberts and Benezra (1993). [c]Calculated from K_{ow} of urushiol I.

lie above 400°C. Attempts to distill them at atmospheric pressure result only in charring or polymerization, and even though vacuum distillation leads to some decomposition, this is still the best means of purification for greater than milligram amounts. Vapor pressure is related to volatility—again, no values have been reported—but given values for the molar refraction and parachor, the boiling points allow their estimation (table 5.4). All of these calculations require assumptions and approximations, so the results probably fall only within an order of magnitude. With vapor pressures of 10^{-7} torr at best, these compounds are not very volatile.

Because no aqueous solubilities have been reported either, they must again be estimated. However, the octanol-water partition coefficient (K_{ow}) of urushiol I is known (Itokawa et al., 1989), so its solubility can be calculated from regression equations to within an order of magnitude (Lyman et al., 1990). Despite the polar nature of catechol, solubilities average only about 0.3 µg/L for urushiol I and 3 µg/L for urushiol III—very low. The K_{ow} confirms that urushioids are very hydrophobic, and the values of more than 10^8 are among the highest on record.

One practical consequence of low vapor pressure and aqueous solubility is that the Henry's constant (H')—a measure of volatility from wet surfaces—may be comparatively high. Although an H' below 10^{-6} discounts appreciable volatility for urushiol I, that of $\sim 6 \times 10^{-4}$ for urushiol III should allow it to vaporize slowly but surely where it occurs on wet leaves; laccol III must be even more volatile. Although these values fail to explain the negative results of early attempts to steam distill the allergens—the distillates apparently were never actually analyzed—they do lend credence to frequent complaints by especially sensitive persons that they develop an allergic reaction "just walking past" a stand of poison oak or poison ivy on a warm day.

A practical consequence of the high K_{ow} values is that skin absorption of the liquid urushioid mixtures must be extremely rapid and efficient, and simply washing with cold water may not dissolve away the poisons or affect their entry through skin. Within a homologous series of 3-alkylcatechols, log K_{ow} increases steadily from 3.59 for the C_7 congener to 7.75 at C_{13} and 9.27 at C_{15} (Urushiol I) (Itokawa et al., 1989). Because the unsaturated forms have only slightly lower calculated values, the allergens of T. radicans and T. diversilobum should all be equally well absorbed. Another consequence of high K_{ow} values is that urushioids will physically bind to the surface of soil or clothing because of equally high sorption coefficients—10^6 or more—and persist there.

Photodegradation

Substituted catechols are expected to be sensitive to light, and the sole reference states, without evidence, that urushiol I is strongly influenced by air, light, and moisture (Balint et al., 1975). However, UV absorption by the urushiols reaches a maximum near 275 nm and then declines sharply until there is virtually none above 290 nm (appendix C). The UV component of sunlight does not extend much below 290 nm at the earth's surface, and little if any energy would be available. However, urushiols are easily air-oxidized even in the dark, and the corresponding quinones show absorption maxima near 400 nm in the visible spectrum. The practical consequence is that urushiol degradation on surfaces may indeed be increased by sunlight and even by incandescent illumination indoors.

Biodegradation

There is little information on the actual biodegradation of urushioids. Kouakou (1991) did not detect them in the milk or urine of goats fed leaves of T. diversilobum, most of the ingested amount being excreted in feces. However, congener ratios changed to favor the laccols, suggesting that a reduction of olefinic double bonds had occurred in the rumen. Tzeng (1993) later showed that the saturated congener indeed increased in isolated rumen fluid at the expense of triolefin. Unfortunately, urinary metabolites were not investigated.

Despite this, certain metabolic pathways are fairly predictable (fig. 5.3). One should expect oxidative transformation in any type of catechol. Bacteria generally cleave the aromatic ring between the hydroxyl groups to form substituted cis, cis-muconic acids, which are further degraded into small

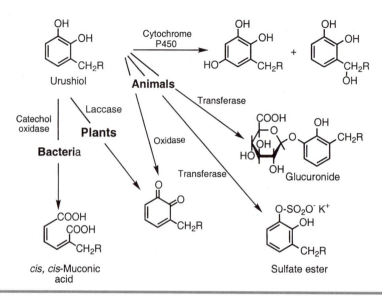

Figure 5.3 Proposed metabolism of urushiols and laccols.

fragments. Fungi oxidize catechols via either the enzyme, phenol oxidase, that converts them to the *ortho*-quinones, or the copper enzyme laccase, a blue oxidase that converts hydroquinones to quinones. Animals hydroxylate catechols on either the ring or side chain via the almost ubiquitous oxidase, cytochrome P450 (Parke, 1968), and urushioids should be no exception. Most organisms also epoxidize side-chain double bonds as they do the natural unsaturated fatty acids.

Animals protect one catechol hydroxyl group with glucuronic acid or sulfate so rapidly that there is little time for the other, more hindered one to react (see Williams, 1959), and the water-soluble conjugates are then voided in the urine. Conjugates are not susceptible to oxidation to ACD-producing quinones, so this may be how excess urushioids are detoxified in the body. Plants convert the hydroxyl groups to β-D-glucosides rather than glucuronides, yet urushiols and laccols do not appear to occur as sugar derivatives in *Toxicodendron*.

Because both glutathione-*S*-transferase and quinone reductase are found in skin (Mukhtar, 1992), one might expect that the proposed quinone metabolites could be either reduced to the hydroquinone and conjugated with glucuronic acid or converted into mercapturic acids or other sulfur-containing metabolites. Unfortunately, these common and predictable metabolic routes must remain largely speculative for urushioids, as their metabolic fate apparently remains unknown.

5.5 Reactions with Proteins

Skin sensitization and an allergic response require that urushioids combine with cellular proteins to form an antigen (section 9.5). There is little evidence that catechols and other benzenediols can combine with protein directly, but they are easily oxidized to quinones capable of the reaction (Byck and Dawson, 1968). Indeed, Dawson and his coworkers showed that the oxidation proceeded in dilute solution and the products were reasonably stable. Although air alone was sufficient for complete the conversion, it seems likely that some sort of oxidases are involved in vivo: laccase (Zhan et al., 1990) or perhaps the widely occurring cytochrome P450.

The combination of protein -OH, -SH, and -NH groups with quinones is to be expected (Finley, 1988). This is called a Michael-type reaction. A true Michael addition is slightly different; according to March (1992), it is a conjugate addition in which the nucleophile adds across the quinone's conjugated double bond system to form an intermediate enol that is in equilibrium with the keto (or quinoid) form (display 5.3).

$$RNH_2 + C{=}C{-}C{=}O \longrightarrow RNH{-}C{-}C{=}C{-}OH \rightleftharpoons RNH{-}C{-}CH{-}C{=}O \qquad 5.3$$

It is thought that the reaction takes place on the external surface of the epidermal cell's membrane. Membrane proteins generally are oriented with their hydrophobic backbone arranged in an α-helix in the membrane's interior and their polar functional groups protruding into the hydrated epidermis. The rate and selectivity depend on the nucleophilicity of the particular side-chain functional group, the strongest being the secondary amine of histidine and the cysteine sulfhydryl, followed by lysine's primary amino group, the tyrosine phenolate, and finally the guanidino group of arginine (Ross, 1962). Stauffer (1972) found that amines were the reactive species, and that 3–4 quinone molecules added to each molecule of human serum albumin.

The quinone, too, offers electronic and steric restrictions. Liberato et al. (1981) found that the sulfhydryl of acetylcysteine reacted only at the 6-position of 3-pentadecylquinone (corresponding to hydrourushiol), whereas the simple aliphatic pentylamine added exclusively at the 5-position (display 5.4). Further oxidation, even by air alone, restored the quinone form.

Pentylaminoquinone

Proteins, too, including bovine γ-globulin and human serum albumen, reacted with the quinone formed in situ from urushiol I or laccol I (Stauffer, 1972) in the presence of air, but no reaction occurred when the 4- or 5-positions were blocked by a methyl group.

Despite the evidence supporting quinones as haptens, an alternate mechanism has been proposed that involves reaction of a catechol free radical with the protein (Schmidt et al., 1990). The argument is not convincing, but shows that other means of antigen formation might be possible. The matter could be settled by an experiment, possibly with isotope-labeled urushiol, where the protein allergen is isolated and degraded to determine whether a urushiol-substituted amino acid is present; no such experiment has been reported.

5.6 Synthetic Urushioids

Synthesis verifies the identity of a natural product and allows preparation of structural analogs for biological testing. The first reported synthesis of urushiol I (Majima and Tahara, 1915) was rather complex and has not been used since then, but most of the recent routes still utilize classical organic chemistry: (1) Grignard reactions, (2) lithium alkylations, and (3) the Wittig ylide synthesis (fig. 5.4).

The Grignard reaction of dimethoxybenzaldehyde with an alkylmagnesium halide has seen the most use, and the intermediate alcohol need not be isolated. However, the ylide reaction permits synthesis of urushioids containing unsaturated side chains of known configuration, and the discovery that veratrole (o-dimethoxybenzene) adds metallic lithium at its 3-position led to what is now perhaps the most straightforward of the methods (Dawson and Ng, 1978). Long-chain resorcinols also have been prepared using these methods (Cirigottis et al., 1974).

For sheer elegance, the prize must go to T. Miyakoshi and H. Togashi (1990). Where other methods required eventual, rather inefficient removal of O-methyl groups to reach the urushiol, theirs involved construction of a novel tetrahydrofuran, which, when boiled with dilute acid, provided high yields of the catechol directly (fig. 5.4). Laccol and a number of purely synthetic analogs also were obtained in this way.

Over decades, the structures of the major urushiols and laccols have been confirmed by synthesis. However, most other urushioids have been made to study structure-activity relations. In addition to ethers and esters, ring-methyls in various ring positions, various lengths and branching of side chains, halogenation, and additional rings are included (for example, Keil et al., 1944; Baer et al., 1967; Kurtz and Dawson, 1971a,b; ElSohly et al., 1986; Fraginals et al., 1991).

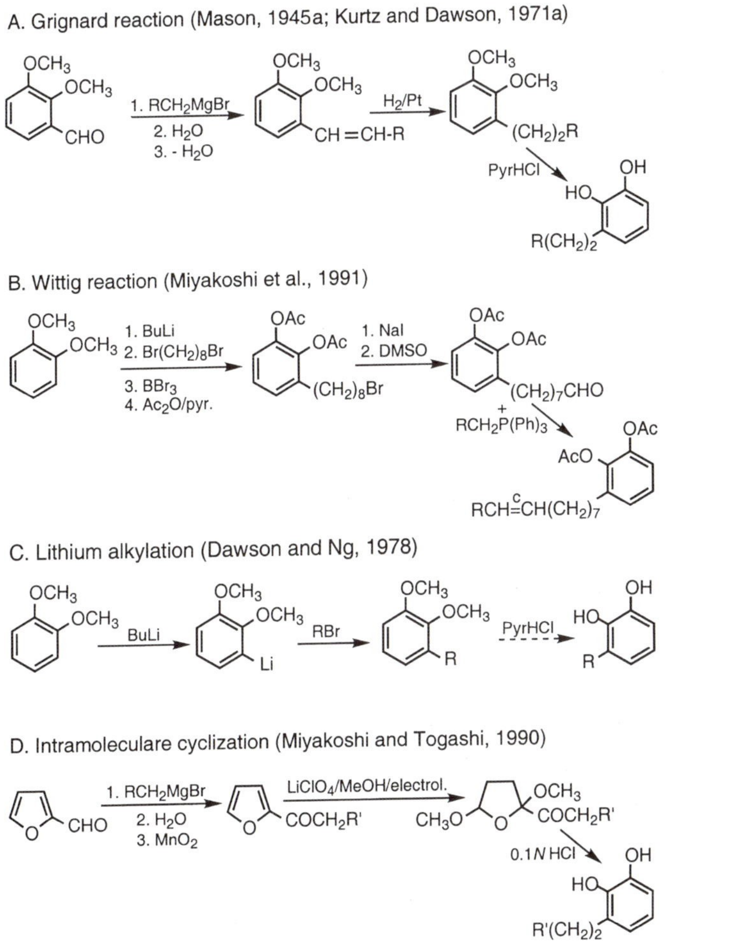

A. Grignard reaction (Mason, 1945a; Kurtz and Dawson, 1971a)

B. Wittig reaction (Miyakoshi et al., 1991)

C. Lithium alkylation (Dawson and Ng, 1978)

D. Intramoleculare cyclization (Miyakoshi and Togashi, 1990)

Figure 5.4 Synthesis of urushiols. R = alkyl or alkenyl.

5.7 Natural Urushioids

The natural urushioids represent urushiols, laccols, and other plant substances that share certain chemical and immunological properties with
them, including a hydroxylated benzene ring, a long-chain alkyl substituent, allergenicity, and cross-reactivity with each other (section 8.6). In
addition to other substituted catechols, a number of resorcinols (1,3-
dihydroxybenzenes) and phenols are included, but, strangely, the allergenic
hydroquinones (1,4-dihydroxybenzenes) appear not to cross-react with
urushiol. The known natural urushiols and laccols are listed in appendixes
A and B, but one can expect that each plant will produce a mixture of saturated and mono-, di-, and triunsaturated congeners.

Biosynthesis

Despite the toxicological importance and unique structures of urushioids, there seems to be no published data on their biosynthesis. However, several early investigators reported the isolation from cashew nut oil of "anacardic acid," a mix of 2-hydroxy-6-alkylbenzoic acids whose side chains correspond to those of urushiols (table 5.3). The name now refers only to the parent of the group, 2-hydroxy-6-*n*-pentadecylbenzoic acid (3-pentadecylsalicylic acid); the pentadec-8-enyl analog is ginkgoic acid, its source the Ginkgo tree (*Ginkgo biloba*).

The biochemical route to anacardic acid apparently has not been established either. Although resorcinols (*m*-dihydroxybenzenes) are common in the plant kingdom, simple catechols (*o*-dihydroxybenzenes) are not. Many natural phenols are known to be biosynthesized by internal condensation of an acyl coenzyme-A (polyketide synthesis), which could provide both urushiols and resorcinols (fig. 5.5). This route has been confirmed for the

Figure 5.5 Proposed biosynthesis of urushioids. ESH = 6-methylsalicylic acid synthase, M = malonyl. See Abell and Staunton (1984).

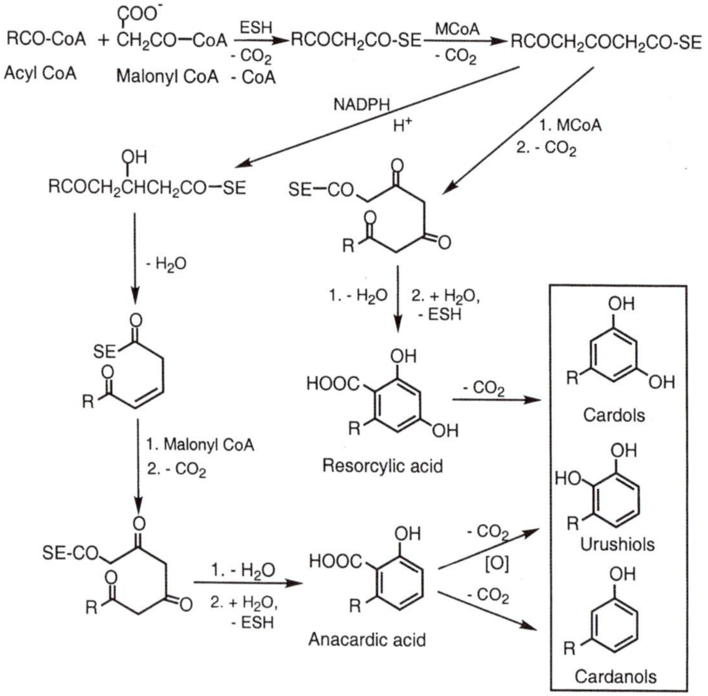

biosynthesis of an anacardic acid relative, 6-methylsalicylic acid (fig. 5.5, R=CH$_3$) (Abell and Staunton, 1984).

An enzyme, 6-methylsalicylate synthase (6-MSS) from *Penicillium patulum*, catalyzes the condensation of acetyl CoA with malonyl CoA. This is repeated to provide a diketohexanoyl enzyme, which subsequently is reduced, dehydrated to an olefin, combined with one more malonyl CoA molecules, and finally aromatized to provide 6-methylsalicylic acid. The entire synthesis occurs on the enzyme surface without release of any intermediates (Abell and Staunton, 1984). Based on the detection of traces of cardanols (3-alkylphenols) in *Toxicodendron* extracts, Tyman and Lam (1978) suggested that urushiols might be derived by oxidation of cardanol rather than from anacardic acids, but the new hydroxyl actually would go into the 6- rather than the 2-position as proposed.

The side chains of anacardic acids and urushiols surely must be derived from common long-chain fatty acids. Palmitoyl CoA would lead to the 15-carbon side chain of anacardic acid and on to urushiol I (fig. 5.5), and the saturated C$_{17}$ side chain of poison oak laccol would arise from stearic acid. The common 9Z,12Z-octadecadienoic (linoleic) acid would provide 8'Z, 11'Z-Laccol III, 9'Z-hexadecanoic acid (palmitoleic) acid the observed 8'Z-urushiol II, and so on.

The presence of two other closely related constituents, cardol (5-pentadecylresorcinol) and cardanol (3-pentadecylphenol), in cashew oil supports anacardic acid as a product of polyketide synthesis and offers a biosynthetic route to other 5-alkylresorcinols as well. The discovery by Gross et al. (1975) of traces of 3-heptyl-, 3-nonyl-, and 3-tridecylcatechols among the urushiols of toxic Anacardiaceae species suggests that any of the common fatty acids may participate.

Resorcinols

There are a lot more natural resorcinols than one might expect. Many are listed in table 5.2, and typical structures are shown in figure 5.1. The side chains, generally in the 5-position, are the usual mix of saturated and singly or multiply unsaturated C$_{11}$—C$_{17}$ congeners, although cereal grains provide congeners of up to C$_{27}$, and the weakly allergenic orcinol has only a methyl substituent. 5-Alk(en)ylresorcinols in cashew nutshell liquid are accompanied by corresponding 2-methyl-5-alk(en)yl compounds (Tyman, 1973).

As 1,3-benzenediols, resorcinols share many of the chemical characteristics of catechols (1,2-benzenediols), such as acylation, etherification, and ring-nitration. However, with hydroxyls in this *meta-* configuration, they cannot be oxidized to quinones directly, leading several authors to doubt the significance of quinone intermediates in the allergenic process. Unlike corresponding catechols, one cannot simply mix solutions of resorcinols and proteins in air and expect conjugates.

However, in vivo, widely occurring oxidases such as laccase, tyrosinase, and no doubt cytochrome P450 can hydroxylate the resorcinol ring to form benzenetriols capable of further conversion to the quinone. An example is the oxidation of orcinol (5-methylresorcinol) by the fungus *Aspergillus niger*, as shown in display 5.5 (Sahasrabudhe et al., 1986). Even in vitro, 5-tridecylresorcinol (grevillol) is easily oxidized to the corresponding benzoquinone (Hausen, 1981). The analysis and proposed biosynthesis of resorcinols and phenols were described earlier in this chapter.

5.5

Phenols

Several plant species produce allergenic long-chain monophenols (table 5.3), and improved separation methods undoubtedly will reveal others. They most likely are formed by decarboxylation of the corresponding anacardic (salicylic) acids (fig. 5.4). Phenols were first detected in the highly corrosive and allergenic nutshell liquid from cashews (*Anacardium occidentale*), but modern chromatographic techniques have detected them in a variety of other plants (Tyman et al., 1984; Du et al., 1986). Like resorcinols, phenols are hydroxylated in the same manner as the tyrosinase-catalyzed oxidation of tyrosine (4-hydroxyphenylalanine) to DOPA (3,4-dihydroxyphenylalanine) and then to the corresponding quinone (Zubay, 1986).

5.8 Conclusions

Urushioids are a class of plant allergens that contain a hydroxylated benzene ring and long alkyl side chain, and that cross-react immunologically with urushiol. They are best known in the form of long-chain catechols (1,2-benzenediols), now well characterized, that are suggested to arise from the corresponding fatty acids via anacardic acids. Their high fat solubility and very low water solubility ensure rapid skin absorption, and they are easily oxidized to quinones and then to black polymers; the quinones are thought to bind covalently to skin proteins to form allergens. Long-chain resorcinols and phenols do likewise, and, all together, the known urushioids are surprisingly large in number and structural diversity. For most people, this combination of widespread occurrence, easy skin absorption, and oxidation to reactive quinones means trouble.

SIX

"There are over 300 publications on Primula *allergy, which is the most common form of plant dermatitis [in Europe]. Primin may not be the sole cause, as screening tests with extracts from over 80 Primulaceae species showed that the great majority contained [quinone-type] compounds, while primin was detected in only twenty ..."*
—R. H. Thompson, 1987

6.1 Other Kinds of Allergens

Certainly not all plant allergens are urushioids—far from it. Many other structural types are represented, including quinones, lactones, acetylenes, terpene alcohols, aldehydes, and esters (table 6.1). However, like urushiol, they all serve as haptens and, to an extent, react with skin proteins to form allergens. Many kinds of plant constituents cause ACD in humans (Mitchell and Rook, 1979), and a review of their structures (figs. 6.1 and 6.2) reveals that, improbable as it may seem, they all appear capable of Michael additions. The significance of this will be discussed in section 9.8.

6.2 Quinones and Hydroquinones

Literally hundreds of plant quinones have been isolated, and from a wide range of species (Thompson, 1971, 1987), as seen in table 6.2. A good example of this is 2,6-dimethoxybenzoquinone (DMB), which is found in wheat (*Triticum vulgare*, Graminaceae), tree of heaven (*Ailanthus altissima*, Simarubaceae), red oak (*Quercus rubra*, Fagaceae), sugar maple (*Acer saccharum*, Aceraceae), and at least two dozen other species from a broad cross section of plant families (Hausen, 1978b). Some of their structures are quite complex (fig. 6.1), but they all share certain chemical traits.

Quinones are very reactive (fig. 6.2), adding mercaptans and other nucleophiles in typical Michael fashion (section 5.5). They are hydroxylated by the addition of water, undergo epoxidation, and are easily reduced to

Table 6.1 Allergens from Familiar Plants

Allergen	Source	Species	Chemical Class
Ambrosin	Ragweed	*Ambrosia* spp.	Ketolactone
Anthocotulide	Mayweed	*Anthemis cotula*	Ketolactone
Arteglasin A	Chrysanthemum	*Dendranthema* × *grandiflorum*	Epoxylactone
Cinnamaldehyde	Cinnamon	*Cinnamomum cassia*	Aralkene aldehyde
Cynaropicrin	Artichoke	*Cynara scolymus*	Ester-lactone
Falcarinol	English ivy	*Hedera helix*	Acetylenic alcohol
Lactucopicrin	Lettuce	*Lactuca sativa*	Ketolactone
Limonene	Orange (peel)	*Citrus sinensis*	Terpene hydrocarbon
Menthol	Peppermint	*Mentha piperita*	Terpene alcohol
Primin	Primrose	*Primula obconica*	Quinone
Protoanemonin	Buttercup	*Ranunculus* spp.	Lactone
Taraxin acid	Dandelion	*Taraxacum officinale*	Acid lactone
Tulipalin A	Tulip	*Tulipa* spp.	Hemiterpene lactone
Vanillin	Vanilla	*Vanilla planifolia*	Aromatic aldehyde

hydroquinones. For more detail on these reactions, see Finley (1988). Quinones act like alicyclic compounds: They are colored (DMB is bright yellow), exhibit strong ultraviolet or visible spectra useful in their identification and analysis, and have very high reduction potentials. They form crystalline charge-transfer complexes (quinhydrones) with hydroquinones, which can complicate their isolation and identification. Hydroquinones, however, generally behave like the benzenoid compounds they are, their phenolic hydroxyls forming the usual alkyl and acyl derivatives but being readily oxidized to quinones.

In particular, 1,2-quinones (*o*-quinones) tend to be especially reactive and are seldom found as such in plants (e.g., urushiol quinones), although examples include Macassar quinone from *Diospyros celebica* (Macassar ebony) and a series of mansonones from *Mansonia altissima* and *Ulmus* (elm) species (table 6.2). Although *o*-quinones almost always occur in reduced form as the corresponding catechols, *p*-quinones and their corresponding hydroquinones sometimes may be obtained from the same plant. For example, primin (2-pentyl-6-methoxyquinone) and 2-farnesylquinone are found together in *Primula* species along with their hydroquinones (Aregullin and Rodriguez, 2000).

In addition, *Primula obconica* contains at least eight other related phenols, ethers, and resorcinols (Horper and Marner, 1995), and *Iris* seeds or roots contain over 20 primin relatives with side chains up C_{29} (Marner and Horper, 1992). The isolation of such compounds requires great care, as both catechols and hydroquinones are easily reoxidized to the corresponding quinones by oxidases, chemical oxidants, or even by air alone (section 5.3).

Table 6.2 Allergenic Quinones and Their Precursors

Compound[a]	Species	Common Name (Family)
Acamelin[b]	*Acacia melanoxylon*	Australian blackwood (Fabaceae)
Bowdichione[b]	*Bowdichia nitida*	Sucupira (Fabaceae)
Coleone O[c]	*Coleus blumeii*	Coleus (Lamiaceae)
Cordiachrome A[b]	*Cordia goeldiana*	Cordia (Boraginaceae)
Cypripedin[d]	*Cypripedium calceolus*	Ladyslipper (Orchidaceae)
Deoxylapachol[b]	*Tectona grandis*	Teak (Lapacho) (Verbenaceae)
*Dietchequinone[d]	*Cyperus dietrichae*	Papyrus (Papyraceae)
2,6-Dimethoxyquinone,[b,e]	*Bowdichia nitida*	Sucupira (Fabaceae)
	Swietenia macrophylla	Honduras mahogany (Meliaceae)
	Cymbidium cultivars[f]	Cymbidium (Orchidaceae)
Dimethoxydalbergione[b]	*Machaerium scleroxylon*	Pao ferra (Fabaceae)
	Dalbergia spp.	Rosewoods (Fabaceae)
Farnesylhydroquinone[g]	*Wigandia caracasana*	Wigandia
2-Geranylquinone[g]	*Phacelia crenulata*	Desert heliotrope (Hydrophyllaceae)
2-Geranylhydroquinone[g]	*Phacelia crenulata*	Desert heliotrope (Hydrophyllaceae)
Irisquinone[d]	*Iris pseudacorus*	Yellow flag (Iridaceae)
Lapachenol	*Tectona grandis*	Teak (Lapacho) (Verbenaceae)
Lapachol (Tecomin)[b]	*Tectona grandis*	Teak (Lapacho) (Verbenaceae)
*Lapachonone	*Tecoma peroba*	Peroba do Campos (Bignoniaceae)
Macassar Ii[b]	*Diospyros celebica*	Macassar ebony (Ebenaceae)
Mansonone A[b]	*Mansonia altissimoa*	Mansonia (Sterculiaceae)
Mansonone X[b]	*Thespesia populnea*	Milo (Malvaceae)
Melacacidin[b]	*Acacia* spp.	Australian blackwood
4-Methoxydalbergione[b]	*Dalbergia* spp.	Rosewoods (Fabaceae)
Obtusaquinone[b]	*Dalbergia obtusa* (*retusa*)	Cocobolo (Fabaceae)
Oxyayanin A[b]	*Distemonanthus benthamianus*	Ayan (Fabaceae)
*Oxofarnesylhydroquinone[g]	*Phacelia campanularia*	Desert bluebells (Hydrophyllaceae)
*Plumbagin[h]	*Plumbago* spp.	Plumbago (Plumbaginaceae)
Prenylquinone[h]	*Phagnalon purpurescens*	Mecha (Asteraceae)
Primetin[i]	*Primula* spp.	Primrose (Primulaceae)
Primin[i]	*Primula* spp.[j]	Primrose (Primulaceae)
Thymoquinone[b]	*Calocedrus decurrens*	Incense cedar (Cupressaceae)
	Thuja plicata	Western red cedar (Cupressaceae)

[a]Structures are in figure 6.1, except *. [b]See Hausen (2000a). [c]Hausen et al. (1988). [d]Thompson (1987). [e]Hausen (1978b) lists 43 species. [f]Hausen et al. (1984). [g]See Aregullin and Rodriguez (2000). [h]See Thompson (1971). [i]See Christensen (2000). [j]Hausen (1978a) lists 21 species.

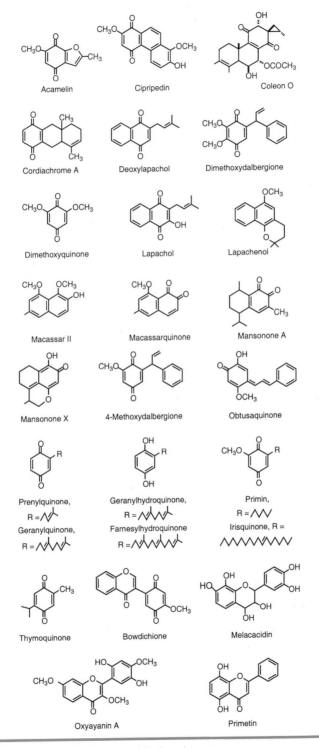

Figure 6.1 Structures of quinones and hydroquinones.

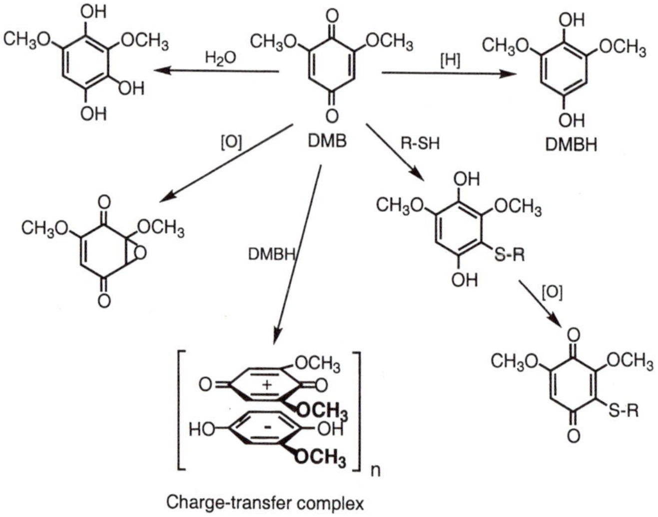

Figure 6.2 Reactions of 2,6-dimethoxybenzoquinone.

Among the allergenic quinones and hydroquinones are several that are classified as flavonoids (fig. 6.1). Flavonoids are a venerable group of plant products—yellow dyes used long before the advent of organic chemistry. They are oxygen heterocycles (benzo-4-pyrones) substituted with a phenyl group in the 2-position (as in primetin) or in the 3-position in isoflavonoids (such as bowdichione). However, where most of the dyes are *meta*-dihydroxyflavones, the allergenic ones are monosubstituted or show *ortho*- or *para*-hydroxylation. For example, primetin (from primroses) has two hydroxyl groups *para* to each other and so is easily converted to the corresponding primetin quinone isolated along with it from the plant extracts (Hausen et al., 1983). The wide occurrence of flavones in nature suggests that others may yet prove to be dermatotoxic.

Hydroquinones usually precede quinones in biosynthesis and often exist in the plant as glycosides. They originate from shikimic acid (Bolkart and Zenk, 1968; Horper and Marner, 1996) rather than from acetyl coenzyme A as do catechols (fig. 5.4); natural naphthoquinones, too, are at least partly derived from shikimate (Bolkart and Zenk, 1969). Geranylhydroquinone and other phaceloids from desert heliotrope (*Phacelia crenulata*) bear side chains of two, three, or even four isoprene units derived from mevalonate (fig. 6.1; Reynolds and Rodriguez, 1986). The Michael addition of mercaptan, amine, or water to a quinone results in a corresponding hydroquinone after enolization (display 5.3), but the product soon is reoxidized to the quinone form by air or oxidases.

Prenylated quinones occur in *Wigandia* (Reynolds and Rodriguez, 1989). Both quinones and hydroquinones can be strongly allergenic. Among ten quinones tested, thymoquinone (2-methyl-5-isopropylquinone) was the most active, followed by obtusaquinone, Macassar quinone, and 2,6-DMB (Hausen, 1978b). The allergenicity of some, such as miconidin (2-pentyl-6-methoxyhydroquinone; Horper and Marner, 1995), remains undetermined, but despite the presumption of a common mechanism of action, neither quinones nor hydroquinones appear to cross-react with urushioids.

Another type of quinoid—not really a quinone by the classical definition—is the quinone methide exemplified by obtusaquinone from cocobolo (*Dahlbergia obtusa*). In this case, one quinone carbonyl is replaced by an unsaturated side chain to form a carbon–carbon rather than a carbon–oxygen bond (fig. 6.1). However, methides undergo the usual quinone reactions such as Michael addition, and obtusaquinone might become a normal quinone simply by demethylation of the methoxyl. Mansonone X (from *Thespesia populnea*, or milo) also qualifies as a methide.

Some nonallergenic substances, too, may be converted to quinones. *Coleus*, a popular houseplant notable for its brightly multicolored leaves, is not particularly allergenic (Hausen et al., 1988), but the coleon O isolated from its extracts causes ACD due, perhaps, to isomerization and dehydration of the substance during or after extraction. Related examples include lapachenol from teak (*Tectona grandis*) and Macassar II from Macassar ebony, *Diospyros celebica* (fig. 6.1). Not all long-chain quinones need be allergenic—vitamin K and the energy intermediate ubiquinone are not—but the dermatotoxicity of most of the known long-chain quinones has not actually been tested.

6.3 Lactones

The largest class of substances to cause ACD are cyclic esters called lactones (Perold et al., 1972; Connolly and Thornton, 1973). They occur in many familiar plants (table 6.3): chrysanthemums from the flower garden; vegetables such as endive and lettuce; trees like oak, acacia, and fir that harbor scale mosses and lichens; and common weeds, from dandelions to giant ragweed. Of over 1000 lactones identified from the Asteraceae alone, at least 180 are considered potentially allergenic, and 31 are reportedly allergenic (Mitchell and Dupuis, 1971; Mitchell et al., 1972). Structures of some allergenic ones are shown in figure 6.3.

Most allergenic lactones are sesquiterpenes, abbreviated to STLs, C_{15} alicyclic esters composed of three 5-carbon isoprene units assembled in various configurations (display 6.1). The most reactive site is the methylene

Table 6.3 Allergenic Sesquiterpene Lactones[a]

Allergen[b]	Species[c]	Common Name
Alantolactone	*Inula helenium*	Elecampane
Ambrosin	*Ambrosia* spp.	Ragweed
Anthocotulide	*Anthemis cotula*	Mayweed
Arbusculin A	*Tanacetum vulgare*	Tansy
Arteglasin A	*Dendranthemum* spp.	Chrysanthemum
Carabron	*Arnica longifolia*	Arnica
Coronopilin	*Parthenium hysterophorus*	Wild feverfew
Costunolide	*Saussurea costus*	Costus
Cynaropicrin	*Cynara scolymus*	Artichoke
Desacetylmatricarin	*Matricaria chamomilla*	German chamomile[d]
Frullanolide	*Frullania dilatata* (Frullanaceae)	Frullania
Helenalin	*Inula helenium*	Elecampane
Isabelin	*Ambrosia psilostachya*	Western ragweed
Lactucin	*Chicorium endiva*	Chicory
Lactucopicrin	*Lactuca sativa*	Lettuce
Laurenobiolide	*Laurus nobilis* (Lauraceae)	Grecian laurel
Ludovicin A	*Artemesia* spp.	Sage
Niveusin A	*Helianthus annuus*	Sunflower
Nobilin	*Chamaemelum nobile*	Roman camomile
Parthenin	*Parthenium hysterophorus*	Wild feverfew
Parthenolide	*Tanacetum parthenium*	Feverfew
Protoanemonin	*Ranunculus* spp. (Ranunculaceae)	Buttercup
Pyrethrosin	*Chrysanthemum cinerariaefolium*	Pyrethrum daisy
Taraxin acid	*Taraxacum officinale*	Dandelion
Tulipalin A	*Tulipa* spp. (Liliaceae)	Tulip
Thapsigargin	*Thapsia gargarica* (Apiaceae)	Thapsia
Xanthinin	*Xanthium pennsylvanicum*	Cockleburr

[a]For more extensive lists, see Evans and Schmidt (1980) and Seaman (1982). [b]For structures, see figure 6.3. [c]Asteraceae unless indicated. [d]Also spelled camomile.

group (circled) next to the ester carbonyl; without it, there is no allergenicity. The isoprene units form six basic patterns known respectively as ambrosanolide, xantholide, eremophilanolide, eudesmanolide, germacranolide, and guaianolide—named for their type genera (fig. 6.4)—but many variations exist within each. Alantolactone represents the eudesmanolides, for example, and parthenin the ambrosanolides. Several numbering systems have been applied to these lactones, but we will use the most common one that also specifies the ring system. Thus, alantolactone becomes 3β-hydroxy-4αH-eudesm-5-en-12-oic acid lactone, and parthenin is 1α,6β-dihydroxy-4-oxo-10αH-ambrosa-2,11-dien-12-oic lactone; α and

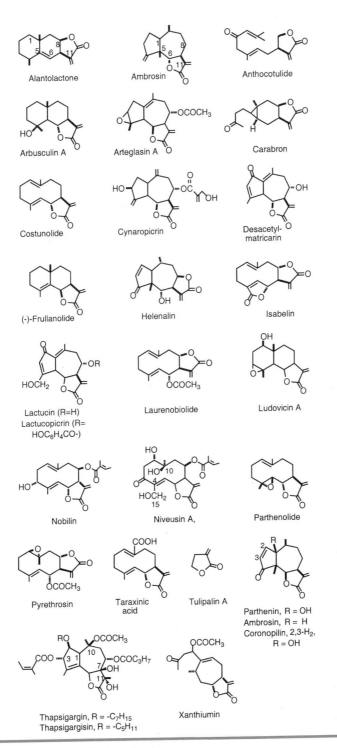

Figure 6.3 Sesquiterpene lactone structures.

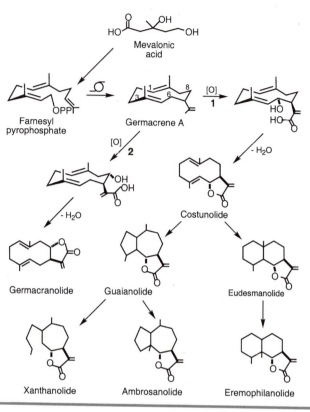

Figure 6.4 Biogenesis of sesquiterpene lactones.

β denote a group below or above the plane of the ring, respectively, as shown in display 6.1.

The common names of most lactones are now distinguished by the suffix -olide (e.g., costunolide), but this is not true of those like helenalin first isolated many years ago. An STL may exist in several stereoisomeric forms: Helenalin is the 6α,8β form of the structure shown in figure 6.3; epihelenalin is 6α,8α, the 6β,8α is called mexicanin I, and 6β,8β is balduilin. Both structure and stereochemistry now are identified mostly by nuclear magnetic resonance (NMR) spectrometry, and Yoshioka et al. (1973) provide an extensive catalog of pertinent NMR spectra.

The simplest allergenic lactone, tulipalin A (2-methylenebutanolide), is not an STL but a hemiterpene representing only a single isoprene unit. It occurs in both tulips (*Tulipa* spp.) and Peruvian lilies (*Alstroemeria* spp.), largely as glucosides called tuliposides (display 6.2). There are several other tulipalins and tuliposides, all less allergenic than tulipalin A. Tulipalin B and its glycoside have a hydroxyl group in the lactone's 3-position, whereas tuliposide D is a diester of the α-hydroxyethylacrylic acid (Christensen et al., 2000). The readily hydrolyzed 1-tuliposides first isolated by Tschesche et al. (1969) quickly rearrange to more stable 6-tuliposides, the ones generally detected in plant extracts. Reversed-phase HPLC shows that tuliposide A occurs throughout the Alstroemeriaceae and in some Liliaceae, but tuliposide B is found only in the latter. The glucosides are too water-soluble to enter the skin unless subjected to prior hydrolysis and lactonization (display 6.2), but because both the tuliposides and tulipalins are strongly allergenic, hydrolysis may be occuring on the skin surface.

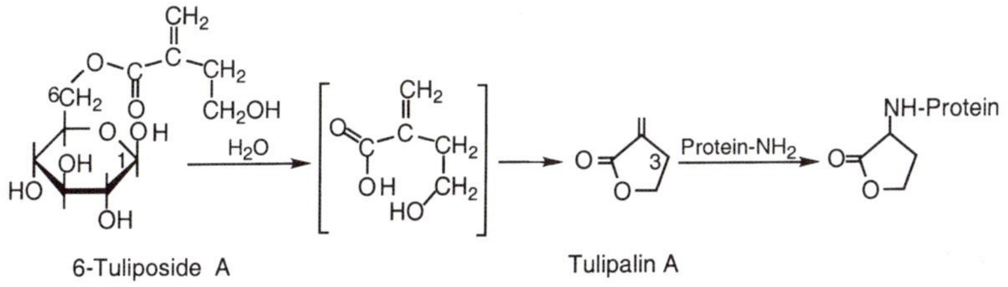

6-Tuliposide A   Tulipalin A

6.2

The tulipalins illustrate the importance of having an α-methylene group adjacent to the carbonyl for the lactone's allergenicity; the γ-methylene relative, protoanemonin (5-methylenebut-2-enolide) from *Ranunculus* species, is a powerful skin irritant but is not allergenic, and γ-butyrolactone, with no methylene at all, is completely nontoxic (display 6.3).

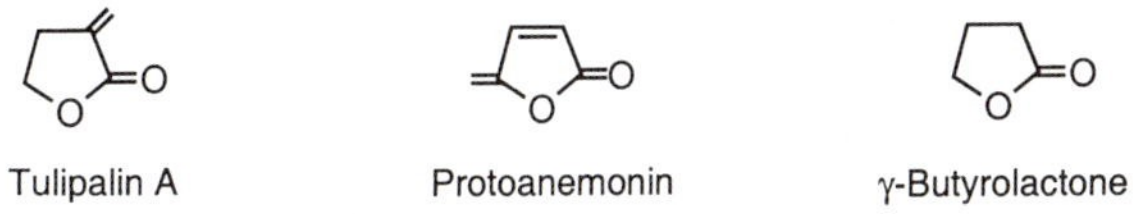

Tulipalin A   Protoanemonin   γ-Butyrolactone

6.3

Like *o*-quinones (section 5.5), α-unsaturated lactones are thought to undergo a Michael-type addition of protein nucleophiles deemed essential for their toxic action (Dupuis et al., 1974). Display 6.2 showed how a nucleophiic amino group on a protein surface adds to a methylene conjugated with the lactone carbonyl in the typical style of 1,4-conjugate addition to form the required allergen. Sulfhydryl compounds behave similarly (Lee et al., 1977).

Other than this, lactone chemistry is not unusual (Herz, 1977). The lactone carbonyl also reacts with nucleophiles such as -NH- and -OH; the ring is opened slowly under base-catalyzed hydrolysis but closes rapidly upon reacidification. In most allergenic lactones, the junction of the lactone ring is *cis* to the plane of an adjacent carbocyclic ring (display 9.6), and such rings generally take the chair form (Fronczek et al., 1989). Other aspects of lactone chemistry are discussed by Yoshioka et al. (1973). The lactones occur most often in Asteraceae (table 6.3), and extensive lists have been provided by Evans and Schmidt (1980), Hertz (1977), and especially by Seaman (1982).

Sesquiterpene lactones are thought to arise biosynthetically from mevalonate via farnesyl pyrophosphate (Herz, 1977; fig. 6.4), although tulipalin biosynthesis starts with the self-condensation of pyruvate with acetylcoenzyme A (Hutchinson and Leete, 1970). The pyrophosphate can then cyclize to form the 10-member germacrane ring (germacrene A) that becomes oxidized sequentially to germacranolides by hydroxylation at either position 6 or 8 (reactions 1 and 2 of fig. 6.4). In addition, (+)-germacrene A has been isolated as an intermediate in the synthesis of guaianes and eudesmans (De Kraker et al., 1998), reactions catalyzed by the enzyme germacrane cyclase. Anthocotulide, the allergen from mayweed (*Anthermis cotula*; Baruah et al., 1985) represents a precyclization inter-mediate. Other biosynthetic sequences have been proposed to account for structurally unusual lactones (Seaman, 1982), but definitive proof for them is lacking and the stereochemistry often is inconsistent.

Sesquiterpene lactones come in an intriguing variety of structural styles (fig. 6.3), and the requisite three isoprene units are apparent if one looks closely (display 6.1). Normally, a number of related lactones occur together in the plant, for example, sunflower (*Helianthus annuus*). Hausen and Spring (1989) identified seven allergenic STLs in dichloromethane extracts of sunflower leaves, and extracts of excised trichomes gave the same re-sults. All of them are derivatives of niveusin A (display 6.4; R denotes the 1-methylbutenoyl ester), and the most strongly allergenic were designated STL IV (8% of total trichome lactones) and STL II (7%).

Niveusin A   STL IV   STL II   6.4

The sesquiterpene lactone skeletons have been verified by chemical synthesis. Starting from the readily available (nontoxic) eudesmanolide lactone santonin, a simple ring cleavage led to elemanolides and germacranolides, whereas solvolysis produced guaianolides (Ando, 1992). Many STLs are unstable when exposed to light, and parthenin (from *P. hysterophorus*) was dehydrated and also rearranged under UV radiation (Saxena et al., 1991). An elegant synthetic route, starting from a purely synthetic derivative of cyclobutenecarboxylic acid, generated the germacranolide, elemanolide, cadinanolide, and guaianolide skeletons stereospecifically (Lange and Lee, 1987).

6.4 Acetylenic Alcohols

Natural polyacetylenes occur in at least eight plant families, primarily the Araliaceae, Apiaceae (Umbelliferae), and Asteraceae (Compositae). Some acetylenic alcohols, such as the neurotoxic cicutoxin from water hemlock (*Cicuta* spp.), are known for their extreme oral toxicity, but others like falcarinol are allergenic or irritant. They all are derived biosynthetically from oleic acid via linoleic and crepenynic ($C_{17}H_{29}COOH$) acids (Hansen and Boll, 1986; Barley et al., 1988).

Falcarinol, a C_{17} acetylenic allergen from English ivy (*Hedera helix*) and other Araliaceae species is typical (Boll and Hansen, 1987). Generally, it is accompanied in the plant by a number of related compounds—up to 18—including falcarinone, falcarindiol, and the falcarinol enantiomer panaxynol (display 6.5). Both (−)- and (+)-falcarinol have been isolated (from different species), and their absolute configuration was long controversial. It has now been established by an unambiguous synthesis from D-gulonolactone (Zheng et al., 1999); (−)-falcarinol is designated as 3R.

3R-(9Z)-Falcarinol,
3S-(9Z)-Panaxynol,

Falcarinone

3R,8S-Falcarindiol,

6.5

Falcarinol and its relatives are also highly fungicidal, often functioning as phytoalexins equivalent to the antibodies of mammals. Among other places, they occur in carrot roots (Bentley and Thaller, 1969; Crosby and Aharonson, 1967), where their levels increase with prolonged storage (Lund and Bruemmer, 1991). Among eight common commercial carrot varieties, the normal falcarinol levels averaged 24.1 mg/kg, with 65.1 mg/kg for falcarindiol. Although not usually found in tomato plants (*Lycopersicon esculentum*, Solanaceae), the substances have been detected in tomato fruit and stems infected by fungi, including *Cladosporium fulvum, Verticillium albo-atrum,* and *Alternaria solani* (De Wit and Kodde, 1981).

The falcarinol in carrots can cause ACD in humans (Murdoch and Dempster, 2000). One victim patch tested strongly positive to carrot, celery, and English ivy, and the symptoms disappeared when all contact with the plants was avoided. Regarding a biochemical mechanism for the allergenic action, falcarinol is easily oxidized to falcarinone, which readily undergoes Michael additions (Bohlmann et al., 1973). However, Hausen et al. (1987) reported that the ketone was not a sensitizer. An alternative mechanism would allow the allylic hydroxyl to be displaced by nucleophiles if it were first converted in vivo to its sulfate ester (display 6.6), a suitable leaving group and one that is well known in mammalian metabolism (Josephy, 1997). Falcarinol is known to be just this kind of biological alkylating agent (Hausen, 2000b).

Falcarinol, R = C_7H_{15}

6.6

The mechanism is supported by the strong allergenicity of any falcarinol relative in which a secondary alcohol is activated by allylic double and triple bonds, whereas those lacking these features—including falcarinone and cicutoxin—show none. Unfortunately, the formation of falcarinol sulfate has not yet been reported.

6.5 Essential Oils

Essential oils are volatile plant extractives that possess an odor (essence). They have been used since ancient times in perfumes and flavorings, and some of the most delicate of them still are extracted by layering flower petals or other plant parts with odorless fat followed by reextraction into an organic solvent—a process called *enfleurage*. The more stable oils often are separated from their plant matrix by steam distillation, sometimes right in the field, but many of today's flavor or fragrance substances are synthetic. Naves and Mazuyer (1947) offer an interesting account of both historic and "modern" production methods.

Some allergenic essential oils were listed in table 3.7, but their toxic constituents are given in table 6.4. Most of the oils are complex mixtures (Srinivas, 1986) in which aliphatic and alicyclic compounds—most often terpenes—predominate, but others tend toward the aromatics, that is, benzene derivatives (fig. 6.5). For example, oil of geranium (from

Table 6.4 Allergenic Flavor and Fragrance Substances

Compound[a]	Original Source	Typical Use
Carvone	Spearmint (*Mentha spicata*)	Toothpaste
Cinnamaldehyde	Cinnamon (*Cinnamomum zeylanicum*)	Toothpaste
Geraniol	Geranium (*Geranium* spp.)	Skin cream
Hydroxycitronellal	Rose (*Rosa* spp.)	Ointments
γ-Methylionone	Violet (*Viola odorata*)	Cosmetics
Limonene (*d-* and *l-*)	Orange (*Citrus sinensis*) peel	Cleaners
Linalool	Bergamot (*Monarda* spp.)	Perfume
l-Menthol	Mint (*Mentha piperita*)	Toothpaste
Santalol	Sandalwood (*Santalum album*)	Incense
α-Terpineol	Longleaf Pine (*Pinus palustris*)	Perfume
Thujone	Oakmoss (*Evernia prunastri*)	Perfume

Data from de Groot and Frosch (1997). [a]See figure 6.5 for structures.

Pelargonium graveolens) is composed of the terpene alcohol geraniol (17%), its close relative citronellol (26%), their formate and acetate esters (22%), 7% menthone, and over 40 other components, whereas 85% of clove oil is the benzenoid eugenol. All together, hundreds of components have been identified, and the major components from the three oils detailed in section 3.5 are typical.

Like their respective fruits, lemon oil is pale yellow and orange oil is yellow to deep orange; both are fluorescent and highly refractive. A cyclic terpene hydrocarbon, *d*-limonene, (fig. 6.5), constitutes 90–95% of both oils (the limonene in the oils of citronella and lemongrass is almost entirely the *l*-, or S-, form). The limonene isomers are common constituents of many plant species as well as foods (IARC, 1993). Acyclic terpene aldehydes such as citral make up another 4% of both the citrus oils, but lemon oil also contains citronellal and geranyl acetate, whereas orange oil contains linalool and the nonterpenes decanal and methyl anthranilate (O'Neill, 2001). Both oils contain phototoxic furocoumarins (section 7.2).

Tea tree oil, steam distilled from *Melaleuca alternifolia* and other *Melaleuca* species, comes from Australia. Its composition has been controversial (Carson and Riley, 2001), but Brophy et al. (1989) identified 62 constituents of which the allergenic terpinen-4-ol (α-terpineol) comprised up to 58%; the limonene isomer γ-terpinene provided another 28%, with cineol making up much of the remainder (fig. 6.5). Cineol (eucalyptol), the main constituent of oil of eucalyptus, is often referred to as an "epoxide" (by definition, a 3-membered ring containing oxygen); instead, it must actually be considered a pyran (a 6-membered oxygen-containing ring) or

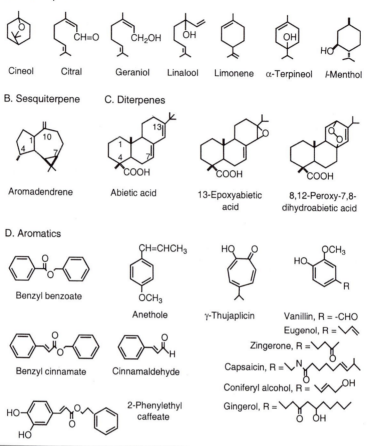

A. Monoterpenes

Cineol Citral Geraniol Linalool Limonene α-Terpineol *l*-Menthol

B. Sesquiterpene   C. Diterpenes

Aromadendrene   Abietic acid   13-Epoxyabietic acid   8,12-Peroxy-7,8-dihydroabietic acid

D. Aromatics

Benzyl benzoate   Anethole   γ-Thujaplicin   Vanillin, R = -CHO
Eugenol, R = ⌇

Zingerone, R = ⌇

Capsaicin, R = ⌇

Coniferyl alcohol, R = ⌇

Gingerol, R = ⌇

Benzyl cinnamate   Cinnamaldehyde

2-Phenylethyl caffeate

Figure 6.5 Sensitizers from essential oils.

else a boat form of cyclohexane in which the oxygen-containing bridge connects the opposite ends (display 6.7).

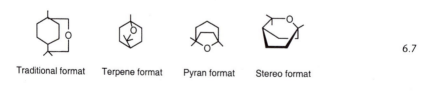

Traditional format   Terpene format   Pyran format   Stereo format

6.7

On the other hand, oil of cinnamon is low in terpenes. The bark oil (section 3.5) is up to 85% cinnamaldehyde and the leaf oil over 81% eugenol. Cinnamyl alcohol and cinnamyl acetate also can be present at significant levels, depending on the oil's source, but limonene makes up only 1–4% (Srinivas, 1986). Eugenol and its relative, vanillin, occur widely in essential oils; eugenol is the principal flavor substance of oil of cloves, whereas vanillin, once extracted only from "beans" (seed pods) of the tropical vanilla orchid, *Vanilla planifolia,* now comes from wood pulp.

Vanillin also occurs in "balsams" such as balsam of Peru, balsam of Tolu, and the Siam benzoin from which tincture of benzoin is derived. A balsam is "an aromatic, resinous substance that flows from a plant," the sticky stuff left on your hands after you handle a Christmas tree (a balsam fir). Typical of the genre, balsam of Peru (section 8.5) is a complex mixture in which analysis and patch testing show cinnamein (a mixture of benzyl cinnamate and coniferyl benzoate) to be the main allergenic constituent (Benezra et al., 1985). Tolu balsam is about 40% cinnamate and benzoate esters (5–13% cinnamein), but Canada balsam (balsam of fir) is at least one-third volatile terpenes.

Eugenol and vanillin are mildly allergenic (Collins and Mitchell, 1975), presumably as a result of demethylation to catechols that are then oxidized to protein-reactive quinones (display 6.8). Similar dealkylation and oxidation also would be required of the esters in propolis and balsam of Peru, although allergens such as cinnamaldehyde already have the necessary conjugated system to undergo the Michael addition of a nucleophile (display 6.9).

Vanillin, R = CH=O
Eugenol, R = CH$_2$CH=CH$_2$

6.8

Cinnamaldehyde

6.9

Aliphatic and alicyclic terpenes like citral and geranial may also provide conjugated systems that allow Michael additions, but the toxicity of other terpenes has been more difficult to explain. For example, turpentine is a mixture of ostensibly nonallergenic α- and β-pinenes, terpene alcohols, and limonene, and skin reactions to turpentine were found to be due primarily to a minor component, Δ^3-carene (Hellerström et al., 1957; Pirilä et al., 1969), the allergenicity being correlated with carene level. Even then, the actual allergens proved to be not the hydrocarbons but rather allergenic hydroperoxides formed from their air-oxidation (display 6.10A). Ketones resulting from dehydration of the hydroperoxide also may participate in Michael additions (Lee and Uff, 1967).

A.

Δ^3-Carene Δ^3-Carene Hydroperoxide

B.

Limonene   Carvone

6.10

Other terpenes, too, react readily with oxygen (Erman, 1985). Like any allylic or tertiary hydrocarbon, their autoxidation leads to hydroperoxides via free-radical hydrogen abstractions that eventually form polymers (essential oils must be protected from light and air). Albert Fisher was the first to observe that people allergic to perfumes often failed to respond to the individual ingredients, and he suggested this might be due to oxidative "aging" of the essential oils (Fisher and Dooms-Goossens, 1976). Further evidence came from the strong allergenicity of air-oxidized d-limonene and the corresponding ketone, carvone (Karlberg et al., 1992; display 6.10B).

The α-terpineol and d-limonene of tea tree oil (from *Melaleuca alternifolia*) behaved similarly (Beckmann and Ippen, 1998), although Knight and Hausen (1994) reported that the carvone in *M. leucadendron* (cajeput oil) was inactive as a sensitizer. The allergenicity of such simple terpenes as linalool, geraniol, and their esters (Kanerva et al., 1995), all widely used in perfumery, must surely be due to oxidative processes. This also explains sensitization by normally unreactive terpenes such as abietic acid (fig. 6.5; Foussereau et al., 1982), because gum rosin (colophony) is a mixture of this acid with pimaric, dehydroabietic, and dihydroabietic acids. The allergens are oxidation products such as 15-hydroperoxyabietic acid (Karlberg et al., 1988), epoxyabietic acids, and 8,12-peroxo-7,8-dihydroabietic acid (Karlberg, 2000) whose radicals react readily with nucleophiles to attach a resin acid to proteins (Gäfvert et al., 1992).

6.6 Lichen Substances

Most allergens from the lower plants known as lichens are phenolic esters. They are called depsides if they are simple phenyl esters such as evernic acid (display 6.11), or depsidones if they are macrocyclic lactones, like protocetraric acid, formed from a benzoic acid on one ring and a phenolic hydroxyl on the adjacent ring (Culberson, 1969). Originally termed lichen acids, they now are referred to as lichen substances because some are not strongly acidic. From the beginning, their structures often have been drawn in a simplified format, like the one shown for evernic acid, that provides little information about steric configuration.

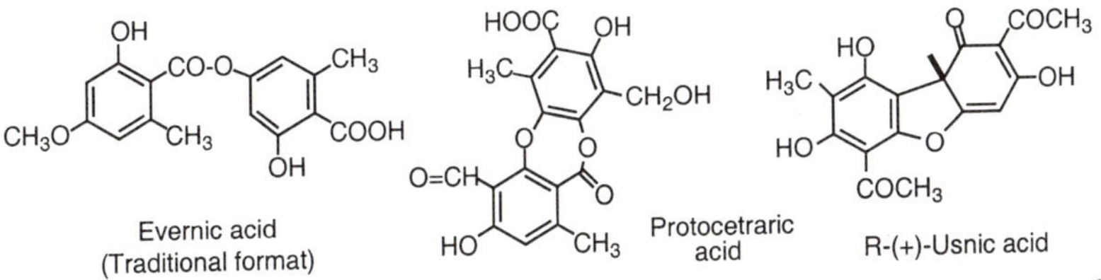

Evernic acid (Traditional format)

Protocetraric acid

R-(+)-Usnic acid

6.11

As a typical depside, atranorin (display 6.12) is found in many lichen species and especially those of the genus *Parmelia*. Atranorin forms white crystals, with a melting point of 195°C and a strong UV absorption; it is soluble in bases and hydrolyzed by them. The biosynthesis of atranorin by the fungus partner of the symbiosis is through a polyketide condensation of four molecules of acetyl CoA (section 5.7), addition of a C_1 piece (possibly from formate), aromatization to DDBA, and esterification with another molecule of the same polyketide precursor (display 6.12; Yamazaki et al., 1965).

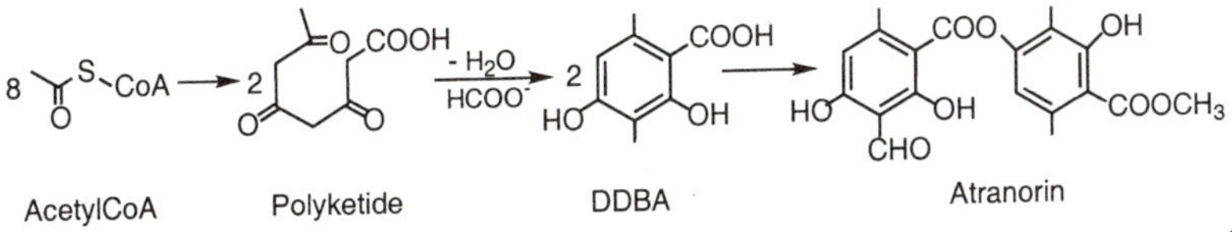

AcetylCoA   Polyketide   DDBA   Atranorin

6.12

Alkaline solutions of depsides are yellow and fluorescent. Being polyphenolic, almost all depside, give a red-violet color with ferric chloride solution. They are easily decarboxylated, so identification is best accomplished by heating to 40°C with potassium hydroxide in methanol to provide the methyl esters of both benzoic acids. Depsidones, found mostly in *Parmelia* and *Usnea* spp., are hydrolyzed to relatively stable diphenyl ethers (Asahina and Shibata, 1954).

A change in condensation pattern produces dibenzofurans like usnic acid (display 6.11), the principal allergen of *Usnea* species, that exists in two natural enantiomeric forms. It is like atranorin biosynthetically, but is formed via 2,4,6-trihydroxy-5-methylacetophenone rather than DDBA. It has been synthesized elegantly in vitro from this intermediate by the same reaction shown in display 6.12 (Barton et al., 1956). Although the lichen substances of display 6.11 seem so structurally different, careful examination shows they are actually very similar.

The mechanism of the (weak) allergenicity remains unknown. As a resorcinol, atranorin is oxidizable at positions *o*- or *p*- to its phenolic hydroxyls, so allergenicity may yet be due to the resulting quinones. However, usnic acid cannot form a quinone, and the reason for its toxicity remains obscure. For over a century, lichens and lichen substances were identified by their color and crystal form (Asahina and Shibata, 1954), but now they often can be identified from the mass spectra of tiny plant fragments (Santesson, 1973).

6.7 Rubber Latex

The Pará rubber tree (*Hevea brasiliensis*) is not usually considered to be allergenic. However, like the sap of poison oak and the lac trees (section 8.1), its fluid latex contains water, protein, sugars, resins, and 30–40% of an emulsified hydrophobic substance, in this case *cis*-1,4-polyisoprene (Rogers, 1974). The stabilized liquid latex can be converted into gloves and condoms, or, after coagulation, into dry sheets later processed into such familiar items as tires and hot water bottles. *Hevea* rubber is responsible for about 90% of the world trade, supplemented with smaller volumes of rubber from *Parthenium argentatum* (guayule, Asteraceae) and *Manihot glaziovii* (Ceara, Euphorbiaceae).

In recent years, increasing evidence indicates that *Hevea* latex is indeed allergenic (Slater, 1994), the allergy generally immediate and IgE-mediated (Type I). Since 1992, there have been frequent reports of latex ACD not associated with rubber-processing chemicals (Gottlieb et al., 2000), but the responsible agent has never been identified. Although *Hevea* belongs to the Euphorbiaceae, the polyisoprene in the latex is not the cause of the allergy. The original sap contains several highly allergenic proteins, among them hevein (molecular weight [MW] 47,000), prohevein (MW 20,000), and rubber elongation factor (MW 14,600), along with a number of others (Turjanmaa et al., 2000). Residues of these proteins remain in the rubber as long as it is not heated above their denaturation point, and they can be transferred to hands or other body parts. However, the mechanism for access of these high molecular weight, polar substances to the body's immune system is not apparent. Additionally, the myriad stabilizers, antioxidants, accelerators, and other additives in processed rubber must be of at least equal importance to any allergenicity.

6.8 Conclusions

Many types of plant constituents other than urushiols can react with proteins to provide allergens. For quinones and substances convertible to them, as well as for unsaturated ketones, lactones, and aldehydes, a Michael-type addition by protein-surface nucleophiles offers the most attractive route; plausible alternatives exist for other lactones, acetylenic alcohols, and resin acids. This reactivity is not always apparent: Vanillin and it relatives require demethylaton, most terpenes must undergo oxidation, and lichen substances probably have to be hydrolyzed. However, such transformation processes are well known in vivo and are usually enzymatic, and some could even be nonenzymatic.

Even such everyday items as perfumes, flavor ingredients, latex rubber, buttercups, and Christmas trees contain identifiable allergens. We seem to live in a world of allergenic chemicals.

SEVEN
PHOTOTOXIC AND IRRITANT CONSTITUENTS

"It is probably safe to say that most people would be reluctant to wax eloquent about stinging nettles. The name says it all, doesn't it?"
—Pamela Jones, 1994

7.1   More Dermatotoxicity

Many dermatotoxic plant products are not allergens. Diterpene esters from euphorbs, sulfur compounds from mustard oils and garlic, and amines from nettles simply irritate the skin; no allergy is involved. Others, such as furocoumarins in fig latex, require sunlight for their toxic effects. In either case, the physical and chemical properties can reveal their toxic action and environmental fate, allow us to predict other chemicals that might affect skin, and, we hope, help us learn how to protect skin from harm.

7.2   Photodynamic Agents

There are three main kinds of photodynamic (phototoxic) plant constituents: thiophenes, furocoumarins, and polyhydroxyquinones. They can be systemic—that is, circulate in the blood after skin contact or ingestion—but not allergenic, although the symptoms of poisoning include erythema and blisters reminiscent of urushioids. However, they are unusual in that they require exposure to sunlight or UV radiation to exhibit dermatotoxicity.

Furocoumarins

In furocoumarins (display 7.1), a furan ring is fused to a coumarin (benzo-2-pyrone) nucleus at either the 6,7-position (psoralen) or the 7,8-position (angelicin). These unusual compounds are derived from the amino acid phenylalanine, which is first deaminated to *trans*-cinnamic acid, then hydroxylated in the 7- and 2-positions, and isomerized to the *cis* (Z) isomer. Next, umbelliferone (7-hydroxycoumarin) is formed by ring-closure, and the furan ring finally is added via mevalonate. Plant furocoumarins are

128

reviewed by Murray (1997). Table 7.1 lists some common plant furo-coumarins, and structures for most of them are provided in figure 7.1.

| Coumarin | Psoralen (Common numbering) | Psoralen (C.A. numbering) | Angelicin | 7.1 |

Coumarin names can be confusing. Originally, each coumarin received a trivial name, often from its plant source—for example, psoralen from *Psoralea*. With the advent of position numbers, the pyrone oxygen was labeled 1, the furan ring was numbered separately, and furocoumarins and coumarins shared a common numbering system (display 7.1). Some of the old names were retained, so 8-methoxypsoralen also continued to be called xanthotoxin. However, the two numbering authorities, IUPAC and *Chemical Abstracts*, then decided to start at the *furan* oxygen and

Table 7.1 Phototoxic Plant Furocoumarins

Common name	Chemical Name (Structure Type)[a]	% Occurrence[b]
1. Angelicin	2*H*-Furo[2,3-*h*]-1-benzopyran-2-one (1)	12
2. Bergamottin	5-Geranoxypsoralen (3)	
3. Bergapten	5-Methoxypsoralen (3)	39
4. Bergaptol	5-Hydroxypsoralen (3)	
5. Byakangelicin	5-Methoxy-8-(2,3-dihydroxyisopentoxy)psoralen (5)	
6. Byakangelicol	5-Methoxy-8-(2,3-epoxyisopentoxy)psoralen (5)	
7. 8-GOP	8-Geranoxypsoralen (4)	
8. Heraclenin	8-(2,3-Epoxyisopentoxy)psoralen (4)	
9. Heraclenol	8-(2,3-Dihydroxyisopentoxy)psoralen (4)	
10. Imperatorin	8-Isopentenyloxypsoralen (4)	29
11. Isobergapten	5-Methoxyangelicin (1)	15
12. Isoimperatorin	5-Isopentenyloxypsoralen (3)	19
13. Isopimpinellin	5,8-Dimethoxypsoralen (5)	25
14. Lanatin	5-Isopentenyloxyangelicin (1)	
15. Oroselone	2'-isopropenylangelicin (2)	
16. Oxypeucedanin	5-(2,3-epoxyisopentoxy)psoralen (3)	16
17. Phellopterin	5-Methoxy-8-isopentenyloxypsoralen (5)	9
18. Pimpinellin	5,6-Dimethoxyangelicin (1)	13
19. Psoralen (Ficusin)	7*H*-Furo[3,2-*g*]-1-benzopyran-7-one (3)	10
20. Sphondin	6-Methoxyangelicin (1)	16
21. Xanthotoxin	8-Methoxypsoralen (4)	16
22. Xanthotoxol	8-Hydroxypsoralen (4)	

[a]For chemical structures, see figure 7.1. [b]Average of 410 species of Apiaceae (Murray et al., 1982).

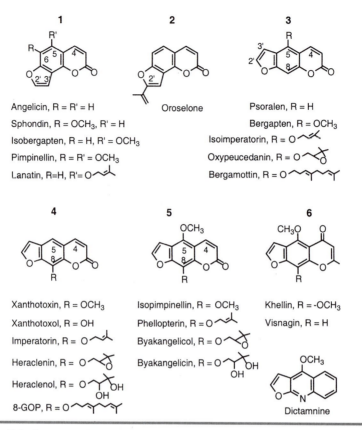

Figure 7.1 Furocoumarin structures.

move consecutively clockwise, so xanthotoxin became 9-methoxy-7*H*-furobenzopyran-7-one. To make matters worse, most of the biochemical literature now numbers the furan double bond as 4′,5′. The original system is retained here because it has been used so widely, although it is not as logical as that of the IUPAC.

Angular angelicin and linear psoralen each give rise to a series of natural derivatives (fig. 7.1). Almost all have 5- or 8-alkoxy substituents: methoxy, isopentenyloxy from isoprene, or geranoxy from two isoprene units are common, and these often occur in the plant accompanied by the corresponding epoxides or diols. Occasionally, the parent phenol is present (e.g., bergaptol, 5-hydroxypsoralen), and a few like oroselone have the isoprene unit bonded directly to carbon rather than to oxygen. Similar heterocyclic series (fig. 7.1) provide phototoxic furochromones (benzopyran-4-ones) such as khellin and furoquinolines such as dictamnine, but other related substances often fail to meet the structural requirements for phototoxicity.

Furocoumarins are reactive, and typical reactions are summarized in figure 7.2. The most diagnostic of them is ring-opening by base—simply an ester hydrolysis (reaction 1)—which is instantly reversed upon acidification. There are also several types of oxidation; for example, the furan ring can be epoxidized at the 2′,3′-double bond (reaction 2), the epoxide rearranges to a carbonyl, and the resulting lactone ring will be opened by base hydrolysis (reaction 3).

Aromatic ring oxidation provides a phenol (reaction 4), and ring-opening allows the coumarin ring to form again but in the alternate configuration (reaction 5)—the psoralen becomes an angelicin. Further oxidation produces the corresponding quinone (reaction 6) and may go further to destroy everything except the furan ring (reaction 7). Catalytic or enzymatic reduction saturates either the 2′,3′- or the 3,4-double bond (reaction 8), depending on the catalyst, although the lactone ring is the more easily reduced. There are few examples of Michael addition at the 3,4-double bond, but it obviously happens. Side-chain reactions are to be expected.

Figure 7.2 Chemical reactions of furocoumarins.

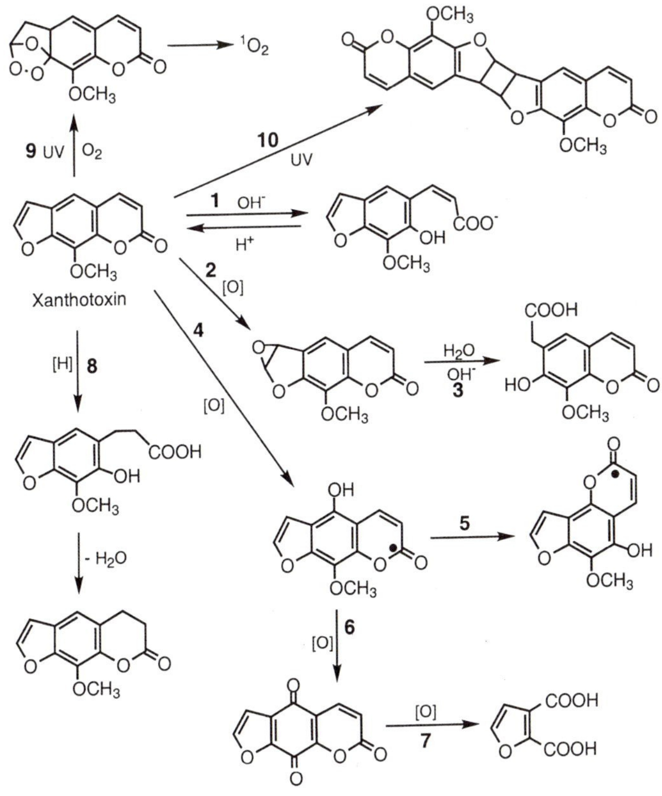

These transformations are reflected in furocoumarin metabolism. All of the major products shown in figure 7.2 were found in the urine of goats dosed orally with ^{14}C-labeled xanthotoxin (Pangilinan et al., 1992), and several were seen in the excreta of dosed chickens. These products of furocoumarin metabolism also were present in the urine of dogs that had received xanthotoxin intravenously (Kolis et al., 1979), proving that they were not due to gut microflora.

Two notable characteristics of the highly unsaturated furocoumarins are their strong UV absorption and intense fluorescence (appendix D). Psoralens usually absorb within four spectral bands: 205–25 nm (log ε ~4.0), 240–55 nm (log ε 4.06–4.45), 260–70 nm (log ε 4.18–4.26), and 298–316 nm (log ε 3.85–4.13); angelicins absorb only in the regions of 242–45 and 260–70 nm (Murray et al., 1982). Under UV radiation, psoralen fluoresces blue, angelicin purple, and their alkoxy derivatives bright yellow, which is useful for quantitation and identification. Consistent with the fluorescence, furocoumarins are planar and rigid—a key to their phototoxicity (section 9.5).

UV absorption leads to characteristic photochemical reactions. Fluorescence is quenched by transfer of the energy to molecular oxygen, which generates highly reactive singlet oxygen ($^1O_2$), often via an intermediate peroxide (fig. 7.2, reaction 9). An excited coumarin may react with oxygen to cleave either or both hetero rings (reaction 6/7; Marley et al., 1995), or the 2′,3′-double bond can generate a diradical that couples with another radical—including a second excited furocoumarin molecule—to form dimers containing a cyclobutane ring (reaction 10). As discussed in section 9.5, these UV-energized reactions form the basis of furocoumarin phototoxicity.

Phototoxic furocoumarins are found in many fruits and vegetables (section 4.1), including carrots, celery, parsley, parsnip, common citrus fruits, and fig latex (SGCAFS, 1996). The highest levels occurred in vegetables: Parsnips contained 40–1740 mg/kg of bergapten and 2500 mg/kg of xanthotoxin; celery root (celeriac) contained 25–100 mg/kg of bergapten and celery stalks 1.3–46.7 mg/kg of psoralen; and parsley contained 11–112 mg/kg of isoimperatorin, all on a fresh weight basis. Dried parsley flakes contained 300 mg/kg of oxypeucedanin.

Cooking reduced these levels, but prolonged cold storage of celery stalks sharply increased levels (Chaudhary et al., 1985). Luckily, only half of the baby foods tested had any furocoumarin at all, and those totaled only 8 mg/kg. Normally, a number of furocoumarins occur together in a particular species. For example, the Tromsø palm (*Heracleum laciniatum*; section 4.2) contains angelicin, bergapten, isobergapten, isopimpinellin, pimpinellin, and sphondin (Kavli et al., 1983), and our local *H. lanatum* contains angelicin, bergapten, imperatorin, isobergapten, lanatin, isopim-pinellin, pimpinellin, psoralen, sphondin, and xanthotoxin (Murray et al., 1982; fig. 7.2)

Hypericins

The sunny yellow blossoms of St. John's wort (*Hypericum perforatum*) belie the trouble it has caused (see section 4.1). The phototoxic constituent, hypericin, is a polyhydroxyquinone found in the dark, foliar oil glands; the highly conjugated system strongly absorbs visible light (appendix D) to result in a deep red-purple color. The combined carbonyl and phenolic groups lead (theoretically) to 16 tautomeric forms (display 7.2), of which the natural 7,14-quinone is the most stable (Etzstorfer et al., 1993), although pure hypericin is thought to exist in the plant as the rapidly isomerized 1,6-quinone. As with furocoumarins, several numbering systems have been applied to hypericin over the years, and we will use that of *Chemical Abstracts* (display 7.2).

| 7,14-Hypericin | 1,6-Hypericin | Fagopyrin |

7.2

Hypericin biosynthesis starts with acetate and goes through a classic polyketide intermediate (Brockmann, 1957) to an anthracene derivative, emodin-anthrone-9, and then to a protohypericin oxidized subsequently to hypericin. Plants also contain pseudohypericin and protopseudohypericin, which possess hydroxyethyl groups instead of methyls in the 10- and 11-positions. Each of these is more soluble in polar solvents than is hypericin (Falk and Schmitzberger, 1992); the 3- (or 4-) hydroxyl is the most acidic, with a pK_a of 11.0 similar to that of phenol, and hypericin exists in sap as a water-soluble potassium salt (Falk et al.,1992).

Like other quinones, hypericin can be reduced to the octahydroxy hy-droquinone but is not readily oxidized or conjugated. It is recovered un-changed from the urine after ingestion and can be detected in the intact skin of orally exposed individuals (Pace, 1942). Similar to the furocoumarins, hypericin is planar, highly light-absorbing, and strongly fluorescent (ap-pendix D; Wynn and Cotton, 1995); unlike them, it passes the absorbed energy directly to molecular oxygen to generate the singlet oxygen re-sponsible for its phototoxicity (Jardon et al., 1987).

The *Hypericum* extracts used in herbal medicine contain a wide variety of constituents—flavones, phloroglucinols, and terpenes—in addition to dianthrones ((Nahrstedt and Butterweck, 1997); hypericin is strictly a minor component. With ten-fold more pseudohypericin than active ingredient, the "hypericin" in commercial St. John's wort generally constitutes no more than 0.3% of total extractives, although levels vary greatly among individual *Hypericum* plants (Southwell and Campbell, 1991).

Fagopyrin, from buckwheat (*Fagopyrum esculentum*), is hypericin's 2,5-di-(2'-piperidinyl) relative (display 7.2; Brockmann and Lackner, 1979), and the light absorption and other properties of the two are almost identical (Brockmann, 1957). However, being an amine confers alkaline properties despite the acidic phenolic groups, and fagopyrin has normal amine reactions.

Di- and Terthienyls

Natural thiophenes are common constituents of the Asteraceae (Bohlmann and Zdero, 1985; Kagan, 1991). Even a decade ago, some 70 already had been identified, most with two thiophene rings joined at the 2-positions (like 3-buten-1-ynyl-2,2'-dithienyl, display 7.3), two thiophene rings separated by an acetylene (a dithienylacetylene), or three rings all joined at their 2-positions, the so-called α-terthienyls.

| 5-(3-Buten-1-ynyl)-2,2'-dithienyl | Dithienylacetylene | α-Terthienyl | 7.3 |

Biosynthesis of these unusual compounds starts with acetate, goes through linoleic acid to an acetylene, crepenynic acid (section 6.4), then to the 13-carbon 1-tridecen-3,5,7,9,11-pentayne (Bohlmann et al., 1973), with final incorporation of the sulfur (Schulte et al., 1968). The first of these compounds to be isolated was α-terthienyl, from marigolds (Zechmeister and Sease, 1947), but further attention had to await eventual investigation of its possible role in the resistance of marigold roots to nematodes. Results remained inconsistent and controversial until the discovery that light was required for its biological activity—that is, it was phototoxic (Gommers, 1972).

As with other phototoxic substances, the highly conjugated polythienyls strongly absorb UV radiation (maximum at 350 nm, log ε 4.33), are brightly fluorescent, and energize the formation of excited singlet oxygen (Bakker et al., 1979; Scaiano et al., 1990). Alternatively, 2-substituted thiophenes can use the absorbed energy to change into the 3-isomer, and, like furocoumarins, 3-(buten-1-ynyl)-2,2'-dithienyl (display 7.3) dimerizes at the external double bond to form a substituted cyclobutane (see Kagan, 1991).

The phototoxicity of dithienyls was discovered by accident when the hands of a worker in Kagan's laboratory were exposed to one inadvertently and later exposed to sunlight—with painful consequences (Kagan, 1991). Pure dithienyls also are phototoxic to microorganisms, plants, and many kinds of animals, but whether people are normally exposed to them remains unknown.

7.3 Irritant Esters

Many plants and plant products only irritate the skin—euphorbs, nettles, chili peppers, buttercups—but the results equal those from allergens. Euphorbiaceae species often contain irritant and vesicant esters of diterpene polyols that include phorbols (display 7.4) and deoxyphorbols, resiniferonols, and ingenols based on the (hypothetical) multiringed hydrocarbons tigliane, the closely related daphnane, and ingenane, respectively (see fig. 7.4). Tigliane esters have remained chemically and medically interesting for the strong cocarcinogenicity they display; ingenanes are the most frequently encountered euphorb irritants (Evans and Kinghorn, 1977); and the daphnane-type resiniferonol esters are the most proinflammatory of all plant substances (Evans, 1986a; Schmidt and Evans, 1979). Over 100 phorbol-type esters have been isolated and identified.

Phorbol
(2-dimensional)

Phorbol (4,10-*trans*)

4α-Phorbol (4,10-*cis*)

TPA, Tetradecanoyl-
phorbol acetate

7.4

Phorbol's structure was determined by classical chemical means (Crombie et al., 1968) and confirmed by X-ray crystallography (Hoppe et al., 1969). As shown by display 7.4, its 3-dimensional shape has a β- (*trans*) configuration at the 4,10-ring juncture that confers biological activity; esters with the 4α, or *cis*, configuration are inactive (Evans, 1986b), as are all the parent polyols. Phorbol contains five hydroxyl groups, but those at C-4 and C-9 are unreactive. Of the rest—one each of primary, secondary, and tertiary—that at C-12 can be oxidized to a ketone by chromic acid. Surprisingly, the C-13 hydroxyl is even more reactive and undergoes oxidation under mild conditions (Fehling's solution, cuprammonium ion) to form an isopropenyl side chain and C-13 carbonyl. The C-20 primary hydroxyl is the most reactive of all and is easily oxidized to its aldehyde. Each hydroxyl is readily etherified, but no oxidation products or ethers are irritant. The 6,7-double bond can be epoxidized, but the 2,3-bond is much less reactive (Evans, 1986b).

The C-12 and C-13 phorbol esters, like TPA, are strongly irritant (display 7.4), but esterification at C-20 destroys irritancy. Although phorbol is easily acetylated in vitro to a 12,13, 20-triacetate, the acyl groups of *natural* esters generally are mixed. Probably the best known is TPA, the 12-O-tetradecanoyl-phorbol 13-acetate used in cancer research. Most euphorbs produce multiple esters, and Evans (1986b) provides an extensive list. Diesters are rapidly hydrolyzed enzymatically or by base to nonirritant phorbol, but 12-deoxyphorbol is less stable, and separation of its esters once challenged both reverse-phase TLC and HPLC (Evans et al., 1975; Berry, 1977). Among this group, 4-deoxyphorbol is the least stable and quickly epimerizes. The UV, NMR, and mass spectra by which phorbols were identified are reviewed by Evans (1986b).

A few phorbol esters are even more highly oxygenated. Irritant mono- and diesters of 16-hydroxyphorbol, where one of the cyclopropane methyl groups is hydroxylated, were isolated from seeds and fruit of *Aleurites* (*Vernicia*) *fordii* (candlenut), *Croton flavens*, and several *Jatropha* species (Evans, 1986b; Adolf and Hecker, 1984). Unusual diterpene ketones—not esters—such as curcusone A (fig. 7.3) also are present, but their biological activity remains unreported.

Despite a somewhat different three-dimensional structure (fig. 7.3), the highly irritant ingenol esters remain closely related to those of phorbol, the principal differences being the C-11 bond to C-10 rather than to C-9, and conversion of the C-9 hydroxyl to a carbonyl (Schmidt, 1986a). In addition to the many known ingenol esters, Schmidt (1986a) listed 28 *Euphorbia* species whose ingenol esters remained unidentified at the time of publication; some of these were known to be exceptionally dermatotoxic (Kinghorn and Evans, 1975). Except in only a few instances, ingenol is esterified solely on the 3-hydroxyl; for example, the common garden weed, *E. peplus*, contains the 3-angeloyl ester of 20-deoxyingenol as well as ingenol 20-octanoate (Rizk et al., 1984).

However, the intriguing daphnane orthoesters (Schmidt, 1986a) are among the most irritant chemicals of the plant world (Schmidt and Evans, 1979). Isolated from such species as February daphne (*Daphne mezereum*) and winter daphne (*D. odora*), they are similar to tiglianes except for the opened cyclopropane ring and unusual orthoester group (fig. 7.3). The orthoester arises from a normal ester carbonyl, in this case as a result of the favorable configuration of the axial hydroxyls at C-9, C-13, and C-14.

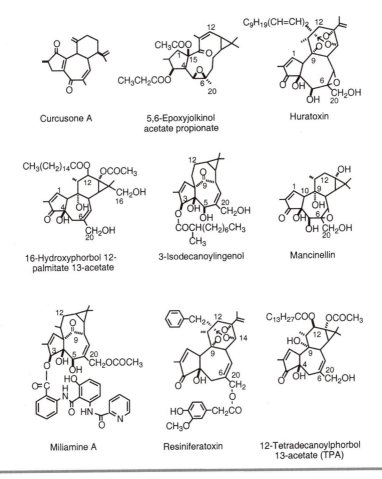

Figure 7.3 Structures of irritant diterpenes.

Among the most irritant of all, resiniferatoxin occurs in *E. resinifera* (not in a *Daphne*) and combines a phenylacetic orthoester and a C-20 ester of homovanillic acid (Adolf et al., 1982). Other unusual euphorb constituents shown in figure 7.3 include isodecanoylingenol from the ancient medicinal "Euphorbium," also from *E. resinifera*; the daphnane huratoxin from the sandbox tree, *Hura crepitans*); miliamine, an ingenane from the crown of thorns, *E. milii*); and the tigliane mancinellin from the Caribbean manchineel tree (*Hippomane* species).

For decades, chemists have attempted to synthesize the polyols and their esters, but only in the past 5 years has this finally been accomplished. In 1997, Wender et al. (1997a, 1997b) reported the total synthesis of phorbol and resiniferatoxin. Winkler et al. (2002) successfully concluded a 16-year effort with the 43-step synthesis of sterically correct ingenol.

All of these diterpene esters are structural variations on the basic tigliane theme, itself derived from the macrocyclic lathyrane ring system in which cyclopentane and cyclopropane rings are first introduced (fig. 7.4). Lathyrane esters, too, can be dermatotoxic, as shown by the group of highly irritant epoxyjolkinol polyesters isolated from the common garden orna-mental, *E. characias* ssp. *wulfenii* (the structure of one is shown in fig. 7.3). However, not all diterpene esters are toxic: For example, the ingenol esters of *E. peplus* are irritant and cocarcinogenic (Rizk et al., 1984), whereas jatrophane esters from the same plant—lathyranes without a cyclopropane ring—are not irritant (Jakupovich et al., 1998) and exhibit *antitumor* activity (Evans, 1986a).

Some irritant esters are not based on diterpene polyols. Of particular interest is a group of guaianolide lactones extracted from Mediterranean weeds of the genus *Thapsia* (Apiaceae; Christensen et al., 1997). They com-prise about 40 derivatives of the (hypothetical) thapsane, as typified by the tumor-promoting thapsigargin and thapsigargicin (fig. 6.3). Each has 6 hydroxyl groups, some represented by long-chain esters with structures

Figure 7.4 Biosynthesis of euphorbia diterpenes.

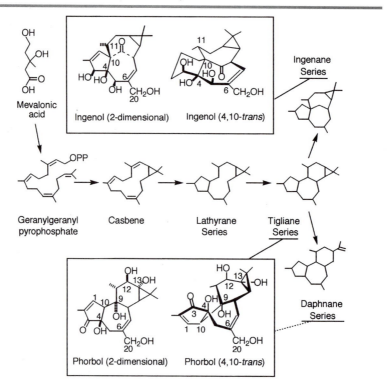

reminiscent of phorbol esters (section 6.5). The accompanying trilobolides lack only the C-2 carbalkoxy group. There is no α-methylene, but the C-11 position is occupied by a tertiary hydroxyl and methyl group that could readily form a double bond by dehydration. The rather complex structure of thapsigargin was verified by X-ray crystallography (Christensen et al., 1982). (See fig. 6.3.)

The constituents of podophyllin, a resin from mayapple (*Podophyllum* spp.), likewise are not diterpenes but are so irritant they are used to kill cancer cells; one drop of resin extract placed on a wart quickly destroys it. The active constituents of *P. peltatum* rhizomes include E- and Z-podophyllotoxin, desoxypodophyllotoxin, and α- and β-peltatins (Hartwell and Schrecker, 1958), all of them present in the plant as β-D-glucosides. Their structures (fig. 7.5) reveal a familiar lactone ring that can still react with a protein amino group even without an α-double bond.

The closely related plicatic acid (Swan et al., 1967) forms 40% of the nonvolatile extractives of western red cedar (*Thuja plicata*) wood and is a major cause of occupational asthma in the United States, Japan, and

Figure 7.5 Structures of other irritants.

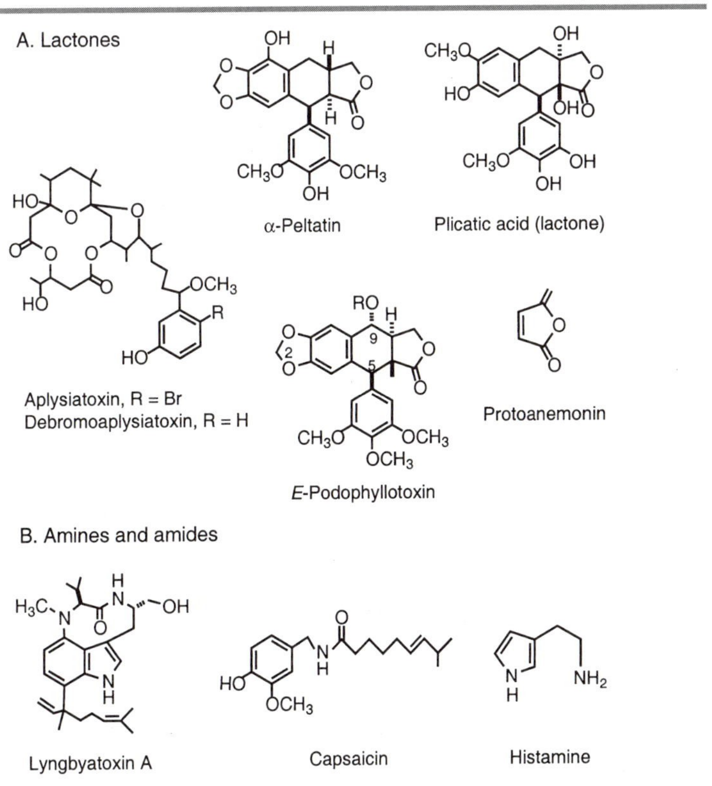

A. Lactones

α-Peltatin

Plicatic acid (lactone)

Aplysiatoxin, R = Br
Debromoaplysiatoxin, R = H

E-Podophyllotoxin

Protoanemonin

B. Amines and amides

Lyngbyatoxin A

Capsaicin

Histamine

anywhere the wood or sawdust is used or produced (Chan-Yeung, 1994). Plicatic acid combines with serum albumin, presumably via its lactone form, and thus is allergenic, whereas the accompanying irritancy of red cedar may be due to thymoquinone.

7.4 Organosulfur Compounds

Several classes of naturally occurring organosulfur compounds have been known for centuries to affect human skin (section 4.2). However, although those from mustard and garlic, especially, also have a long history of use in foods, condiments, and medicines, many people seem unaware that they are dermatotoxic.

Mustard Oils

Isothiocyanates (R-NCS, display 7.5) are the principal toxic constituents of the mustard oils found in many Brassicaceae (Cruciferae) and in a few other families (Kjaer, 1960; VanEtten,1969), as illustrated by familiar cole crops of the genus *Brassica* (table 7.2). As the name implies, they are oily, fat-soluble, distillable liquids (methyl isothiocyanate boils at 119°C) with a pungent odor, and over 70 have now been isolated (table 7.3).

Table 7.2   Glucosinolates and Mustard Oils from *Brassica*

Species	Common Name	Glucosinolate[a]	Isothiocyanate R
B. hirta	White mustard[b]	Gluconasturtiin (R)	2-Phenylethyl-
		Sinalbin (S)	4-Hydroxybenzyl-
B. juncea	Indian mustard	Gluconapin (L)	3-Butenyl-
		Gluconasturtiin (LR)	2-Phenylethyl-
		Sinigrin (S)	Allyl-
B. napus	Rutabaga, rape	Glucobrassicin (S)	3-Indolylmethyl-
		Glucoiberin (S)	3-Methylsulfinylpropyl-
		Gluconapin (S)	3-Butenyl
		Progoitrin (LS)	2-Hydroxy-3-butenyl-
		Sinalbin (S)	4-Hydroxybenzyl-
B. nigra	Black mustard	Gluconasturtiin (LRS)	2-Phenylethyl-
		Sinigrin (LRS)	Allyl-
B. oleracea	Cabbage	Gluconapin (L)	3-Butenyl-
ssp. capitata		Gluconasturtiin (LS)	2-Phenylethyl-
		Sinigrin (RS)	Allyl-
B. rapa	Turnip	Gluconasturtiin (RS)	2-Phenylethyl-
		Progoitrin (RS)	2-Hydroxy-3-butenyl-

Kjaer (1960); VanEtten et al. (1969). [a]L, leaves; R, roots; S, seeds. [b]Also called *Sinapis alba*.

Table 7.3 Mustard Oil Isothiocyanates

Isothiocyanate[a] R-NCS	Glucosinolate R-C(S-Gl)=NOSO$_3$-	Typical Source
CH_3-	Glucocapparin	*Cleome hassleriana* (Spider plant)
CH_3CH_2-	Glucolepidiin	*Lepidium menzii* (Menzies peppergrass)
CH_3CHCH_3	Glucoputranjivin	*Cochleara officinalis* (Scurvygrass)
$CH_3CH_2CHCH_3$	Glucocochlearin	*Erysimum cheiri* (Wallflower)
$CH_2=CHCH_2$-	Sinigrin	*Brassica nigra* (Black mustard)
$CH_2=CHCH_2CH_2$-	Gluconapin	*Brassica napus* (Rape)
$CH_2=CHCH_2CH_2CH_2$-	Glucobrassicanapin	*Brassica oleracea* (Broccoli, cauliflower)
$CH_3SCH_2CH_2CH_2$-	Glucoibervirin	*Iberis sempervirins* (Evergreen candytuft)
$CH_3SOCH_2CH_2CH_2$-	Glucoibirin	*Iberis amara* (Rocket candytuft)
$CH_3SO_2CH_2CH_2CH_2$-	Glucocheirolin	*Erysimum cheiri* (Wallflower)
$CH_3SO_2CH_2(CH_2)_7CH_2$-	Glucoarabin	*Arabis alpina* (Mountain rockcress)
$CH_2=CHCH(OH)CH_2$-	Progoitrin	*Brassica oleracea* (Broccoli, cauliflower)

$C_6H_5CH_2$-	Glucotropaeolin	*Lepidium sativum* (Garden cress);
		    Carica papaya (Papaya); *Tropaeolum*
		    majus (Nasturtium)

p-$HOC_6H_5CH_2$-	Sinalbin	*Sinapis alba* (White mustard)
$C_6H_5CH_2CH_2$-	Gluconasturtiin	*Nasturtium officinale* (Watercress)

Data from Kjaer (1960). [a]See display 7.5 for parent structures.

7.5

The isothiocyanates seldom occur naturally. They are generated upon injury of the plant or during isolation—a freshly cut stem of mustard normally has no mustard odor. Instead, isothiocyanates exist in the plant as thiohydroxamate S-glucosides (known as glucosinolates, display 7.5) and are generated by a hydrolysis catalyzed by acid or by a thioglucosidase called myrosinase. Acidic conditions produce glucose, hydroxylamine, sulfate, and the carboxylic acid, RCH_2COOH, whereas myrosinase yields isothiocyanate and sulfate. Glucobrassicin contains an indolylmethyl group but decomposes to a variety of indole-containing products upon hydrolysis (VanEtten et al., 1969).

Myrosinase has been said to consist of two closely coupled enzymes: a thioglucosidase (EC 3.2.3.1; International Union of Biochemistry, 1979) and a less well-defined sulfatase called myrosulfatase (Roy, 1987). However, there is additional evidence that it actually exists as a glycoprotein group that can hydrolyze both glucosides and sulfates (Björkman, 1976).

Isolation from several *Brassica* species points to a family of enzymes of molecular weight 150,000 containing 2 or 4 equal subunits, about 15% carbohydrate (mostly hexose), with an isoelectric pH of 4.6–6.2; myrosinases have also been isolated from mammals and fungi (Goodman et al., 1959; Björkman, 1976). Subsequent Lossen rearrangement of thiohydroxamate to isothiocyanate is spontaneous and similar in mechanism to the Hofmann rearrangement (Imamoto et al., 1971). By-products include the corresponding thiocyanate, R-SCN and nitrile R–CN, both artifacts from the plant extractions.

The general nature of mustard oils had been known for centuries before sinigrin (allyl glucosinolate) was first isolated in crystalline form in 1831—at the very beginnings of organic chemistry (Bussy, 1840). Typical of the others, it occurs as a monohydrated potassium salt (m.p. of 127–29°C, $[\alpha]_D^{18}$–16.4°) and was first called potassium myronate (*myron* is Greek for "balsam"). Except for sinigrin and sinalbin, glucosinolates are named by adding the prefix "gluco-" to a reduced form of the Latin name of a parent genus or species and the suffix "-in," for example, glucoiberin from plants of the genus *Iberis* or gluconapin from *Brassica napus* (rape).

Protein amino acids are the starting point for biosynthesis of glucosinolates. For example, sinalbin (display 7.5, R=4-hydroxyphenyl) is formed from tyrosine via a series of oxidations, introduction of the divalent sulfur, and a final glucosylation and sulfation by the usual mechanisms. Methylthioalkyl is a common substituent, for example, in glucoibervirin from *Iberis sempervirens* (R=$CH_3SCH_2CH_2CH_2$-). The group does not come from methionine (it has one methylene too many), and other glucosinolates can have four or more extra methylenes. This is due to homologization, a reaction sequence in which acetate is inserted into the α-carbonyl representing the deaminated amino acid, followed by reconstitution of a new amino acid containing one additional methylene group (Kjaer, 1976).

Toxicologically, the most important reactions of isothiocyanates undoubtedly are those with protein nucleophiles. The reaction with an amine can be explosively rapid and generate a stable thiourea; a thiol produces a thioester, and an alcohol a carbamate. (A slower reaction with water forms a thiolcarbamic acid that spontaneously loses carbon oxysulfide, COS, to yield an amine that reacts with excess isothiocyanate to give a thiourea.) Thus, it is not surprising that mustard oils can both react with skin and, being fat-soluble and absorbable, serve as haptens leading to allergy.

Mustard seeds have long played an important role in medicine, and over 300 other kinds of plants—mostly crucifers such as radish, cabbage, candytuft, nasturtium, and cresses—are found to contain one or more glucosinolates that release mustard oils when crushed (table 4.3). The skin's reaction is generally an immediate and short-lived urticaria, especially prominent in food handlers and housewives, that is sometimes accompanied by ACD (Mitchell and Jordan, 1974). Eyes are especially sensitive, and mustard oil was used as tear gas in World War I and is in today's "chemical mace." More complete lists of isothiocyanate-producing plants are provided by Kjaer (1960) and Mitchell and Rook (1979).

Garlic Oils

The bulbs and leaves of garlic, onion, and other *Allium* species are known worldwide for their penetrating odor when cut. The first scientific explanation for this was provided by the German chemist Wertheim in 1848, cited by Koch and Larson (2000), when he detected organosulfur compounds in steam distillates of garlic and coined the term *allyl* (from *Allium*) to describe them. Like mustard oils, the odorous and caustic *Allium* constituents are generated from unusual amino acids such as alliin (*S*-allylcysteine sulfoxide), here by action of the enzyme alliinase or alliin lyase (EC 4.4.1.4). The products are typified by allicin (diallyl thiosulfinate). A thiosulfinate is a disulfide in which one sulfur bears a semipolar-bonded oxygen (SO); see figure 7.6.

First isolated by Stoll and Seebeck (1947), garlic alliinase is a glyco-protein (5.5–6% carbohydrate) composed of two 55,000 molecular weight subunits—that is, 448 amino acid units (Jansen et al., 1989). The enzyme is deactivated by heat, so the popular baked garlic actually has very little garlic taste or odor. When active, the reaction it catalyzes is very rapid, and more than half the alliin in a sample of dried garlic powder is converted to allicin in less than 6 seconds (Lawson and Hughes, 1992). There appear to be several alliinases: One converts alliin to allicin, another forms *S*-methylallicin from *S*-methylcysteine sulfoxide, and probably yet another acts on the 1-propenyl analog.

Allium species biosynthesize alliin from cysteine (fig. 7.6, reactions 1–4). Alliin is high-melting, water-soluble, odorless, and forms an unstable allylsulfenic acid in the presence of alliinase (reaction 5). This acid dispro-portionates spontaneously to allicin (diallyl thiosulfinate), a mild-smelling, yellow, fat-soluble liquid, via reaction 6. However, the familiar and char-acteristic garlic odor actually is due to the allyl sulfides formed by thermal degradation of allicin (reaction 7), as when garlic is steam distilled (ap-pendix E) or simply cut. Garlic also contains the methyl-, propyl-, and 1-propenyl analogs of allicin, and so the nine possible mixed thiosulfinates also are present. However, most of the 1-propenylcysteine is diverted to other products such as unreactive cycloalliin (fig. 7.6), which does not form either thiosulfinate or sulfides.

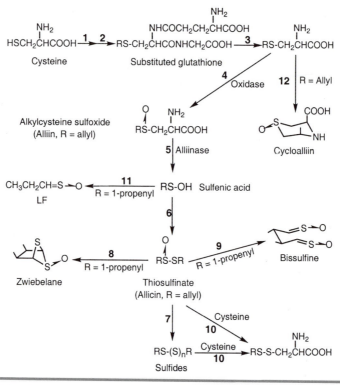

Figure 7.6 Biosynthesis and reactions of thiosulfinates. See Koch and Lawson (2000), R=CH$_3$-, C$_3$H$_7$-, CH$_3$CH=CH_, or CH$_2$=CHCH$_2$-.

The methyl analog of alliin, methiin (*S*-methylcysteine sulfoxide), is the most widely distributed of the congeners, occurring, for example, throughout the Brassicaceae and as one of the most important flavor precursors in the alliums (table 7.4). The 1-propenyl analog (isoalliin) so far is restricted to the genus *Allium,* but still others undoubtedly await discovery (Lawson, 1996). Although the biosynthesis and methylation of glutathione to generate *S*-methylcysteine are normal (reactions 1–3), the means by which the allyl- and 1-propenyl- substituents are incorporated is still largely speculative (Granroth and Virtanen, 1967). It is suggested that the process involves the intermediate *S*-(2-carboxypropyl)glutathiones already identified in garlic extracts (table 7.4), and these would lose glycine and formic acid to provide γ-glutamyl-1-(or 2-)propenylcysteines.

Upon standing or heating, alliin and other thiosulfinates form polysulfides (Lawson et al., 1991), probably via the trisulfide, which can be detected in the air around crushed alliums and in one's exhaled breath after eating them (Laakso et al., 1989). Rather than using steam distillation, the

Table 7.4 Organosulfur Compounds in Garlic (g/kg)

Compound	Whole Bulb[a]	Crushed Bulb[a]
Alliin (S-allylcysteine sulfoxide)	5–14	—[b]
γ-Glutamyl-S-trans-(1-propenyl)cysteine	3–9	3–9
γ-Glutamyl-S-allylcysteine	2–6	2–6
Methiin (S-methylcysteine sulfoxide)	0.5–2	—
Cycloalliin	0.5–1.5	0.5–1.5
Isoalliin [S-trans-(1-propenyl) cysteine sulfoxide]	0.2–1.2	—
γ-Glutamyl-S-methylcysteine	0.1–0.4	0.1–0.4
γ-Glutamyl-S-cis-(1-propenyl)cysteine	0.06–1.5	0.06–0.15
γ-Glutamylmethionine	0.02–0.12	0.02–0.12
S-(2-Carboxypropyl)glutathione	0.09	0.09
Allicin	—	2–6
Allyl methyl thiosulfinate	—	0.3–1.5
Allyl trans-(1-propenyl)thiosulfinate	—	0.05–1
Methyl trans-(1-propenyl)thiosulfinate	—	0.02–0.2
Methyl methanethiosulfinate	—	0.05–0.1

Data from Lawson (1996). [a]g/kg fresh weight by HPLC. [b]— means <0.02 g/kg.

Allium flavor constituents currently are extracted into vegetable oil (more so in Euope than in the United States), resulting in a composition rich in dithiins (appendix E). Perhaps surprisingly, elemental analysis of alliums also reveals volatile selenosulfides, in which one of the sulfur atoms has been replaced by Se (Cai et al., 1995). The health implications of this require consideration because organoselenium compounds generally are quite toxic.

Unfortunately, during the past decade 30-years worth of analytical data have been brought into question; inadvertent overheating during analyses often resulted in serious errors in identification and quantitation (Block et al., 1992a). Most recovery and analysis of *Allium* constituents now are carried out by mild methods such as room temperature distillation and liquid chromatography. It also seems certain that no di- or polysulfides occur in the bulbs themselves, and that several complex constituents such as thiophenes, ajoenes, cepaenes, and dithiins (display 7.6) are actually artifacts generated by heat; see Block and Calvey, 1994.

2-Vinyl-1,3-Dithiin   3,4-Dimethyl-thiophene   (E)-Ajoene   Cepaene   7.6

Our discussion of alliums so far has dealt mainly with garlic. Onions are different. As mentioned in section 4.2, the structue of the onion bulb (layers) is unlike that of garlic (segments). Onions contain no alliin, allii-nase, or allicin; their primary odorant precursor appears to be methiin, so onion odor and taste differ markedly from those of garlic. Perhaps the most noticeable feature is that a freshly cut onion brings on tears. Identification of the lachrymatory factor (LF) occupied some of the world's best food chemists for an extended period, but the compound eventually proved to be derived from isoalliin. Although detectable in onions, some of this compound is converted rapidly to a corresponding 1-propenesulfinic acid, which then isomerizes to the elusive, volatile lachrymator called propylsulfine S-oxide (display 7.7; see Block et al., 1980) or, chemically more correct, (Z)-propanethial S-oxide. Typically, a white onion contains only about 30 μg/g (0.003%) of LF (Block et al., 1992b), but even that represents about half the bulb's total of volatile sulfur constituents and is still plenty to make one cry.

$$CH_3CH{=}CH{-}\underset{\substack{\text{Isoalliin}}}{\overset{\substack{O\\\uparrow\\}}{S}}CH_2\underset{}{\overset{NH_2}{CH}}COOH \xrightarrow{\text{Isoalliinase}} CH_3CH{=}CH{-}SOH \rightleftharpoons CH_3CH_2CH{=}S{\rightarrow}O \qquad 7.7$$

LF

Isoalliin also forms (Z)-1-propenyl thiosulfinates, an LF relative called bissulfine (Block and Bayer, 1990), and unusual (Z)- and (E)-dithiabicyclo[2.1.1]hexanes called zwiebelanes (named from the German word for onion (Bayer et al., 1989). See figure 7.6 for structures and appendix F for the comparative composition of onions and garlics. From this appendix, one can conclude the following: (1) onions and their relatives do not generate anything with allyl subsituents; (2) allyl derivatives are the principal volatile components of garlics; (3) garlics generate far more odorants than do onions; and (4) the perceived "strength" of each type of bulb is directly related to the level of its volatile sulfur compounds.

Alliums have been recognized for centuries as a cause of skin irritation and ACD (Mitchell and Rook, 1979; Papageorgiou et al., 1983). Although there is no information on the exact mechanism of the dermatitis, it seems likely that a reaction of the irritant chemicals (thiosulfinates and sulfides) with nucleophiles again may be involved. These sulfur compounds do react with cysteine (fig. 7.6, reaction 10), and presumably with amines and alcohols as well (Lawson and Wang, 1993), which would account for both the observed irritation and the generation of haptens. A cyclic trisulfide (1,2,3-trithiane-5-carboxylic acid) from a very different source—asparagus (*Asparagus officinalis*, Liliaceae)—is responsible for an allergic contact dermatitis called asparagus scabies long recognized among harvesters and canners (Hausen and Wolf, 1996).

Cysteine reacts rapidly with allicin, the half-life being less than one minute and that with diallyl trisulfide less than two minutes, and allicin is known to react with a variety of sulfhydryl-containing enzymes and other proteins (Papageorgiou et al., 1983). Methyl- and 1-propenyl analogs of allicin react with cysteine in the same manner (Fujiwara et al., 1955), but any participation of zwiebelanes and bissulfines remains unknown.

7.5 Irritant Amines and Amides

Perhaps because of their relative polarity, there seem to be few nitrogen-containing irritants. The capsaicin from pepper is an interesting one, a *trans*-8-methylnonenamide of 4-hydroxy-3-methoxybenzylamine (vanillylamine) related to vanillin, eugenol, and coniferyl benzoate (fig. 6.5). It is one of over 20 structurally related capsaicinoids (Bosland and Votava, 1999) that include the equally irritant dihydrocapsaicin (an 8-methylnonanamide), nordihydrocapsaicin (7-methyl-n-octanamide), and a homodihydro analog (9-methyldecanamide). Thus, the capsaicin side chain can be saturated, lengthened, branched, and the amide NH and CO even reversed without seriously affecting pungency, but any changes in the ring substitution reduce the effect.

Like its vanillin-related analogs, capsaicin is reported to be a skin sensitizer (Benezra et al., 1985). However, it also is related to the diterpene ester resiniferatoxin (section 7.3) and shares many aspects of that ester's irritancy and neurotoxicity (Holzer, 1991).

The superirritants in nettle trichomes are notable, too. Amine mediators released from mast cells—histamine, 5-hydroxytryptamine (serotonin), and acetylcholine—have been detected in *Urtica*, *Cnidoscolus*, and *Laportea* (see Lookadoo and Pollard, 1991). The first two are primary amines that act in protonated form, whereas the third already is cationic (fig. 7.7). Although all three act as neurotransmitters in the mammalian nervous system, injection of a mixture of them into the skin still does not provide the full effect of a nettle sting.

This is not the case with the bicyclic octapeptide, moroidin, extracted from the terrifying gympie bush (*Laportea moroides*) (Leung et al., 1986). Although topical application to skin produced no reaction, intradermal injection of even a few micrograms reproduced most of the pain and redness felt with crude leaf extracts. A structure proposed for moroidin (fig. 7.7) has several peculiar features (at the arrows), including a C–C bond between isoleucine and the 6-position of tryptophan, a C–N bond from the 2-position of tryptophan to an imidazole nitrogen on histidine, and

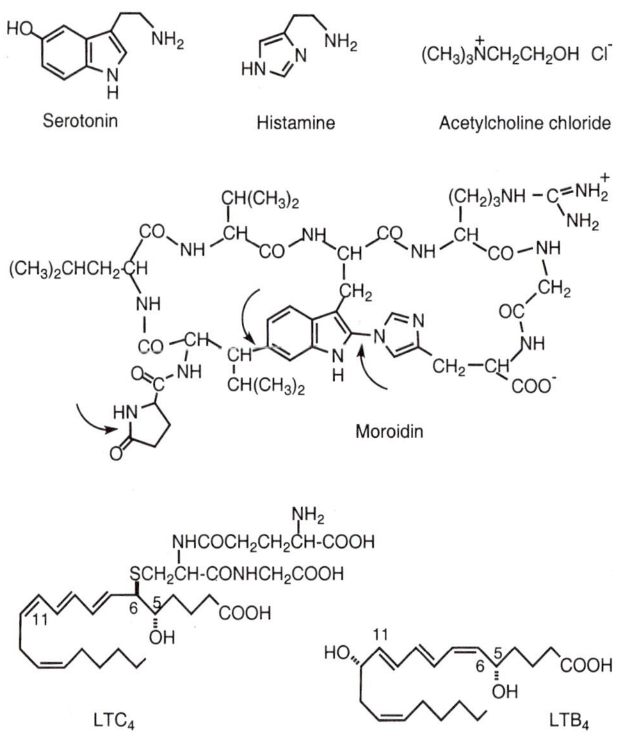

Figure 7.7 Nettle irritants. LT = leukotriene; arrows indicate unusual bonds

cyclization of an extracyclic glutamate sidechain to pyroglutamate. The structure is based on NMR and mass spectra but should be verified by X-ray crystallography; a second dermatotoxic component remains unidentified.

An investigation into the reaction of skin to nettles detected the polypeptide mediator leukotriene C$_4$, its nonpeptide LTB$_4$ mate, and histamine in trichomes and leaves of *Urtica urens* (fig. 7.7; Czarnetzki et al., 1990). The authors point out that these are also constituents of insect venoms and mast cell contents responsible for other forms of contact urticaria. The trichome contents of spurge nettle, *Cnidoscolus stimulosus*, likely are similar to those of *Urtica*, as trichomes of *C. oligandrus* from South America were reported to contain histamine (Cordiero et al., 1983), and Lookadoo and Pollard (1991) found serotonin but no histamine in those of *C. texanus*.

At least three highly irritant substances are found in the blue-green alga *Lyngbya majuscula*: lyngbyatoxin A, aplysiatoxin, and a related debromoaplysiatoxin (Fujiki et al., 1990). Lyngbyatoxin A is a complex indole alkaloid (fig. 7.5), but aplysiatoxin is a bromophenol whose equally irritant debromo analog lacks only the bromine. None are structurally like any other plant irritants except, perhaps, for serotonin (5-hydroxytryptamine), which lyngbyatoxin A somewhat resembles. Aplysiatoxin derives its name from the sea hare (*Aplysia* spp.), which appears to accumulate it from *Lyngbya* as a defense mechanism.

7.6 Calcium Oxalate

At least 250 plant *families* display insoluble calcium oxalate crystals in some form: crystal sand, aggregates (druses), or slender, sharp needles called raphides (Frey-Wyssling, 1981; Khan, 1995). They generally represent a monocliinic monohydrate, $CaC_2O_4 \cdot H_2O$—the mineral whewellite—but sometimes appear also as an unstable tetragonal dihydrate termed weddelite that contains variable amounts of water inclusions $[CaC_2O_4 \cdot (2+x)H_2O]$ within the crystal lattice. The aqueous solubility of calcium oxalate is 6.7 mg/L at 13°C (solubility product constant 1.8×10^{-9}), so it is thought that oxalate concentrations in the cell vacuole must be high enough to suppress dissolution via the common ion effect, and that calcium ions are fed into this solution from the cytoplasm.

Single crystals found in noseburn (*Tragia* spp., Euphorbiaceae) may be as long as 200 μm, sharp at the upper end and blunt at the lower (Thurston, 1976). The double-pointed needles, suspended in bundles inside ejector cells on the surfaces of dumbcane (*Dieffenbachia* spp., Araliaceae) are 60–250 μm long and grooved lengthwise to accomodate the release of toxic cell constituents into the wounds they cause. Other irritants thought to accompany the mechanical injury from the raphides include histamine and other mediators, proteolytic enzymes, and polypeptides (Burrows and Tyrl, 2001), but the concentrated oxalate solution actually might be toxic enough by itself to account for most of the unpleasant effects (Frohne and Pfänder, 1984).

7.7 Conclusions

It seems almost as though any plant that is not allergenic must be either phototoxic or irritant. The irritant esters of the euphorbs are the most dangerous, both for their immediate caustic action, especially on the eyes, and their ability to promote tumors; several are thought to be the most irritant chemicals of the entire plant world. However, phototoxicity is serious, too, and the furocoumarins that commonly cause it are consumed daily in celery, carrots, and citrus products, to be transported into the skin via the bloodstream. Other common foods such as mustard, garlic, cabbage, and onions contain irritant (and often allergenic) organosulfur compounds used since antiquity in medicine, and even latex rubber of the kind used in surgical gloves produces a skin rash in many people, most often health professionals.

Several common chemical features are emerging. Structural components of capsaicin, the chili pepper irritant, are identical to those in the diterpene ester resiniferatoxin and the allergens of balsam of Peru; the dermatotoxic constituents of mast cells are to be found in the stinging hairs of plants and irritant venoms of insects; and the effects of most organosulfur constituents of onion and garlic seem to stem from their reactivity with the protein amino acid cysteine. The stinging cells of nettles inject histamine and other mediators under the skin, whereas those in *Dieffenbachia* inject crystalline needles of calcium oxalate.

One can hardly avoid the photodynamic agents and irritants from plants—there are just too many of them—but it *should* be feasible (and wise) to learn the sources of the worst offenders and then, sensitive or not, to do your best to avoid them.

EIGHT

*"We struggled toughly upward, canted to and fro by
the roughness of the trail, and continually switched
across the face by sprays of leaf or blossom. The last
is no great inconvenience at home; but here in
California it is a matter of some moment. For in all
woods and by every wayside there prospers an
abominable shrub or weed, called poison oak, whose
very neighbourhood is venomous to some, and whose
actual touch is avoided by the most impervious."*
—*Robert Louis Stevenson, 1883*

8.1 Forms of Exposure

The trouble always begins with exposure: no exposure, no dermatitis. Most
often, the exposure is direct—the skin actually contacts a plant or plant
product. Alternatively, exposure can be indirect (secondary), where contact
is made with contaminated fur, tools, clothing, or even your own or someone else's skin. It also can be systemic, when one eats food that contains
phototoxic constiturents and then goes out into the sunlight. Occupational
exposure is very common (table 8.1), but *everyone* is exposed to plant
allergens and irritants at some point.

Sap is usually at fault. The oily allergens or irritants may be emulsified
into a milky latex: *Toxicodendron* latex consists of water (20–25%), carbohydrate (5–7%), soluble protein (1%, mostly the enzyme laccase), but principally (65–70%) toxic resin (Kumanotani, 1983). It is fluid in the spring
but becomes increasingly viscous as the season progresses. Any part of the
plant that contains sap—roots, stems, leaves, flowers, and fruit—also contains allergen. With their sap ducts sealed off by nature, intact fallen leaves
are nontoxic (McNair, 1923), but *cut* parts such as prunings, and even
leafless stems, remain active for a long time.

However, the latex must contact the skin for there to be a toxic effect. In
an interesting experiment (McNair, 1921b), poison oak leaves were steeped
in alcohol such that no cut petioles were included. The resulting yellow

Table 8.1 Occupational Dermatitis from Plants

Occupation or Activity	Principal Exposure[a]
Bakers, confectioners	BOP,[b] essential oils, rye, wheat, vanilla
Construction workers	Composites, exotic woods, Florida holly, nettles, POR,[c] rosin, turpentine
Farmers, stockmen, road crews	Buttercups, composites, cow parsnip, lichens, wild parsnips, POR[c]
Firefighters, linemen, police, arborists	Conifers, lichens, liverworts, POR,[c] silky oak
Food handlers, chefs	Asparagus, chili oil, cinnamon, cloves, essential oils, garlic, lettuce, mustard
Foresters, lumbermen, woodworkers	Cedars, conifers, lichens, liverworts, pine oil, rosin, tropical hardwoods
Gardeners and groundskeepers	Chrysanthemum, dandelion, euphorbs, ivy, Peruvian lily, POR,[c] tulips
Health care providers	Latex rubber, eugenol, lemon oil, pine oil, BOP[b]
Horticulturists, florists, nurserymen	Chrysanthemum, daffodil, euphorbs, ivy, lichens, orchid, Peruvian lily, primrose, tulip
Homemakers, office workers, janitors	BOP,[b] citrus oils, euphorbs, ivy, philodendron, pine oil, primrose, rosin
Sportsmen, surveyors, rangers	Brazilian pepper, buttercups, composites, cow parsnip, *Frullania*, lichens, nettle, POR[c]
Pickers, packers, grocerymen, cooks	Artichoke, asparagus, celery, citrus, endive, figs, lettuce, mangoes

[a]For a discussion of the plants, see chapters 2–4. [b]Balsam of Peru. [c]Poison oak and relatives.

extract proved nontoxic, indicating that leaf surfaces and hairs (trichomes) do not produce ACD; laticifers must actually be broken. Once thought to be the main cause of poison oak and poison ivy rash, trichomes, pollen, and waxy leaf surfaces are the only parts that do *not* contain allergens (McNair, 1921b). Plants such as primrose (*Primula obconica*) confine their allergens largely to the hairs of stem and leaf, and nettles in the Urticaceae outdo normal trichomes by *injecting* the irritant into unprotected skin through quartz needles (fig. 4.1). In other exposures, allergenic or irritant sawdust, smoke, or pollen can be inhaled, and even the runoff of rain or dew from leaves of certain species such as manchineel (*Hippomane mancinella*) is reported to be dermatotoxic. Exposure is multidimensional.

8.2 Direct (Primary) Exposure

Like the writer Robert Louis Stevenson, most people are exposed to allergens and irritants by direct contact. Exposure during outdoor recreation is common, for as McNair (1923) observed, "the desire to gather spring wild flowers is often greater than the fear of *R. diversiloba*" [poison oak] (p. 51). In a classic 1912–18 study of students at the University of California in Berkeley exposed in this way, McNair (1921b) found that the incidence of "*Rhus* dermatitis" observed at the university dispensary generally peaked about March and again in November (fig. 8.1A).

The first surge coincided with expansion of the plant's leaf buds in early spring, when the tender leaflets were easily damaged and outdoor recreation was gearing up. The second peak occurred in late autumn, after most leaves had fallen but bare stems were present and outdoor recreation was still active. Although McNair's study was interrupted by summer vacations

Figure 8.1 The incidence of "*Rhus* dermatitis" among UC Berkeley students (A) and its proportion of total infirmary admissions (B). Monthly totals in A and total *Rhus* dermatitis cases in B are in parentheses. Data from McNair (1923).

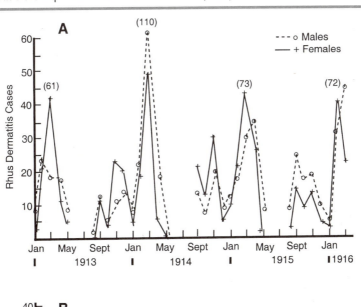

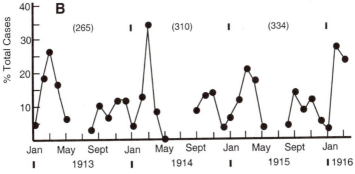

(June and July), others have reported that, as expected, exposure remains especially high during these months.

The Berkeley study revealed several other significant features. Although the young victims represented only 6% of the total student body, the actual incidence of poisoning must have been far higher, because men in particular would tend not to seek medical help. Even so, they provided as much as 35% of the total cases treated by the dispensary in any given month (fig. 8.1B). The results also prove that one need not be a rugged outdoorsman to become exposed and that exposure can occur in any month, with May generally the lowest (studying for final exams?). In fact, poison oak and its relatives are responsible for more cases of ACD in the United States than all other sources combined, both occupational and nonoccupational (Rietschel and Fowler, 2001).

Occupational Exposure

Dermatitis is the principal form of occupational injury in the United States and is high on the list in most other countries. A recent book on occupational dermatitis (Kanerva et al., 2000) records the incidence of contact dermatitis in 90 common occupations, and even though all types of exposures are included, over 40 of the job types involved plants, often toxicodendrons (table 8.1). In fact, plants represent the leading cause of occupational dermatitis in the United States (Guin, 2000).

Poison Oak and Its Relatives

Exposure to toxicodendrons is typical of allergenic exposures to wild plants in general. As suggested by Stevenson's 1883 remark, poison oak and poison ivy cover literally millions of acres of our country, and one or the other can be found virtually "in all woods and by every wayside." Although uncommon in highly urbanized areas, the plants do occur frequently in suburbs where untended open spaces still remain, and occasionally they are seen even in public parks. I "got poison oak" in my urban garden while planting mint purchased in a 4-inch pot from a local nursery but apparently collected by them from the wild.

Although widely distributed in the eastern United States, poison sumac (*Toxicodendron vernix*) fortunately is uncommon, growing mostly in marshy places not normally frequented by people. However, the closely related poisonwood (*Metopium toxiferum*) of Florida and the Caribbean often grows in close proximity to people: Its flowers and foliage are used in wreaths, attractive young specimens transplanted into gardens, and clothing on a wash line rubs against it, all with predictable results (Morton, 1982). The highly allergenic *Schinus terebinthifolius* now occupies large areas of Florida (Florida holly) and Hawaii (Christmasberry), forcing out native species and making the land hazardous to develop.

How much exposure to *Toxicodendron* provides a toxic dose? Contact with only a single freshly damaged poison oak leaf delivers roughly 2.0–2.5 µg of the allergens, and most people in the United States—black, white, yellow, brown, or red—react to doses between 5 and 50 µg (Epstein, 1990). However, 10–15% of the population react to less than 0.5 µg— perhaps just a brush against a plant—while about an equal proportion fail to react to even 1000 µg (1 mg), ordinarily a massive dose. The smallest crystal of granulated sugar one can see unaided weighs about 10 µg.

Although no one seems to keep track of the total number of people afflicted by toxicodendrons, the California Department of Health Services does compile data on lost-time occupational illness and attributes as many as 5000 of them each year to poison oak (Epstein, 1990). Utility workers, police, construction workers, firefighters, and foresters are at greatest risk. The actual number of occupational exposures must be substantially larger than 5000, because most male workers would not report mild cases, and a full third of the thousands of firefighters in western states must retreat from the firelines annually because of "Rhus dermatitis." And significant as they are, exposures to *Toxicodendron* represent only part of the total when considering all the allergenic and irritant plants.

Other Wild Plants

Exposure to sesquiterpene lactones (STLs), especially those from the Asteraceae, is a widespread problem (table 8.2). This plant family is ubiquitous and exposure is common, although the lesions are usually much less severe than those from toxicodendrons. Exposure is mostly occupational

Table 8.2 Exposure to Lactones

Source	Example	Most Likely to Be Exposed
Weeds	Sagebrush (*Artemesia* spp.)	Farmers, outdoorsmen, linemen
Cut flowers	*Chrysanthemum* sp.	Flower cutters, flower handlers, florists
Salad greens	Lettuce (*Lactuca sativa*)	Harvesters, handlers, grocerymen, chefs
Bulbs	Tulip (*Tulipa* spp.)	Growers, handlers, nurserymen, gardeners
Pollen	Ragweed (*Ambrosia* spp.)	Farm workers, gardeners, general public
Herbal medicines	Chamomile (*Anthemis* spp.[a])	Pickers, purveyors, users (e.g., herb teas)
Feed and grain	Buttercup (*Ranunculus* spp.)	Harvesters, handlers, dealers
Forest products	Liverworts (*Frullania* spp.)	Cutters, haulers, millwrights, carpenters
Christmas trees	Lichens (*Usnea* spp.)	Cutters, haulers, sellers, buyers
Firewood	Lichens (*Usnea* spp.)	Cutters, haulers, sellers, buyers

[a]Now the genus *Chamaemelum*.

("weed dermatitis"), the rash generally appearing on the hands, arms, and upper chest where the shirt opens. This disease is largely confined to adult males, with few cases in women and almost none in children.

The most important sources are *Chrysanthemum* species, the chamomiles (especially *A. cotula*), ragweeds (*Ambrosia* spp.), wild feverfew (*Parthenium hysterophorus*), and the sneezeweeds (*Helenium* spp.). Feverfew (*Tanacetum parthenium*) is important in Europe. Australian bush dermatitis is due to these same Asteraceae members as well as to Shasta daisy (*Chysanthemum maximum*), an indigenous wild artichoke (*Cynara cardunculus*), capeweed (*Arctotheca* spp.), and stinkwort (*Dittrichia graveolens*; Burry et al., 1975). Equipment operators and farmworkers most often contact the mowed weeds, but so do hikers, picnickers, and innocent bystanders.

A similar meadow dermatitis is caused by wild carrot or Queen Anne's lace (*Daucus carota*, Apiaceae), buttercups (*Ranunculus acris* called blister plant, Ranunculaceae), and wild parsnip (*Pastinaca sativa* ssp. *pratensis*, Apiaceae). Meadow dermatitis also requires both sunlight and moisture (water or sweat) and is known medically by the rather pretentious name Oppenheim's dermatitis bullosa striata pratensis. The disease is characterized by a crisscross network of ugly blisters a bit like those from toxicodendrons.

Foresters, firefighters, lumbermen, and others involved with trees and wood are exposed to the STLs from lichens such as *Usnea* and the liverwort *Frullania* that grow on trees (section 3.4). The resulting "forester's itch" even extends to cutters and burners of firewood. Conifer pitch and its turpentine and rosin also can be sensitizers.

Cultivated Plants

Of course, people who handle cultivated plants also must deal with many of the same problems—cutting, transporting, and selling Christmas trees, for example. However, they work mostly with a different class of dermatotoxic plants: ornamentals such as chrysanthemums, ivy, euphorbs, and tulips; houseplants that include orchids and philodendron; and lawn weeds like dandelion and spotted spurge. Arborists who trim street trees such as silky oak or rhus are exposed to those allergens, especially in sawdust and sometimes seriously enough to require a trip to the hospital. The public is seldom aware of how hazardous many such professions are.

Floristry actually is considered risky work (Guin, 2000). Florists must personally handle almost every kind of allergenic or irritant plant grown in nurseries, as indicated by such descriptive clinical terms as "tuliip finger" and "florist's dermatitis." Although the incidence of dermatitis is 25% among American florists, it is 30% in Portugal and 50% in Germany

(Guin, 2000). The most offensive species in both the United States and Europe are Peruvian lilies (alstroemerias), tulips, chrysanthemums, and irritant euphorbs such as variegated croton (Lovell, 2000).

Not even office workers and custodians are exempt. They must deal with indoor plants such as philodendron, variegated croton, ivy, and ornamental figs, with citrus and pine oils in cleaners, and with rosin coatings—a leading source of ACD in those who deal with a lot of paper—in other words, most of us. Musical performers such as violinists also are exposed to rosin, and its use on nonslip dance floors suggests that rosin allergy actually helps select those who will become ballerinas from those who will not. Many indoor workers, especially in health fields, regularly don allergenic latex rubber gloves, "to protect themselves."

Food industry workers face a wide variety of allergens and irritants. Pickers, packers, canners, shippers, and grocers must deal with everything from artichokes to yams, including asparagus, endive, lettuce, and mangoes (Guin, 2000). Celery is especially a problem, because everyone from harvesters to grocery clerks to housewives who handle the vegetable suffers from phototoxicity (celery-pickers disease; Birmingham et al., 1961; Seligman et al., 1987). Guin (2000) lists 70 plant-derived foods known to cause acute contact urticaria (see section 9.4).

Restaurant employees endure these same difficulties, but they also may be exposed to such risky items as chili oil, spices and their essential oils, mustard, and horseradish, and the most frequent source of contact dermatitis among chefs is garlic. Bakers add rye, wheat, vanilla, and the pervasive and allergenic balsam of Peru (Adams, 1990), whereas confectioners contend with spices (especially cinnamon), flavor concentrates such as mint, and citrus peel (Lyon, 2000). It's a nasty job, but somebody has to do it.

8.3   Casual (Nonoccupational) Exposure

Although occupational exposure to allergenic and irritant plants obviously is important, it probably is exceeded by casual exposure in the general population. Toxicodendrons are again of prime importance in this country: Extrapolating from the occupational figures, we find that tens of thousands of California residents contract ACD annually just from poison oak, so the U.S. total from all allergenic and irritant plants could easily exceed 100,000 victims each year—year after year.

Exposure from Plants

Apart from Stevenson's particular problem, there are even more extreme forms of exposure to toxicodendrons. With surprising frequency, people use handfuls of poison oak or ivy leaves to clean themselves after defecating in the wild, always with appalling results. The plants have been used in the garden for their attractive foliage and bright autumn color; in what I hope is an extreme example, a presumably unsensitized man planted hedges of poison ivy in his front yard, leaving them for an unfortunate subsequent owner to discover—the hard way (Parsons and Cuthbertson, 1992). A well-intended effort to substitute hand-pruning for herbicides to remove brushy weeds around Northern California conifer seedlings was soon terminated when many of the volunteer workers were hospitalized with poison oak allergy.

In a similar incident (Roberts, 1989), a pair of amateur American wood-turners traveling in Yucatan discovered a beautiful burl from a freshy cut tree referred to by the Mexicans as *Chechén*. "The graining of the wood was great ... white sapwood with chocolate brown heartwood, changing to an almost black center" (p. 28). They tried to bring the piece home but suffered such severe dermatitis that they had to end their vacation, and local Mayans later told them that skin eruptions can occur just from walking underneath that kind of tree. The victims identified it as poison ivy, but its size suggests that the tree-like *Toxicodendron striatum* is more likely.

ACD also results from direct exposure to urushiods in related genera. Handling raw cashew nuts (*Anacardium occidentale*), making wreaths of Florida holly (*Schinus terebinthifolius*), and eating unwashed mangoes (*Mangifera indica*) are all common methods of exposure (see section 3.2). *Semecarpus laxiflora* has been used for folk medicine in Melanesia, but it is considered "the most feared plant in the Bismarck Archipelago" because its corrosive sap "destroys skin and inflicts painful wounds upon even the slightest contact" (Peekel, 1984, p. 328). Even dew falling on one's skin from the leaves of *Semecarpus* or *Lithrea* is said to inflict dermatitis.

The situation is similar for exposure to some members of the Asteraceae. Section 3.4 mentioned that the principal sources of Composite dermatitis in the U.S. Midwest during 1987 were mayweed (*Anthemis cotula*), cocklebur (*Xanthium pennsylvanicum*), wild feverfew (*Parthenium hysterophorus*), and fleabane (*Erigeron strigosum*). An 8-year study in Europe (Paulsen et al., 2001) showed that, of 4386 patients, 81% reacted to feverfew (*Tanacetum parthenium*), 77% to tansy (*T. vulgare*), 64% to German chamomile (*Chamomilla recutita*), 41% to milfoil (*Achillea millefolium*), and 23% to arnica (*Arnica montana*). Further patch tests with oleoresins extracted from common garden plants showed that 72% also were allergic to florist's chrysanthemum, 74% to marguerite (*Argyanthemum frutescens*), 48% to lettuce, and 64% to chicory (*Chicorium intybus*).

Prolonged contact with any dermatotoxic woods is best avoided. These woods are especially hard on hobbyists who work with them, because the allergenic sawdust and shavings get into clothing and under watch bands

(Hausen and Adams, 1990). Even as prosaic an activity as mowing weeds with a power mower—or, worse, a string cutter—produces a shower of leaf particles and sap that is an invitation to a phototoxic disaster, especially if the operator is sweaty and only partially clothed (Reynolds et al., 1991).

With such precedents, it is just common sense to learn the identity of *any* plant your skin is going to contact. Although Oxford, England, seems an unlikely place to find a toxicodendron, several tree cutters and their firewood customers discovered too late that the felled shade trees that turned their skin and clothes black were Japanese lacs (*T. vernicifluum*) planted 20 years earlier (Powell and Barrett, 1986). Although they all suffered from contact dermatitis, fortunately none of the wood had been burned—its smoke could have caused an airborne urban crisis.

Airborne Allergens

Airborne urushioids usually occur in minute liquid droplets or solid particles that are inhaled by the victims, especially firefighters. The ability of allergens and irritants to become airborne—as particles of dry leaf materials and trichomes, fine sawdust (Quirce et al., 1994; Hausen, 2000a), and smoke from burning plant material (table 8.3)—has been controversial in the past but now appears established. Airborne allergens actually are unexpectedly common, their effects easily mistaken for photocontact dermatitis (Rietschel and Fowler, 2001).

Smoke from dermatotoxic leaves or wood is a serious hazard. In addition to frequent wildfires and domestic fireplaces, there seems to be a human tendency to burn brush or fallen leaves. Any toxic agents become attached to smoke particles that can settle on unprotected skin or, worse, be inhaled. There are reports of harm from burning mango, poisonwood, litre, and manchineel, among others (Mitchell and Rook, 1979), and the few deaths ascribed to toxicodendrons have implicated smoke (McNair, 1923).

Fine airborne dusts are a particular problem. Nonvolatile plicatic acid on particles of red cedar (*Thuja plicata*) sawdust is responsible for the most

Table 8.3 Some Plant Sources of Airborne Allergens

Chrysanthemum (*Chrysanthemum* spp.)	Peruvian lily (*Alstroemeria* spp.)
Dahlia (*Dahlia* spp.)	Primrose (*Primula obconica*)
Dandelion (*Taraxicum officinale*)	Rosewood (*Dalbergia nigra*)
Feverfew (*Parthenium hysterophorus*)	Tobacco (*Nicotiana tabacum*)
Japanese lac tree (*Toxicodendron vernicifluum*)	Tulip (*Tulipa* spp.)
Lichens	Western red cedar (*Thuja plicata*)
Orchids	Yarrow (*Achillea* spp.)

Dooms-Goossens and Deleu (1991); Chan-Yeung (1994).

common form of occupational asthma in the Pacific Northwest (Chan-Yeung, 1994), whereas γ-thujaplicin, thymoquinone, and toluquinone are responsible for ACD (Bleumink et al., 1973). Allergy to cedar dust has also been observed in Finland (Estlander et al., 2001), where patch tests identified woodworkers who had become sensitized to teak, palisander (rosewoods), Honduras mahogany, black walnut, and obeche (*Triplochiton scleroxylon*).

Pollen, too, is a possible carrier of airborne allergens. Most pollen allergy is classed as allergic rhinitis (hay fever) caused by Type I antibody-generating proteins, for example the very common allergy to ragweed (*Ambrosia* spp.). This particular pollen appears not to induce ACD, but many others do (Mitchell, 1981a), either from sticky, lactone-bearing oleoresin contacting the skin directly or from contact with pollen-covered surfaces. Many hay fever plants contain highly allergenic lactones, and a connection between the two seems very likely, but poison oak and ivy pollens are not allergenic (McNair, 1923). Selected references for the period 1986–2000 have been reviewed by Dooms-Goossens and Deleu (1991) and Huygens and Goossens (2000).

The possibility remains that a certain amount of exposure actually results from vapor. After all, most aromatic substances volatilize easily, and it is the vapor we smell. Volatility is a function of a chemical's vapor pressure (section 1.3): The *d*-limonene that gives citrus oils their aroma has a vapor pressure of 1.98 torr (Howard and Meylan, 1997)—about as volatile as kerosene—and the substance was detected at levels up to 32 μg/m^3 in all 150 air samples from a 1974 pollution study in Houston, Texas (IARC, 1993). Thus, it should not be surprising that some even more allergenic chemicals also vaporize easily.

For example, mango blossoms (*Mangifera indica*) release volatile dermatotoxic chemicals that produce facial burning and rash in sensitive individuals (Morton, 1982). The allergenic quinone primin from *Primula obconica* volatilizes from intact primrose leaves and flowers (Christensen and Larsen, 2000), and Christensen (1999) detected the lactone tulipalin A in the air around both intact and cut Peruvian lilies (alstroemerias). Despite urushiol's low vapor pressure, many hypersensitive people maintain that they cannot even be in the vicinity of poison oak or ivy without feeling the effects. Indeed, *every* chemical has a finite vapor pressure (section 1.3) and thus a defined concentration in the air, and the absorption of vapors by skin is well documented (McDougal et al., 1990).

Perfume ingredients must rank high for exposure to dermatotoxic vapor, but there still is remarkably little evidence of their effects (Freeman, 1990). Dooms-Goossens (1993) refers to a terpene-sensitive young woman who broke out in a rash each time she passed a perfume counter. Most perfumes rely heavily on volatile monoterpenes, including the linalool, geraniol, and limonene found by Christensen et al. (1999) to be released as vapor from feverfew (*Tanacetum parthenium*) plants and later associated with its ACD (Paulsen et al., 2002).

Flavors and Fragrances

Flavors and fragrances are significant, near-ubiquitous sources of both occupational and nonoccupational allergens (de Groot, 2000). Although once limited to perfumes, cologne, and soap, fragrances today appear in numerous everyday items (table 8.4), and it is striking how many such products come into direct contact with the skin—sometimes extremely sensitive skin. For instance, Keith et al. (1969) reported ACD from scented toilet paper, facial tissue, and sanitary napkins. Most cosmetics contain fragrance chemicals as well as rosin (colophony); adhesive tape and bandages once utilized colophony, too (Cronin and Calnan, 1978), although most now employ hypoallergenic acrylate polymers instead. Fragrances and people's adverse reactions to them have been reviewed by de Groot and Frosch (1997).

In that 1997 review, the allergen linalool was found in 90% of 400 cosmetic and toiletry products used in the United States, 2-phenylethanol appeared in 82%, and geraniol in 43%. In a 2001 survey, Rastogi et al. (2001) reported linalool in second place, behind limonene, possibly reflecting the explosive growth of citrus oils in cleaning products (table 8.4). An entire issue (Supplement 3) of *Contact Dermatitis* in the spring of 2002 was devoted to contact allergy from fragrances (Duus Johansen, 2002), which indicates the growing recognition of a worldwide health problem. The survey showed that 17% of patients in China reacted to the standard allergist's fragrance mix (table 10.1), whereas the figure was 10% for Germany, 11% for North America, 13% for Singapore, and 14% for Switzerland. Surely this qualifies as an epidemic!

Flavor substances, often the same chemicals found in fragrances, are added today to most prepackaged foods (the label generally states "contains

Table 8.4 Typical Exposure to Allergenic Fragrance Substances

Aftershave lotion	Fabric softeners	Polishes
Antiperspirants	Fabrics	Rubber
Body lotion	Facial tissue	Sanitary napkins
Cleaners	Feminine sprays	Shampoo
Cosmetics	Hair gel	Shaving cream
Deodorants	Insect spray	Suntan lotion
Detergents	Lipstick	Toilet paper
Diapers	Plastics	Waxes

natural and artificial flavoring"). They are also added to nonfood items such as mouthwash, toothpaste, throat lozenges, chewing gum, and tobacco (don't forget menthol cigarettes). The tingling sensation in the mouth from cinnamon gum and candy is actually an irritant reaction to cinnamaldehyde. Additives also may supplement the allergens already present in food; for example, they can aggravate an existing allergy to balsam of Peru by spices (Dooms-Goossens et al., 1990).

For most of us, the flavors and fragrances we encounter daily are generally quite dilute. However, several opportunities for more concentrated exposure warrant attention. The increasing popularity of aromatherapy means that more people are exposed to chemicals applied directly to their skin or as a vapor (Alanko, 2000). As a form of alternative medicine, this field has received relatively little regulatory attention, and its materials—primarily essential oils—largely avoid the food and drug laws by qualifying as "natural products" that are GRAS (Generally Regarded as Safe); see Opdyke (1975b).

The oils are incorporated into bath liquids, skin lotions, and massage oils, or distributed as vapor and aerosols from heated aroma lamps, assuring massive skin exposure. Of course, any dermatotoxicity will depend on the constituents of the particular oil. Although it would seem risky to rub *any* unknown chemical into the skin, one should be especially cautious about oils that have become oxidized by exposure to air for long periods (section 6.5).

Another area of rapidly growing public interest is herbal medicine (Hobbs, 1998). Local pharmacies, health food stores, and even grocery stores often carry herbal extracts and dried plant material intended mostly for internal use as infusions or teas. A recent tour of a nearby grocer's revealed costly little bottles of extracts like "Rhus toxicodendron 30X" and "Podophyllum peltatum 30X," but the 30X turned out to indicate 30 successive 10-fold dilutions of the original extract; after about 14X, the presence of even a single molecule of active ingredient seems unlikely! Capsules of St. John's wort (*Hypericum perforatum*) actually did contain systemically phototoxic hypericin (0.9 mg per caplet), accompanied by a phototoxicity warning on the label, and even at a recommended three caplets per day, hypericin intake is well below the demonstrated phototoxic threshold of 5.6 mg/day (Brockmöller et al., 1997).

However, other herbal products are applied directly to the skin (Hobbs, 1998). Most of those known to cause dermatitis are essential oils (table 8.5), some used in substantial amounts. One popular analgesic preparation to relax sore muscles contains 30% methyl salicylate, 10% menthol, and 4% camphor, and another contains 0.025% capsaicin (from chili pepper). Hobbs (1998) suggests placing a small amount of any such oil on a small patch of

Table 8.5 Some Dermatotoxic Herbal Remedies

Name	Source	Intended to Remedy[a]	Action[b]
Benzoin oil	*Styrax tonkinensis*	Rash, itch, dry skin	ACD
Bergamot oil	*Citrus bergamia*	Acne, eczema, psoriasis	Photo
Camomile	*Matricaria chamomilla*	Sore muscles, rash, burns	ACD
Camphor	*Cinnamomum camphora*	Sore muscles, arthritis, congestion	CD
Cinnamon oil	*Cinnamomum cassia*	Sore muscles	ACD
Clove oil	*Syzygium aromaticum*	Sore muscles, arthritis	ACD
Eucalyptus oil	*Eucalyptus globules*	Coughs, boils, wounds	Irrit
Lavender oil	*Lavandula angustifolia*	Insect bites	ACD
Lemon oil	*Citrus limon*	Facial blemishes	Photo
Peppermint oil	*Mentha piperita*	Skin rash	Irrit

[a]Hobbs (1998). [b]Benezra et al. (1985). ACD, allergic contact dermatitis; CD, contact dermatitis; Photo, phototoxicity; Irrit, skin irritation.

skin overnight to test for a reaction and, even if it appears safe, to dilute it at least 20-fold with a safe solvent such as almond oil and retest.

Of even greater concern are the do-it-yourself plant extracts that may involve relatively little dilution, especially when made into creams and ointments. Those made from arnica (*A. montana*), chamomile (*Matricaria recutite*), and St. John's wort (*Hypericum perforatum*) are used on bruises and sore muscles; cedar oil (*Juniperus* spp.) claims to alleviate skin problems such as acne; and tea tree oil (from *Melaleuca*) is said to control athlete's foot (Hobbs, 1998). However, there are surprisingly few scientific publications regarding the hazards of such products in herbal medicine.

8.4 Indirect (Secondary) Exposure

Indirect exposure to allergens and irritants is the norm wherever people and dermatotoxic plants are in proximity. In her 1996 book, Susan Hauser (1996) writes of her first (or, with sensitization, perhaps her second) contact with poison ivy after having kneeled in a patch of it:

> In the several days before I washed my jeans, I had sat in them in every chair in the house. After that, whenever I sat down wearing shorts or a short nightgown, I sat on a little bit of poison ivy oil. It was a full six weeks before the adventure whimpered to a close.

Although laccase should have provided rapid oxidation of urushiols when the sap was exposed to air (Zhan et al., 1990), it seems to act more slowly when the enzyme is on a surface such as cloth. Transfers of allergen from contaminated clothing to skin are commonplace: I once discovered a large spot of poison oak sap on my trousers (and paid an allergic penance for it), but when the pants were worn again, weeks and several washings later, itching was renewed in the skin beneath where the spot had been. Deactivation of the enzyme may even allow the allergen to remain unchanged for months or years. In an extreme case, a jar lacquered with *T. vernicifluum* sap gave an archeologist dermatitis even after it had been buried for 10 centuries (Toyama, 1918).

The most frequent vehicles of secondary exposure are the hands (eyes and cheeks are the usual recipients), and it is common for lesions to form as finger- or hand-shaped streaks. A man can contract ACD by holding his penis with contaminated fingers when urinating, and women suffer similar hazards (McNair,1923; Gochfeld and Burger, 1983). In one instance, a man's badly contaminated hands led to ACD on his wife's breasts and inner thighs; in another, a woman who had cleaned herself with poison oak leaves instead of toilet paper transferred the allergens to her partner's genitals during later lovemaking, even though she had showered. Such events fit the category of *connubial contact dermatitis* and are common (Morren et al., 1992), although the more accurate term *consort dermatitis* removes the implication of marriage. Such adventures are not funny at best and very serious at worst, but they undoubtedly will continue.

Pet fur, knife handles, water faucets—*any* contaminated surface contacted by human skin can provide exposure (table 8.6). My wife contracted a serious case of ACD when she collected mail at a mailbox located under a Christmasberry tree (*Schinus terebinefolius*) in Hawaii; British soldiers in India developed ACD on their necks from black laundry marks made in ink from the markingnut tree (*Semecarpus anacardium*); and incompletely cured black lacquer on eating utensils, toilet seats, and rifle stocks (chapter 2) has produced ACD at embarrassing moments.

Table 8.6 Indirect Exposure to Poison Oak and Ivy

Automobile steering wheels	Human hands and other skin
Bicycle handlebars and tires	Hunting and fishing equipment
Christmas wreaths	Knife handles
Clothing	Pet fur
Croquet balls	Pillows (of a contaminated person)
Doorknobs	Rain drip from the leaves
Firewood	Shoes and shoelaces
Garden tools	Smoke from burning brush
Gloves	Tobacco products (cigarettes)
Golf clubs and balls	Water bottles and drinking cups
Herbarium specimens	Water faucets and hoses

Partly from data of McNair (1923).

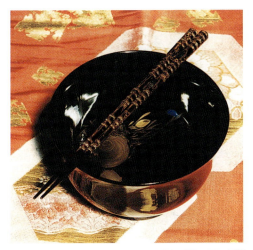

Plate 1
A lacquered bowl from the Edo
period (1603–1867) in Japan.

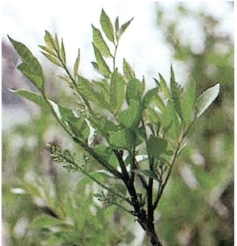

Plate 2
Poison sumac (*T.vernix*), courtesy
of the Eastern Cereal and Oilseed
Research Center, Agriculture and
Agri-Food Canada.

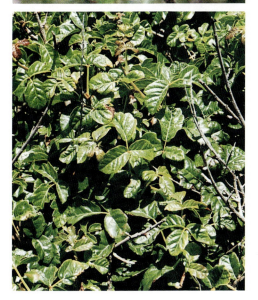

Plate 3
Poison oak (*T. diversilobum*) in
a sunny location, Yolo Co., CA.

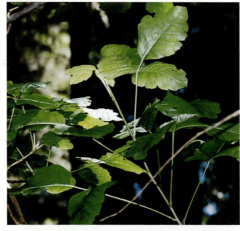

Plate 4
Poison oak (*T. diversilobum*) in a
shady location, Sonoma Co., CA.

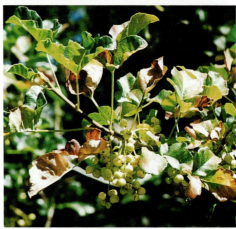

Plate 5
Poison oak (*T. diversilobum*) fruit,
Yolo Co., CA.

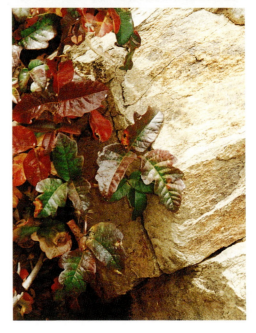

Plate 6
Poison oak (*T. diversilobum*) fall
coloration, Marin Co., CA.

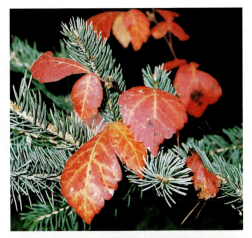

Plate 7
Poison ivy (*T. radicans* ssp. *radicans*), Ontario, Canada.

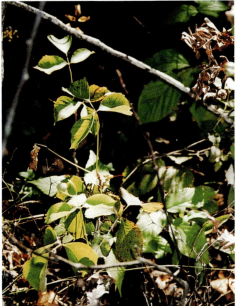

Plate 8
Rydberg's poison ivy (*T. rydbergii*), Ontario, Canada.

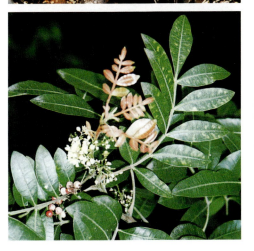

Plate 9
Florida holly (Christmasberry, *Schinus terebinthefolius*), Hawaii Co., HI. Courtesy of Rick Crosby.

Plate 10
Heart-leaf philodendron
(*Philodendron scandens*),
Davis, CA.

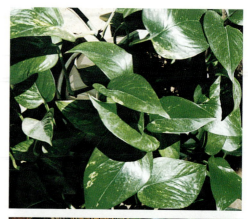

Plate 11
Silky oak (*Grevillea robusta*),
Yolo Co., CA.

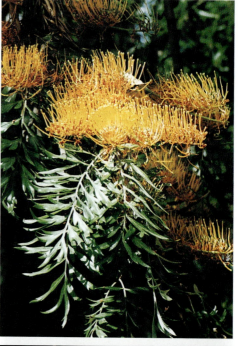

Plate 12
German primrose (*Primula obconica*), Yolo Co., CA.

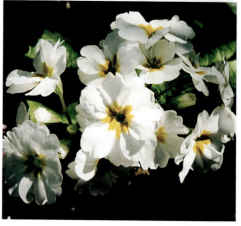

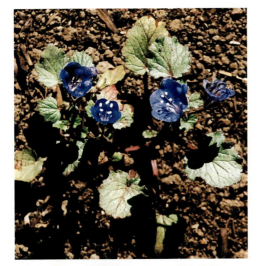

Plate 13
Desert bluebell (*Phacelia companularia*), San Diego Co., CA.

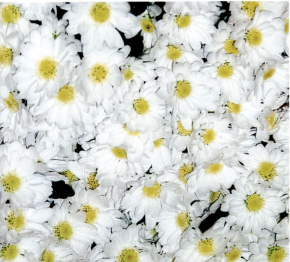

Plate 14
Florist's chrysanthemum (*Dendranthema* × *grandiflorum*), Davis, CA.

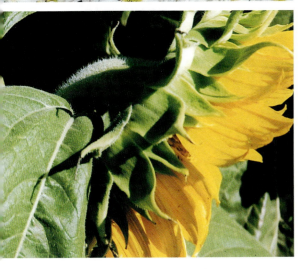

Plate 15
Sunflower (*Helianthus annuum*), Solano Co., CA. Note trichomes.

Plate 16
Alstroemeria hybrid (*Alstroemeria spp.*), Davis, CA.

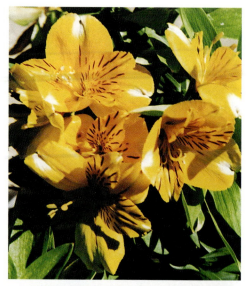

Plate 17
Cow parsnip, hogweed (*Heracleum lanatum*), Marin Co., CA.

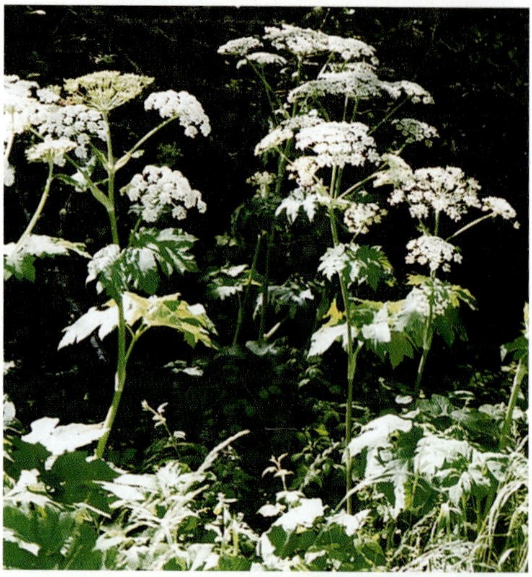

Plate 18
Pencilbush (*Euphorbia tirucalli*), Davis, CA.

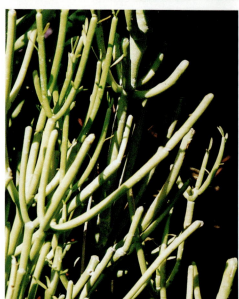

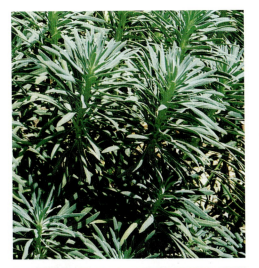

Plate 19
Euphorbia characias wulfenii,
Davis, CA.

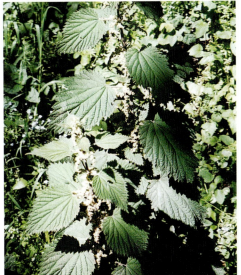

Plate 20
American stinging nettle (*Urtica dioica*), Marin Co., CA.

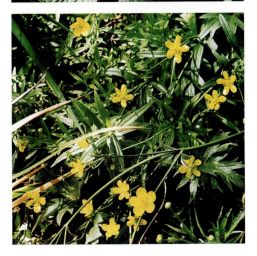

Plate 21
Creeping buttercup (*Ranunculus repens*), Yolo Co., CA.

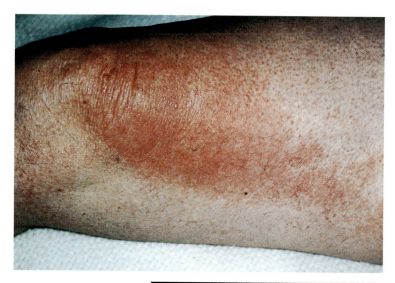

Plate 22
Poison oak ACD: The prodrome stage.

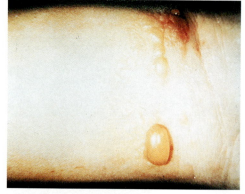

Plate 23
Poison oak ACD: The outbreak stage.

Plate 24
ICD caused by *Euphorbia characias wulfenii*.

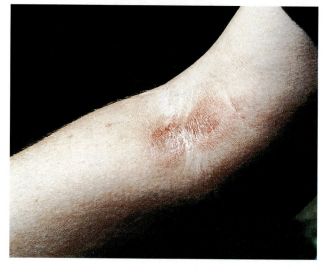

Outside the Anacardiaceae, examples include the rash on a woman's neck in the shape of the rosewood cross she wore on her necklace (Benezra et al., 1985) and the hand dermatitis suffered by a dairy farmer who milked cows pastured in a meadow rich in plants of the Asteraceae. Allergy to latex rubber gloves is most often seen in health care providers, but it also can occur in anyone who contacts latex products such as baby-bottle nipples, contraceptive diaphragms, condoms, or toy balloons (Rietschel and Fowler, 2001). Allergy to fragrance chemicals often appears in children, who develop it from the perfumes and cosmetics worn by overaffectionate relatives.

8.5   Individual Characteristics

It may seem by now as though contact dermatitis is inescapable. However, most exposure and its consequences are highly individual and rely on age, occupation, locale, and many other variables. Occupation is a prime factor, especially for high-risk jobs such as florist, gardener, baker, woodcutter, or outdoorsman (Guin, 2000). Section 8.2 and table 8.1 summarize the dermatotoxic plants and plant products associated with various occupations or activities, and a recent book addresses the subject (Kanerva et al., 2000).

The reduced incidence of *Toxicodendron* allergy in the elderly may be due largely to lack of exposure, and infants escape for the same reason (Rietschel and Fowler, 2001); see further discussion in section 9.7. Poison oak and its relatives remain the principal source of ACD in North American children over age three. Buttercups (*Ranunculus* spp.) and other meadow plants are high on the list of irritants, and *Heracleum* and citrus oils lead in phototoxicity. This is not to say that babyhood is free of risk from plant products: The perfumes and cosmetics of caregivers can rub off, and analgesic salves, chewing gum, and candy are all rich in allergenic essential oils. Balsam of Peru, a frequent sensitizer, is present in many baby products and nonprescription skin medications, and a quarter of older children remain allergic to it (Fregert and Möller, 1963). Skin color seems to make little difference (DeLeo et al., 2002), but susceptibility to ACD is increased by moisture (including sweat), and some types of phototoxicity require moist conditions.

8.6   Cross-Reactions

Medical tests on the skin provide a unique form of exposure. A patch test (section 9.2) is the most common tool of dermatologists in seeking the source of an allergy. A dilute solution of the suspected allergen is applied to a small area of skin in a standardized way, and any resulting dermatitis is scored between 48 and 96 hours later. This has largely replaced the more qualitative test where leaves of suspect plants were placed directly on sensitive skin (Adams and Fischer, 1990).

Patch test results must be interpreted with careful regard for the individual's history of exposure, because cross-reactions are common. In a cross-reaction, a different but structurally related allergen, from perhaps a completely different source, provokes an allergic response in a sensitized individual (Benezra and Maibach, 1984). Chemicals of similar structure, size, and K_{ow} often have about the same effect, regardless of their source. By definition, different urushioids can cross-react—a person sensitized to one becomes allergic to the others, making such interesting cross-reactive partners as poison ivy and philodendron!

Important and useful as they are, patch tests present the risk of a potentially sensitizing exposure that might cause an otherwise unexposed individual to become allergic. According to Benezra et al. (1985), two dermatologists each accidentally sensitized all their patients to the primrose allergen, primin, by testing it at too high a concentration. Psoriasis, scarring, and powerful allergic reactions are other potential responses to an excessive dose. For additional discussion, see section 9.2.

Composites and other lactone-bearing plants likewise tend to stand in for each other's allergenicity: Quinone-containing species, from primroses to tropical hardwoods, also behave this way, and so cross-reactions occur among balsam of Peru, cinnamon, cloves, orange peel, and vanilla (table 8.7). However, the oils of geranium, ylang ylang, and lavender used in perfume and soap cannot be said to cross-react because they contain the *same allergen*—geraniol. In other instances, the seeming lack of cross-reactivity is surprising, for example, among different species of *Grevillea* and between urushioids and the alkenylquinones and hydroquinones of, say, *Phacelia* (Benezra et al., 1985).

Table 8.7 Cross-Reactions to Balsam of Peru

Allergen	Typical Source
Benzyl benzoate	Insect spray, nail polish
Cinnamon (cinnamaldehyde)	Baked goods, chewing gum, colas, toothpaste
Cloves (eugenol)	Candy, chewing gum, linament, mucilage (stamps), soap
Gum benzoin (cinnamates)	Cosmetics, inks, medications, throat lozenges
Orange oil (terpenes)	Baked goods, candy, citrus, marmalade, sherbet, soft drinks
Resorcinol benzoate	Plastics (sunglasses, steering wheels, ballpoint pens)
Rosin (abietic acid)	Chewing gum, cosmetics, glue, ink, linoleum, paper, tape
Tea tree oil (limonene)	Cleaners, toothpaste, soap, body lotion, deodorant
Vanilla (vanillin)	Baked goods, ice cream, perfume, soft drinks, tobacco

Data from Benezra et al. (1985) and Rietschel and Fowler (2001).

The significance of cross-reactions in exposure is evident in table 8.7. Originally sensitized to balsam of Peru, the infants mentioned before were actually sensitized to a mixture of specific chemicals and in the future would respond to *any* of them. Thus, they will react to any item on the list and many more! Although most of the small victims will outgrow their allergy—only 6% of adults are allergic to the balsam—the others are doomed to react forever to everyday items the rest of us accept as harmless. In other words, they already have been sensitized to substances of which they are completely unaware and perhaps have never encountered before.

8.7 Economic Significance

Poison oak, poison ivy, and most other *Toxicodendron* species are economic losers. Their effects cost citizens millions of dollars annually in lost work time; in California alone, up to 5000 cases of occupational dermatitis from poison oak are reported each year (Epstein, 1994), and losses elsewhere from poison ivy must surely be as great. In Washington state, dermatitis due to vegetation was responsible for over 8% of all workers compensation claims for 1990–97 (Zug and Marks, 1999), and plant dermatitis in California's agricultural workforce amounted to 52% of compensation claims in 1978–83 (O'Malley and Mathias, 1988). Few occupations really win.

However, toxic Anacardiaceae species do have a few economic features in their favor. *Toxicodendron* sap provided the lacquers and dyes for Oriental bowls for over 3000 years (plate 1), and by 1900, annual production reached over a million pounds from the Japanese lac tree (*T. vernicifluum*) alone, with additional amounts from *T. succedaneum* in India and Southeast Asia. The trees generally are grown in plantations, tapped by V-shaped grooves cut into the trunk in the same way rubber latex is collected, and the gray translucent sap is held in small bamboo tubes (Casal, 1961).

Stored away from light and air, this liquid can remain unchanged for years, but when painted in thin layers on the surface of a bowl, it polymerizes to a black film that is the hardest and most durable of all natural organic coatings (Kumanotani, 1983). A well-cured finish is not toxic, but raw or poorly cured resin is highly caustic and allergenic. So is the dye made from the poison ivy and poison oak that is used in Native American folk art. Authentic oriental lacquerware has become highly prized in Western markets, and although the use in Native American basketry is still small, a resurgence of interest in it might literally put this cottage industry "in the black." In both cases, the lingering danger of ACD demands thorough curing.

Cashew (*Anacardium occidentale*) is one of the most important export crops of the tropics (Prodi et al., 1994). The nuts are a prized food, and the oil (CNSL, section 3.2) is used in plasticizers and lubricants. World production of cashew nuts, grown largely on plantations in India, Brazil, and Africa, exceeds 1 million tons and is worth over $350 million; the 70,000 tons of CNSL is valued at an additional $10 million. The cashew "apple" contains 18–27% CSNL, primarily anacardic acids and phenols (see section 5.7), and, needless to say, the oil is highly allergenic and a serious hazard during both production and utilization. However, the raw nuts also can have a health impact: An epidemic of ACD in Pennsylvania was traced to Little Leaguers who had sold hastily roasted nuts (Marks et al., 1984).

As for other dermatotoxic plants, the market in cut flowers—Peruvian lilies, chrysanthemums, tulips, daffodils—is large and lucrative, despite the hazard to anyone who handles them. The same is true for common houseplants such as philodendron, ivy, variegated croton, and various euphorbs. Although the spice market is not as profitable as it once was, that for essential oils and flavor ingredients continues to grow, as does the multi-billion-dollar fragrance industry. Even though some say the best hardwood trees have been harvested, interest in exotic woods remains high, and the use of citrus and pine oils in cleansing products has increased sharply.

Despite the high value of the land, the difficulty, expense, and hazards of clearing it when it is infested with allergenic species must be added to its cost. This applies especially to poison oak and poison ivy, but Florida holly and poisonwood (*Metopium*) in Florida and, Christmasberry in Hawaii present similar problems. Similar hazards from forest trees harboring *Frullania*, phototoxic cow parsnips (*Heracleum*), and Asteraceae species that cause weed- and meadow-dermatitis cannot be ignored, either.

8.8 Limiting Exposure

Unless one is a hermit on a desert island, there is no way to be absolutely safe from allergenic and irritant plants—and perhaps not even then. However, Epstein (1990) lists four ways to minimize exposure to poison oak and poison ivy that can extend to most other noxious species: avoidance, protection, destruction, and immunization, in order of increasing futility (but bioavailability and *laissez-faire* must be included, too). They are discussed in more depth in chapter 10.

Avoidance

Avoidance provides the best and surest course, but not necessarily the easiest. Irritant or allergenic plants are widely distributed in temperate climates. Their variable form can make quick identification difficult, but universities and extension offices in many states provide informative booklets that describe the worst of them (DiTomaso and Lanini, 1996). For example, useful guidebooks such as *Poisonous Plants of California* (Fuller and McClintock, 1986) are available at bookstores. Unless you already are familiar with the toxic plants around you, some investigation is advisable, and it is preferable to have someone actually point out the plants to you. Learn to spot them—make it a game, if you like—and to stay away.

Allergenic plant products are another matter. They now form part of modern life (tables 8.3 and 8.6) and are found everywhere. If you are prone to skin rash, try to define the causes (with medical help if necessary) so exposure can be minimized. This book is meant to help as well.

Destruction

Destruction is not as simple as one might think. Toxicodendrons, for example, are relatively insensitive to most herbicide treatments, particularly because their rather waxy foliage can be difficult for spray to penetrate. Using the proper chemical and formulation are very important, but DiTomasi and Lanini (1996) list three other factors that control herbicide effectiveness: appropriate growth stage of the plant, adequate spray coverage, and correct herbicide concentration.

So far, glyphosate (also called Roundup) seems to provide the best chemical control. I have had satisfactory results from applying an aqueous spray containing 4 ounces of 48% glyphosate concentrate and 1 ounce of liquid detergent per gallon of water—that is, a 1.6% glyphosate solution—on poison oak foliage to the point of runoff. Leaves must be fully expanded (April–June in Northern California), just before or while the plants flower. Certain plants may only be stunted and will resprout, so spraying becomes a regular spring task—the plants will be largely eradicated within several years. Despite the great temptation, spraying at other times of year is almost useless, and birds will see to it that seeds are redistributed unless the shoots are sprayed *before* the fruit is ripe.

Glyphosate is considered safe for people and wildlife (EPA, 1993), but it is very toxic to other plants, so spray must be closely controlled. It is absorbed only through the foliage and is inactivated by soil, so it is not environmentally persistent. Of course, the common precautions that apply to any pesticide spraying should be observed: *Read and obey the instructions on the label.*

Another toxicodendron killer is trichlopyr (Garlon), usually sold as a 0.7% aqueous solution or 8% concentrate of its amine salt. It, too, is safe when used as directed by the label and with adequate eye protection (EPA, 1998). The most effective ester formulation of 2,4-D and 2,4,5-T is no longer available, and its replacement, a dilute mixture of 2,4-D, MCPP, and dicamba, does not work against poison oak in my experience. Most other kinds of plants absorb this group of herbicides directly from soil as well as from foliage, so only limited spot treatments can be recommended in any case.

Herbicides like glyphosate serve for small areas and spot treatments, but they may be impractical for clearing large areas. However, goats offer a very effective large-scale alternative (Spurlock et al., 1980): They will eat almost any kind of vegetation, and they remain unaffected by the allergens. (Contrary to popular belief, they do not eat tin cans—only the labels.) In California, at least, some herdsmen rent out their goats for brush removal, because the animals actually like the plants, and the allergens are not transferred to the goat's milk (Kouakou, 1991).

Digging or cutting poison oak and poison ivy plants is dangerous and only marginally effective. If even one small rhizome is missed, it will soon sprout again. Also, the root system often is extensive, so removing plants from one spot only causes them to emerge nearby. Even with protective clothing, contact with the sap is almost inevitable, and, in larger stems, the sap is under enough pressure that droplets fly all over when the cut is made. Cut brush is still very toxic, even when leafless, and should be buried or piled away from human contact and allowed to decompose. Considering the potential lethality of smoke inhalation, *under no circumstances* should allergen-containing brush be burned intentionally.

Protection

Physical barriers are fairly effective—and strongly advised—but are far from foolproof. Long trousers, a long-sleeved shirt, and a hat provide a good start. Wash them often, preferably with bleach; wipe or wash tools with dilute bleach, dry, and oil them; wear gloves, plastic rather than rubber, and treat them with bleach afterward. Spots of sap turn black with this treatment.

Several barrier lotions are available: Ivy Block and Oak-N-Ivy Armor are two. Wash the barrier off in cool water every few hours and apply a new batch. Simply washing exposed skin, even with soap, is not very effective unless done immediately—most of the allergen already has penetrated the skin within a few minutes—but even plain water may be better than nothing. I have found the petroleum emulsion called TecNu to be effective in removing the allergen even hours after exposure. More details on prevention are provided in chapter 10.

Bioavailability

For a substance to be toxic, it must survive skin penetration and degradation so as to be available at the site of action. Biotransformation (metabolism) in the skin is a major determinant of bioavailability, but no data exist for *any* major dermatotoxic plant constituent except a rather minor flavoring agent, methyl salicylate (Bronaugh et al., 1999). Although it seems reasonable that reactive urushiols, laccols, quinones, and phorbol esters should be converted enzymatically to nontoxic metabolites (section 1.4), there still is no published evidence for that, so it is better not to rely on biodegradation. Take every reasonable precaution to keep away from dermatotoxic substances in the first place.

An Alternative

Still another approach in dealing with poison ivy and poison oak is to follow the adage: "Leaflets three, *let it be*." Birds and small animals like these species, they provide summer forage for deer and have pretty fall foliage, and the prospect of trying to eradicate a solid acre of "the poysoned weede" is daunting. My property once claimed a poison oak vine that climbed 40 feet into a tree and had a trunk over 8 inches across at the base. While I struggled to eradicate the smaller surrounding plants, the "big one" was protected as a prized specimen. It died.

8.9 Conclusions

Exposure to urushioids, sesquiterpene lactones, and other plant allergens and irritants is remarkably widespread, both directly by contact and indirectly through contaminated clothing, tools, pets, and especially via hands. Human susceptibility varies with occupation, age (less in the elderly), and lifestyle, but apparently not with race. Cross-reactions add to the problem. Eradicating offending plants with herbicides or goats is effective on a small scale, but digging, cutting, or burning is always risky. Protective clothing, plastic gloves, and barrier lotions help sensitive people, but the best strategy is to learn to recognize sources of trouble and to stay out of the way.

Table 1.1 listed the most dangerous dermatotoxic plants, most of which are avoidable. However, exposure to dermatotoxic plant products in the form of citrus oil cleaners, fragrances such as lavender oil, skin care products containing tea tree oil, homemade herbal remedies from arnica or chamomile, flavorings such as cinnamon oils, latex rubber, and even peppermint-flavored toothpaste is now so widespread that it may simply have to be endured.

NINE
ADVERSE EFFECTS

"Poison ivy does not spare age, sex, color of skin, or race."
—*Alexander A. Fisher, 1986*

"Only God can make a tree, but almost anything can make a rash."
—*Donald M. Vickery, 1990*

9.1   Intoxication

Intoxication means poisoning, and it is not restricted to alcohol. In the usual intoxication process (section 1.6), a substance absorbed through a body surface enters the bloodstream, circulates to a distant site of action, often metabolically activated or deactivated along the way, and finally interacts with some specific biochemical target to elicit an effect considered adverse.

Dermatotoxic substances may behave somewhat differently. They usually act directly on subsurface cells close to the point of exposure, and even the more complicated immunological processes they often initiate lead to the same end: a release of pharmacologically active substances such as histamine that produce the symptoms of contact dermatitis.

9.2   Penetration

The dermatotoxic chemical must be absorbed before any action can occur. Section 1.4 showed that this absorption is related to uptake of the chemical into fat, as measured by a partition coefficient, usually K_{ow}. However, absorption is an equilibrium process, whereas penetration is the *rate* at which a substance moves through successive layers of the skin, allowing for removal by binding and metabolism, before entering the bloodstream and eventually the urine (fig. 9.1).

This movement, often termed transport, usually occurs by simple diffusion, the rate being governed by Fick's law as applied here to skin penetration (display 9.1):

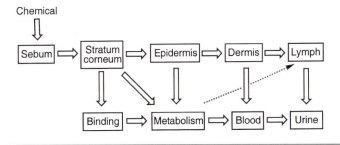

Figure 9.1 Path of a chemical from skin surface into urine.

$$dQ/dt = (D \cdot K_P) \cdot \Delta C/h = K_{perm} \cdot A \cdot \Delta C \qquad\qquad 9.1$$

That is, the quantity of chemical penetrating during a unit of time, called the mass transfer rate (dQ/dt), can be equated to the difference in concentration ΔC across a membrane of thickness h, multiplied by a constant (the diffusion and skin-vehicle partition coefficients, D and K_p). It can also equal the product of a so-called permeability coefficient, K_{perm} (the rate of movement in cm/hr) and the concentration difference across a barrier of area A. The rate depends on the temperature and degree of hydration, supporting the observation that one is more likely to contract dermatitis if one is warm and sweaty rather than cool and dry.

Although less than 20 μm (1/10,000 inch) thick, the stratum corneum (SC) presents the main barrier, so penetration through it mirrors that through the whole skin. The outermost surface of the SC normally is coated with a film of water-repellent sebum, beneath which lies dead, horny keratin (fig. 1.2). This protein is partially hydrated, but its interstices are filled with lipid, so two means of transport through the SC are available—one aqueous (hydrophilic) and the other through fat (hydrophobic). More water-soluble compounds such as cinnamaldehyde move via the protein surface, whereas fat-soluble ones like urushiol diffuse through the interstices.

The preference of a particular chemical for one or the other route changes abruptly near a K_{ow} of 2.4 (fig. 9.2; Roberts et al., 1977). The epidermis and dermis provide easy access to the capillaries for substances of moderate K_{ow} but increasingly inhibiting that of more hydrophobic substances. Figure 9.2 refers to the penetration of a series of phenols, but neutral substances such as aliphatic and aromatic alcohols give almost the same results.

A different approach (Roberts et al., 1995) takes into account the hydrogen bonding of the penetrant to SC protein (measured by α and β) as well as its molecular size (measured by the volume, V; display 9.2), where K_{perm} is the permeability from display 9.1.

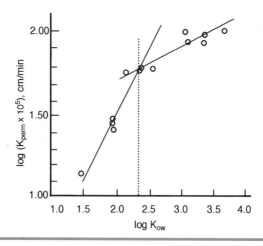

Figure 9.2 Relation of K_{ow} to the penetration of skin by phenols. Data from Roberts et al. (1977)

$$\log K_{perm} = 0.020V - 1.37\alpha - 4.5\beta - 1.35 \text{ cm/hr } (N = 24, r^2 = 0.93) \qquad 9.2$$

The dual polar-nonpolar pathway is thus replaced by one that is only aqueous. A review of this process has been provided by Pugh (1999).

Beneath the SC, the highly hydrated epidermis resists penetration by nonpolar chemicals such as DDT and urushiol that have a very large K_{ow}. For our purposes, it may not matter. The epidermis is also the seat of contact dermatitis, where such substances are made reactive by metabolism and bind to epidermal Langerhans cells, ACD and ICD are initiated (section 1.6), and symptoms appear. Below that, the collagen-rich dermis allows even moderately hydrophobic allergens to enter its capillaries and be disposed of eventually in the urine.

The data for figure 9.2 came from sheets of skin removed from the human body. What about penetration through *intact* skin? In rats, the total amount of penetrated chemical, as measured in urine, reflects the amount originally in the SC (Rougier et al., 1983), but there is no consistent relation between results in rats and those in man (Feldman and Maibach, 1970). This should not be surprising, as skin permeability varies greatly according to species, body locus, age, gender, and skin condition; the skin of a 71-year-old man was seven times more permeable than that of a 25-year-old. Although no penetration data were found for dermatotoxic plant constituents, observation indicates that most of them penetrate skin—at least the SC—rather rapidly, because the symptoms of dermatitis often appear within minutes or at most a few hours after exposure.

9.3 "Toxicity"

Previous chapters referred to the "toxicity" of urushioids, lactones, and other dermatotoxic chemicals. Although this certainly is not incorrect, dermatitis is not commonly part of the definition of toxicity, which is more often associated with systemic poisoning due to an interference with some key biochemical process (section 1.6). Poisoning may be fatal, but this is seldom the case with skin-applied allergens or irritants. However, dermatotoxic agents may still be toxic in the usual sense: For example, poisoning of the kidneys (nephrotoxicity) has been reported in people suffering from poison oak dermatitis and was fatal in at least one instance.

Acute toxicity refers to the harmful effect of a single dose of a chemical. In the standard assay for acute toxicity in mammals, groups of laboratory animals (normally mice, rats, or guinea pigs) are given increasing doses of a toxicant, the number of dead animals counted after a day or two, and the mortality graphed at various dose levels. The median lethal dose, the amount in milligrams of toxicant per kilogram of body weight required to kill a *statistical* 50% of the test species, is termed the LD_{50} (table 9.1). The lower the LD_{50}, the greater the liklihood of toxicity. Dosing may be by mouth (oral), injection into a vein (intravenous, i.v.) or abdominal cavity (intraperitoneal, i.p.), or application onto the skin (dermal). Injection avoids losses due to faulty absorption or intestinal metabolism and gives the lowest LD_{50}, but it is also the least realistic.

Dosing male mice i.p. with poison oak extract containing 6.8% urushiol II, 10.2% urushiol III, and 83% urushiol IV (but surely mostly laccols, as

Table 9.1 Acute Oral Toxicity of Some Plant Allergens and Irritants

Chemical	Animal	LD_{50} Dose (mg/kg)	Reference
Allyl isothiocyanate	rat	339	Jenner et al., 1964
Benzyl benzoate	rat	2800	Opdyke, 1973
Benzyl cinnamate	rat	3280	Opdyke, 1973
Cinnamaldehyde	rat	2220	Jenner et al., 1964
Citral	rat	4960	Jenner et al., 1964
Eugenol	rat	2680	Jenner et al., 1964
Helenalin	mouse	150	Witzel et al., 1976
Podophyllotoxin	rat (i.p.)[a]	15	Phillips et al., 1948
TPA[b]	mouse (i.v.)[c]	0.31	Sweet, 1987
Urushiol	mouse (i.p.)[a]	74	Murphy et al., 1983
Vanillin	rat	1580	Jenner et al., 1964
Xanthotoxin	rat	791	Apostolou et al., 1979

[a]Intraperitoneal injection. [b]Tetradecanoylphorbol acetate. [c]Intravenous injection.

shown in table 5.1) gave a 14-day LD_{50} of 74 mg/kg (Murphy et al., 1983), in the moderately toxic category along with many common drugs and insecticides. However, dosing rats orally with 4 mg/kg three times a week for 24 weeks produced neither gross nor microscopic lesions and no damage to the kidneys, although the dose was proportionately far greater than any human would ever receive. Most of a group of sensitized human volunteers that received a total of up to 300 mg of urushiol orally over a 3–6 month period became hyposensitive (less sensitive), but almost all developed itching and skin rash eventually (Epstein et al., 1982).

Acute toxicities for a few plant allergens and irritants have been reported (table 9.1) and most were not particularly high. However, some results could be obtained only by injection because of the severe reaction to oral dosing; even a few drops of croton oil taken orally would be enough to cause blistering of the mouth and violent evacuation of the bowels.

9.4 Symptoms of Contact Dermatitis

The most obvious and alarming aspect of being around allergenic and irritant plants must surely be the symptoms of contact dermatitis. They take the form of allergic contact dermatitis (ACD), irritant contact dermatitis (ICD), contact urticaria (CU), and phototoxicity (table 9.2).

Allergic Contact Dermatitis (ACD)

Captain Smith of the ill-fated Virginia Colony said it all: "reddness, itching, and lastly blysters," unless one is unfortunate enough to add a bacterial infection. However, the very first contact with the "poysoned weede" and its ilk produces few if any symptoms because the hapten is absorbed, activated, and combined with protein, thus setting in motion what is known as the sensitization stage.

Table 9.2 Comparison of Toxic Responses in Skin

Action	ACD	ICD	ICU	NICU	Phototoxicity
Affected area	diffuse (IV)[a]	local	diffuse (I)[a]	local	local irradiated
Sensation	itch	burn, sting	itch	itch	burn, pain
Symptoms	E, Ed, B[b]	E, P, V	E, Ed	E	E, Ed, B, H, V
Dose/response	independent	dependent	independent	dependent	dependent
Onset	delayed	rapid	rapid	immediate	delayed
Duration	a week	days	hours	minutes	months, years
Cross-reactions	yes	no	yes	no	no

[a]Allergy type. [b]B, bullae; E, erythema; Ed, edema; P, papules; V, vesicles.

The next contact *does* produce effects, but only after what McNair (1923) calls a "latency stage" of one to several days. The students at the University of California (section 8.2) showed latencies of 1–8 days (average of 3.5 days), although many people, including my wife and I, react within 24 hours and enter the "prodrome stage" of evident skin irritation, itch, and erythema. The lesions often appear first on the eyelids, forehead, ears, wrists, ankles, or other places where the skin is thin (plate 22).

Within a few more hours, the reaction reaches the outbreak stage (rash) and often does not go much beyond it, although the local increase in skin temperature (inflammation) and roughness (papules) may persist for several days (plate 23). However, in cases of extensive exposure, blood pressure goes up, breathing becomes difficult because of pulmonary congestion, and there is a sensation of fullness, headache, and disturbed vision. Inflammation and swelling (edema) increase, and blisters, skin eruptions (pustules), or bullae (large blisters) may appear. For one highly exposed, this stage can last up to several weeks and even require a trip to the hospital, although the disease seldom is life-threatening. Intense local exposure may lead to so-called black spot dermatitis in which a dark stain of oxidized urushioid appears on the skin—ICD imposed on top of ACD (Hurwitz et al., 1984). Other unusual symptoms have been summarized by Guin et al. (2000).

High concentrations of white blood cells (leucocytes) appear in the affected skin (McNair, 1923), and otherwise nomal urine may contain increased albumin. Contrary to popular myth, serum from the blisters is sterile and not allergenic—the disease is not contagious—but spreading unreacted surface urushiol to other parts of the body or to other people is likely unless the skin is thoroughly cleansed. Symptoms gradually subside, although the danger of microbial infection remains. In the "convalescence stage," a severely poisoned person still will not feel quite right for several more weeks, and skin rash may even return briefly. The stages overlap, and transition from one to the next may be nearly imperceptible.

The same general symptoms are produced by other urushioids, quinones, and lactones. Eating mango fruit commonly results in dermatitis on the chin and corners of the mouth in the unwary—a condition sometimes referred to as a Florida grin. Protoanemonin, the lactone from buttercups (*Ranunculus*), causes second-degree burns, blisters, and ulceration of the skin (Rudzki and Dajek, 1975). To escape service during World War I, some Italian recruits would apply crushed buttercups to their legs to produce gross-looking blisters (DeNapoli, 1917). Mayweed (*Anthemis cotula*) was observed to cause severe erythema and blisters on the arms, legs, and abdomens of agricultural workers pulling weeds in a California sugarbeet field (O'Malley and Barba, 1990).

Ordinarily, plant dermatitis is annoying and even temporarily incapacitating but not lethal. However, inhaling urushiol-laden smoke has proved fatal, and eating poison oak or poison ivy or even exposing the skin to them extensively has brought death from kidney failure (Rytand, 1948).

Irritant Contact Dermatitis (ICD)

The symptoms of ICD usually are very similar to those of ACD—redness, swelling, blisters, oozing—but they arise more rapidly and may not last as long. The distress caused by *Euphorbia* latex is typical. Morton (1982) describes the painfully caustic results of even brief contact with sap from the crown of thorns (*E. milii*), candelabra cactus (*E. lactea*), and pencilbush (*E. tirucalli*), all of them widely sold houseplants and ornamentals. In one instance, a Florida housewife's forehead barely touched a broken branch of a pencilbush, but although she washed immediately, she still suffered blisters for a week. In another, an arboretum worker carried garden trash containing cuttings of *Euphorbia characias wulfenii* in her bare arms and quickly developed a severe rash wherever the cuttings had rested (plate 24).

The eyes are in particular danger. A woman accidentally got latex droplets on her face, and within a half-hour she experienced swelling, intense burning in her eyes, and sinus inflammation (Morton, 1982). This was followed by chills and fever, loss of vision for 7 hours, and impaired sight for several days. A man planting *E. lactea* absently put his fingers to his mouth and later suffered inflammation and swelling of his lips, a burning tongue and eyes, and palate ulcers.

Not all euphorbs are that dermatotoxic. Table 9.3 lists the relative inflammatory potential (irritancy to mouse ears) of the latex from common euphorbs. Note that in the measure used in the table—the threshold dose for irritancy in half of the test animals (ID_{50})—the smaller the number, the greater the potency. One sees that pencilbush latex is 30 times more irritant than that of the crown of thorns but only half as active as latex of Canary Island spurge. Fortunately, extremely irritant species such as *E. poissonii* are not sold commercially (Cornell University, 1976) and even lack common names. Many contain superirritant resiniferonol esters (fig. 7.3) that are over 100 times stronger than the most irritant phorbol ester, TPA.

Perhaps the most striking toxic action of the irritant esters is their promotion of tumors, discussed in section 9.6. The irritants lyngbyatoxin A and the aplysiatoxins from marine and freshwater algae (so-called seaweed) are equally cocarcinogenic; see section 7.5.

Table 9.3 Proinflammatory Activity of *Euphorbia* Latex

Species	Common Name	ID_{50}[a]
E. canariensis	Canary Island spurge	0.9
E. coerulescens	Blue spurge	7.1
E. cooperi	Cooper's spurge	1.4
E. coralloides		0.5
E. cyparissias	Cypress spurge	1.6
E. helioscopa	Sun spurge	1.6
E. lactea	Candelabra tree	2.0
E. lathyrus	Gopher plant	4.5
E. milii	Crown of thorns	50.0
E. poissonii		0.1
E. resinifera	Euphorbium	0.2
E. tirucalli	Pencilbush	1.6
E. wulfenii (E. characias)		1.3

Data from Kinghorn and Evans (1975) from 51 species tested. [a]4-hour median irritant dose, μg/mouse ear.

Contact Urticaria (ICU and NICU)

Urticaria takes its name from *Urtica*, the nettle. Contact urticaria has two forms: immunological (ICU) and nonimmunological (NICU). Unlike ACD, the onset of ICU, complete with erythema and rash, occurs within minutes, and the symptoms are gone within a day except in chronic exposures. Such prolonged exposure is common among florists and plant propagators who handle tulips, Peruvian lilies (*Alstroemeria*), and some other ornamental plants, and it leads to "tulip finger"—painful, thickened, and cracked fingertips—whose symptoms can even spread to hands, arms, and face (Hjorth and Wilkinson, 1968).

Symptoms of NICU appear within seconds after contact and range from mild irritation to severe pain, swelling, and itching. Most people are acquainted with the unforgettable "sting" of nettles (*Urtica* species, section 4.2), a peculiar, almost instantaneous pain at the point of contact that sets one's teeth on edge to the point of nausea. Fortunately, the distress from most nettles is short lived, although Australian stinging trees of the genus *Dendrocnide* (*Laportea*) cause extreme pain that may last for weeks; pain peaks in the presence of moisture, as when taking a shower, and results in swollen lymph nodes under the arms and in the groin (Wrigley and Fagg, 1988).

An extreme form of contact urticaria is anaphylaxis, a Type I allergic reaction that involves not just the skin but other organs and sometimes the entire body. Symptoms often are felt within seconds or minutes of contact, and they start with flushing skin, itching, breathing difficulties, and generalized hives as a result of the sudden release of histamine and other mediators throughout the body (see section 9.5). Leakage of blood vessels may lead to anaphylactic shock, a drastic drop in blood pressure accompanied by rapid pulse, weakness, and unconsciousness, sometimes followed quickly by cardiac collapse and death. Although anaphylaxis is generally associated with food allergy and insect stings, rubber latex also has been identified as a culprit, and there is no reason there cannot be others.

Phytophotodermatitis

Ancient Egyptians applied the colorless juice of bishop's weed (*Ammi visnaga*) to return color to brown skin spotted white by vitiligo, an example of *phytophotodermatitis*. In another instance, a 1572 description of the folk medicine known as rue (*Ruta graveolens*) stated that "when it is in flower and one cuts it to preserve it in brine, it causes blisters and pimples on the hands and reddens them" (quoted in Murray et al., 1982). The symptoms of this type of phototoxicity—redness, swelling, and blisters—are very similar to those elicited by toxicodendrons, but they tend to appear immediately, do not involve the immune system, and do not appear until the dosed skin is exposed to sunlight.

In what has become a classic example, workers harvesting celery (*Apium graveolens*) may develop "celery itch" or "celery picker's disease," that is, erythema, vesicles, and bullae on hands and forearms from contact with celery juice (Birmingham et al., 1961). The symptoms are especially prominent where the plants are infected with pink rot fungus (*Sclerotinia sclerotiorum*), which causes a sharp increase in furocoumarin levels (Scheel et al., 1963) that is thought to be a defensive response (see section 4.1). Latex of the common fig (*Ficus carica*) produces not only blisters but also a dark pigentation that may last for years (Benezra et al., 1985), and even the ordinary limes used in cooking and drink mixing are severely phototoxic (DeLeo, 1992).

Weeds of the genus *Heracleum* (cow parsnip) are especially dangerous: Their furocoumarins produce not only giant blisters up to 2 inches (5 cm) across but also a similar long-lived pigmentation (Camm et al., 1976). Children playing among the plants, especially after meadows and roadsides have been mowed, can suffer tremendously if they were only scantily clothed, as is often the case in summer (Kavli et al., 1983; fig. 9.3).

In addition to phototoxicity, there is a related *photoallergic* dermatitis, an immune response produced only after the sensitized skin is subjected to sunlight. In practical terms, it differs from phototoxicity primarily in that sensitization must occur some days beforehand and the effects generally extend beyond the irradiated area. The symptoms of photoallergic

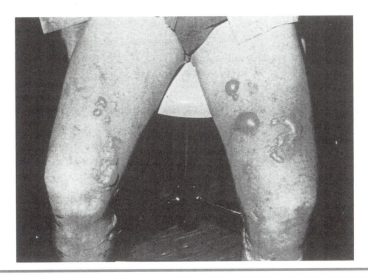

Figure 9.3 Phototoxicity of *Heracleum laciniatum* in a child. From Kavli et al. (1983), by permission of Blackwell Publishing Ltd.

dermatitis are the same as those of ACD, but the disease is uncommon and seldom due to plants or plant products (section 3.6). Epstein (1991) provides more information.

9.5 Mechanisms

Skin responds to foreign chemicals in several ways, each with its own sequence of events or mechanism. Although many types and gradations of effects are recognized by dermatologists (Marzulli and Maibach, 1991), we will discuss only the principal ones caused by plant constituents: allergic contact dermatitis (ACD), irritant contact dermatitis (ICD), immunologic and nonimmunologic contact urticaria (ICU and NICU, respectively), and phytophotodermatitis (table 1.4).

ACD

ACD is considered a true allergy, the body's immunologic response to a specific allergenic substance. This substance penetrates the stratum corneum and becomes metabolically altered, if necessary, to a more reactive form, such as when urushiol is oxidized to a quinone. The hapten then combines with membrane proteins of particular epidermal cells to form an antigen to which the body later reacts. Epidermal Langerhans cells (LC, fig. 1.2) have an especially strong affinity for small haptens and are considered essential for sensitization.

The protein reaction also may occur at the surface of epidermal keratinocytes (section 1.4), which then release biochemical messengers known as cytokines (Interleukins and TNF-α, for example) that generate cellular adhesives at the original point of contact to attract and bind inflammatory cells. Meanwhile, carrying fragments of the allergen, the hapten-activated LC migrate into the dermis by means of collagen-hydrolyzing enzymes, enter lymph capillaries, and migrate to nearby lymph nodes. There, they directly confront, and transfer the antigen to, specialized effector cells—the T-lymphocytes. During the next 7–10 days, these activated T-cells multiply, circulate in the blood, and home in on the inflammation site by recognizing adhesion molecules stimulated there by the keratinocytes' cytokines. The process is summarized in figure 9.4. Detailed reviews of the ACD mechanism are given by Kalish (1995) and Basketter et al. (1999).

Figure 9.4 The mechanisms of ACD and ICD, from exposure to symptoms

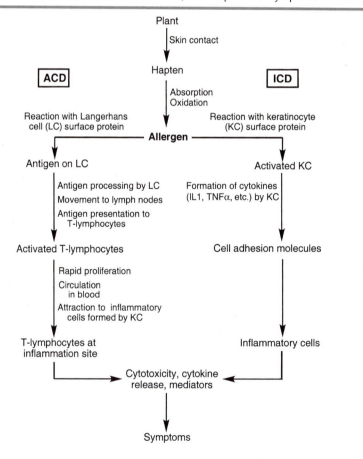

At this point, one is sensitized to the allergen but may be unaware of it, because there often are no noticable symptoms—yet. However, weeks, months, or years later, the *next* encounter with that particular allergen causes rapid T-cell proliferation and the release of inflammatory mediators such as histamine, serotonin, prostaglandins, and others that produce the inflammation, cytotoxicity, and cell destruction familiar to ACD sufferers. One now has a full-blown case of poison oak or poison ivy, that is, allergic contact dermatitis. Furthermore, urushioids cross-react, so that a person sensitized to, say, poison oak will react similarly to poison ivy, mango sap, or silky oak sawdust. STLs cross-react even more among themselves, but not with urushioids.

Even in a sensitized individual, all this may require several days between allergen absorption and allergic reaction, so the symptoms and their possible treatment are delayed; the term for the disease is delayed hypersensitivity. Some types of T-cells even act as supressor cells to reduce or deactivate the immune response, so it is the balance between suppression and activation that determines the severity of the dermatitis. Further, various subsets of T-cells, for example, so-called CD4+ and CD8+ lymphocytes, are now implicated in the allergic process, and Kimber and Dearman (2002) suggest that T-cell responses and mechanisms actually may vary, according to the specific chemical allergen and individual characteristics of the sensitized victim, in influencing the form and severity of the allergic reaction.

ICD

Like ACD, ICD starts with skin penetration by the irritant and its binding to some membrane protein of epidermal cells. However, in this process keratinocytes are the key actors. The stimulated cells liberate a number of proinflammatory cytokines leading to a dose-dependent, nonspecific attraction of leucocytes to the exposed area. Langerhans cells are involved very little, and the irritant does not induce the cytokine IL-1β necessary for their migration to lymph nodes. However, the final stage of ICD is the same as that of ACD: The histamine and other toxic agents released, and the erythema, edema, and lesions produced, are indistinguishable. In addition, ICD and ACD sometimes are superimposed (Hurwitz et al., 1984), and, at the very least, the way is paved for later ACD at the same site.

Esters of phorbol, ingenol, and resiniferonol are among the most powerful of all plant irritants (section 7.3), but their exact mechanism of irritancy is still uncertain. The vesicant effect is ascribed to activation of protein kinase C, a regulatory enzyme discovered in 1977 (Aitken, 1986). This enzyme catalyzes phosphorylation of the serine and threonine hydroxyl groups on proteins and in this way mediates neural and hormonal control over a wide variety of metabolic processes. The enzyme ordinarily is activated by Ca^{++} and also by diolein (glycerol dioleate, or diacylglycerol), which phorbol esters replace. The enzyme represents the phorbol ester receptor (Parker et al., 1984), but it is also activated by urushiol. Alkylation of membrane proteins by their Michael addition to phorbol's unsaturated ketone is another possible mechanism (Evans, 1986b).

Thus, phorbol esters not only promote tumors and platelet aggregation directly, but they also stimulate prostaglandin production, lymphocyte mitogenesis, interleukin (IL-2) release by T-cells, and degranulation of mast cells to release the histamine that produces inflammation (Aitken, 1986). Actually, there appear to be two separate phorbol ester receptors, one governing inflammation and the other tumor promotion. The evidence that urushiol, too, activates protein kinase C (Weissmann et al., 1986) offers an alternate mechanism of urushioid action.

ICU and NICU

Nonimmunological contact urticaria (NICU) is a common skin ailment. No prior sensitization is required, and the reaction can be caused by such diverse things as pine oil, turpentine, cinnamon, and balsam of Peru. The absorbed irritant causes an immediate release of inflammatory mediators, so the response is rapid, proportional to exposure, and soon over with. One need only suck on a piece of cinnamon candy to feel a mild NICU, the tingling sensation on the tongue caused by the irritant cinnamaldehyde.

A more extreme effect is caused by the needle-shaped calcium oxalate crystals (raphides) found in houseplants like *Dieffenbachia* (Araceae). The single crystals in *Tragia*, or noseburn, can be over 200 µm long, sharp at the upper end and blunt at the lower (Thurston, 1976). The 60–250-µm double-pointed needles of *Dieffenbachia* are suspended in bundles inside ejector cells at the surfaces of leaves and stems. It is thought that the raphides penetrate and rupture mast cells, which respond by leaking histamine and other mediators to elicit the observed symptoms.

In addition, the crystals are grooved lengthwise into an H shape to accomodate the movement of toxic cell constituents into the wounds they cause. Among the variety of irritants suggested to accompany the mechanical injury are histamine and other mediators, proteolytic enzymes, and polypeptides (Burrows and Tyrl, 2001), but the concentrated oxalate solution has been said to be toxic enough by itself to account for most of the unpleasant effects (Frohne and Pfänder, 1984). However, Fochtman et al. (1969) offer evidence that a trypsin-like proteinase and additional histamine are the active constituents of the irritant solution.

A nettle sting is different. Histamine and other bioactive amines are literally injected into the skin, causing an immediate triple response: a red spot due to enlargement of blood-filled capillaries, then inflammation from their increased permeability, and finally a welt (wheal) resulting from stimulation of nearby nerve endings. Itching, too, comes from the irritation of epidermal nerves, and pain from those in the dermis. The amines lead to the formation of diolein and thus activation of protein kinase C (Brown and Roberts, 2001). Part of capsaicin's painful effects may also be due to direct stimulation of histamine release (Monsereenusorn et al., 1982).

Immunological contact urticaria (ICU) is a Type I, IgE-mediated hypersensitivity reaction (section 1.6). Once through the epidermis, the hapten reacts with specific IgE antibodies on the surface of dermal mast cells, triggering a release of granules that contain inflammatory mediators. Typical haptens include menthol (from mint), rubber latex, perfume ingredients, spices, and a wide variety of common foods. For more information on all four of these mechanisms, see Basketter et al. (1999) and Gebhardt et al. (2000).

Phytophotodermatitis

This form of dermatitis depends on a combination of chemical and light. Many furocoumarins are phototoxic (section 7.2), and the flat, planar molecules are of the right size to intercalate (fit into) the double-stranded helix of DNA. Subsequent UV radiation causes formation of a cyclobutane (at A in display 9.3) by connecting the double bonds of the furocoumarin and a DNA base (thymine). This monoadduct irreversibly alters the DNA structure, and it also may lead to a similar subsequent *cross-linking* of two DNA strands via the furan double bond (shown at B) to form a diadduct. The resulting inhibition of DNA synthesis is slow but inevitable.

Thymine   Psoralen   Monoadduct   9.3

A second mechanism is more general. As mentioned in section 7.2, light absorption by furocoumarins, hypericin, and other phototoxicants generates singlet molecular oxygen that can react with key biomolecules such as unsaturated lipids in membranes and with protein amino acids. Both UV and visible radiation actually penetrate skin to a surprising depth; 300-nm radiation goes ~0.1 mm through the stratum corneum into the epidermis, whereas that at 400 nm reaches the dermis down to 3 mm and even the fatty subcutaneous tissue below that (Kornhauser et al., 1996).

Thus, when a phototoxic substance in the skin encounters sunlight, singlet oxygen forms in situ exactly where it can do the most damage. Disruption and leakage of membranes cause the swelling and blisters, and the redness and inflammation must result from the release of histamine and especially prostaglandins from injured mast cells and keratinocytes, although the exact mechanism is unclear (Kornhauser et al., 1996). Skin exposure is not required, and furocoumarin-containing foods such as celery cause phototoxicity by being carried to the skin in the bloodstream.

The related photoallergenicity has been ascribed to the photochemical transformation of the hapten into an allergen on or in the skin, or to the formation of an intermediate that can react with protein. From there, the course is that of a typical Type IV, T cell-mediated allergy, but it is too rare to be of much importance to plant dermatotoxicity (section 3.6).

9.6 Tumorigenesis

Unpleasant as acute ICD may be, chronic ICD can cause something far worse. Diterpene esters responsible for *Euphorbia* burns are most notorious for their tumor-promoting ability (Hecker, 1981); repeated or prolonged exposure may lead to skin cancer. A single low dose of carcinogen (initiation) does not produce tumors, but subsequent doses of a noncarcinogen "promoter" such as TPA does so. Achieving an initiating dose is not too difficult today, especially from the almost ubiquitous polycyclic aromatic hydrocarbons (PAH) from petroleum and coal as well as from irritation from mechanical or solar damage. Only minute doses of initiator and promoter are needed—μg levels of TPA will do—but the insult must be continuous or repeated (Kinsella, 1986).

Most promoters cause both irritation (inflammation) and cellular proliferation (hyperplasia), but not all irritants are promoters. Promotion starts with the induction of dark (basal) cells in the dermis of damaged skin and is followed by cellular proliferation. Phorbol ester promotivity is correlated with both, as well as with an increased synthesis of protein, DNA, phospholipid, prostaglandin, and other associates of protein kinase C (Kinsella, 1986). Fortunately, few plant constituents are promoters, and so far none are known to act in humans; the evidence is still primarily from the skin of tumor-prone strains of mice.

Sunlight itself is actually the major cause of nonmelanoma skin cancer, especially in those whose occupation (or recreation) involves being outdoors a lot (Epstein et al., 1990). Males with fair skin are most at risk, especially those of Celtic origin who sunburn easily. These tumors, too, can be promoted if the skin already is damaged (Urbach, 1991), most notably by furocoumarins such as xanthotoxin (8-MOP) and bergapten (5-MOP) in citrus oils. Mouse skin treated with either of these two did not produce tumors except in the presence of UV-A (365 nm), in which case the incidence exceeded 85% (Zajdela and Bisagni, 1981). Again, there is not yet enough evidence to say that the furocoumarins are photocarcinogenic in humans (IARC, 1986).

9.7 Sensitivity Differences

Common laboratory rodents—mice, rats, rabbits, and guinea pigs—can be sensitized to urushiol and develop a rash on reexposure if the hair has been removed. Shaved dogs, too, can be sensitized, for the hair seems to provide an effective barrier to skin exposure, and dogs can enter a poison oak thicket seemingly without harm. Birds, deer, cows, horses, and especially goats can even eat *Toxicodendron* fruit and foliage with impunity, something that would be disasterous for a human. Dairy cows deliberately fed substantial amounts of poison oak leaves showed no signs of distress (Kouakou, 1991).

In humans, there is some evidence that female skin may be more sensitive to irritants and allergens than that of males (Leyden and Kligman, 1977), and black skin may be somewhat more resistant than white or brown (McDonald, 1973), although DeLeo et al. (2002) could detect little difference. In any case, the variations are slight and perhaps are due in part to experimental difficulties such as estimating redness (erythema) in black skin. However, one thing is clear: People with light-colored skin, especially those from Northern Europe, are much more prone to photodermatitis than those whose skin is darker.

When it comes to age, infants are thought to have a low susceptibility to ACD, although Straus (1931) was able to sensitize 73% of 119 newborns. However, children become sensitive above age 3, and by age 12, most of them in this country already are sensitized to urushioids (Kligman, 1958). In a group of young people 21 ± 7 years of age, 61% reacted to poison ivy urushiols and another 31% became sensitized (Jones et al., 1973). ICD occurs at any age, as witnessed by diaper rash in infants exposed to fragrance chemicals in lotions and baby powder. Older kids tend to contract ICD from such things as buttercups, pine resin, and even some constituents of decongestant chest rubs, but this gradually improves after about age 8 (Fisher, 1986).

In fact, susceptibility to ICD and ACD declines with age, and although the elderly still suffer from airborne ragweed oleoresin and from photodermatitis due to dietary furocoumarins, skin contact with such menaces as urushioids and lactones is greatly reduced. Once lost, sensitivity is not regained, due, perhaps, to the general decline in immune responses with age

(Lejman et al., 1984; Kwangsukstith and Maibach, 1995). Skin anatomy also changes over one's life span, and although skin permeability stays the same from ages 20 to 55, it is down by a factor of four by 65 (Rougier et al., 1989). Contact dermatitis is controlled by genetics (Walker, 1967), but this subject still is not well understood. These factors, as well as genetic variability, existing skin conditions, occupation, and lifestyle, simply confirm our individuality regarding contact dermatitis.

9.8 Relation of Structure to Activity

Participation in the Michael reaction is thought to be important for ACD. Thus, for a urushioid to form the required antigen with cell-surface proteins, it would go through a quinone stage: It must be an oxidizable diphenol (catechol or hydroquinone) or be capable of metabolic hydroxylation to such a diphenol (e.g., 3-heptadecenylresorcinol from *Grevillea*).

To ensure skin absorption, a substance must be lipophilic, and a C_{13}-C_{17} side chain or other bulky group is optimal for phenols. Side-chain double bonds inexplicably alter allergenicity: Tests in human volunteers (Johnson et al., 1972) indicate that di- and triolefins such as urushiols III and IV are almost equivalent, over twice as active as the mono-olefin urushiol II, and over three times more active than the saturated form, urushiol I (fig. 9.5). Replacing the phenolic hydroxyl with methoxyl essentially destroys allergenic activity (Keil et al., 1944).

Alternatively, the allergen may already exist as a lipophilic quinone such as primin (2-pentyl-6-methoxybenzoquinone) or a substance such as

Figure 9.5 Relation of urushiol structure of allergenicity in human volunteers. Adapted from Johnson et al. (1972), by permission of Mosby Publishers

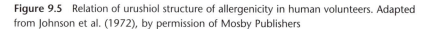

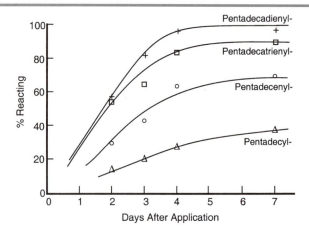

lapachenol that is convertible to one (fig. 6.1). The size of the lipophilic substituent can be as small as methyl (toluquinone) or as large as C_{18} (dietschequinone), but C_{11}-C_{12} seems optimal (Hausen et al., 1995). Quinones take part in Michael additions (display 9.4) in which protein amino groups react primarily at the 5-position and sulfhydryls (SH) at the 6-position (Liberato et al., 1981).

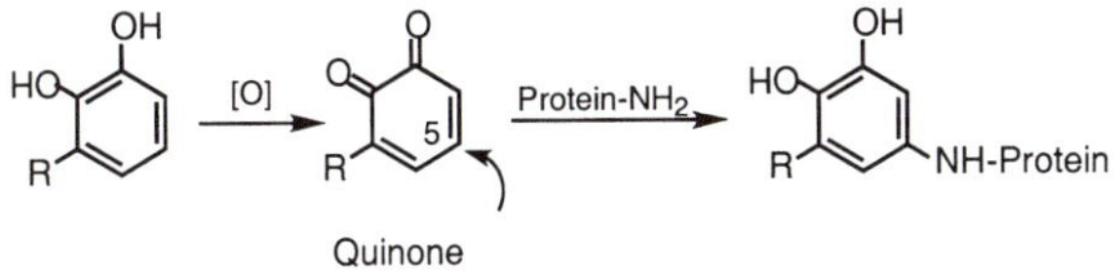

9.4

Quinone

Blocking these positions should preclude any reaction, chemical or biological. Among the 4-, 5-, and 6-methyl-3-pentadecylcatechols, the 4- and 6-methyl isomers were sensitizers in mice, but the 5-methyl was not (Dunn et al., 1982), indicating that amines play a major role in antigen processing. However, pretreatment of the mice with the 5-methyl isomer also suppressed sensitization by urushiol or laccol, whereas the 6-methyl analog was much less effective and the 4-methyl did not suppress at all. ACD-producing urushioids always have either an *o*- or *p*-ring position open; this location must influence substantially the action a particular allergen has in the broad range of ACD responses.

Sesquiterpene lactones are especially prone to Michael addition, and frullanolide (from the liverwort *Frullania*) is a good example. The arrow in display 9.5 shows the point of attack by the nucleophile.

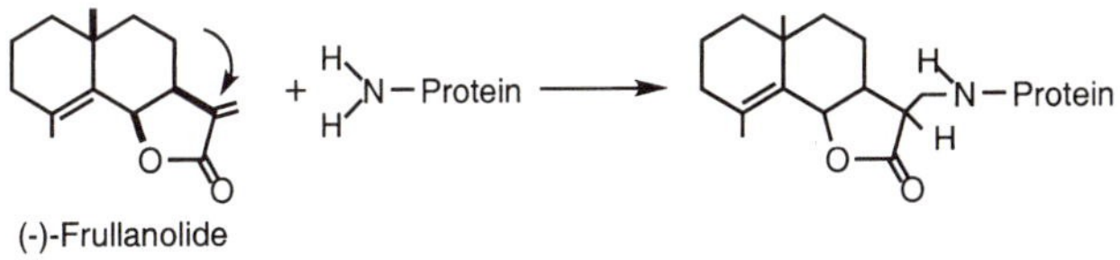

9.5

(-)-Frullanolide

Although natural lactones assume a wide variety of forms (fig. 6.3), the major structural requirement for allergenicity is the exocyclic double bond adjacent to the ester carbonyl (Mitchell et al., 1970). Although generally present, a long side chain or fused ring structure apparently is not essential to form a hapten; tulipalin A (display 9.6) contains a *total* of only five carbons.

However, the same is not true for cross-reactions. For instance, (−)-tulipalin B cross-reacts with tulipalin A but with neither its own (+)-isomer (Papageorgiou et al., 1988) nor any of the other STLs tested (Stampf et al., 1978); stereochemistry is all-important. Alantolactone and its isomeric isoalantolactone (display 9.6) differ in the location of a double bond but fully cross-react—a person sensitized to one is also sensitive to the other (Stampf et al., 1978). Parthenin cross-reacts with the similar damsin and coronopilin but not with its own optical isomer, hymenin (Picman et al., 1982). Similarly, the optical isomers of frullanolide do not cross-react (Barbier and Benezra, 1982) but do so with some unrelated STLs. There is some evidence for the importance of a *cis* configuration at the juncture of the lactone ring (Schaeffer et al., 1990), as shown by a lack of cross-reaction between *cis*- and *trans*-forms of the bicyclic lactone I (display 9.6), but data for allergic cross-reactions among the many examples of *trans*-STLs is lacking. Thus, there is still no unified structure–activity relation for STLs except the requirement of an α-methylene group.

Tulipalin A

Alantolactone

Parthenin, R = *trans*-OH
Hymenin, R = *cis*-OH
Damsin, R = H
Coronopilin = 2,3-dihydro-

cis-I

(-)-Tulipalin B

Isoalantolactone

trans-I

9.6

This steric specificity also is exhibited among the lichen substances. (+)-Usnic acid is a strong sensitizer, but its (−)-isomer is weak (Mitchell and Shibata, 1969; Salo et al., 1981). The chiral center is noted in display 6.11; X-ray crystallography shows the absolute configuration of (+)-usnic acid to be R (Huneck, 1981).

Many irritants are also allergenic, but not the diterpene esters from *Daphne* and *Euphorbia* (section 7.3). They do not appear to attach covalently to enzymes like protein kinase C (Evans and Edwards, 1987) but instead rely on their tertiary structure (display 7.4). Key dimensions of tiglianes, ingenanes, and daphnanes are virtually the same, but there are certain functional group requirements. An ester group at C-12 and/or C-13 in the tigliane series is essential for irritant and cocarcinogenic activity—ethers will not serve—and it is best if there are at least 10 carbons, as is the case with TPA (12-tetradecylphorbol 13-acetate). However, etherification or acylation of the C-20 hydroxyl *always* destroys irritant activity.

On the other hand, the widely distributed 12-deoxyphorbol esters (with no substituent at C-12) remain highly irritant, as do those of natural 4-deoxyphorbol, but a C-13 ester and C-20 hydroxyl are still required. Also, 16-hydroxy-12-deoxyphorbols exhibit skin irritant activity, and the unusual 12-deoxy-13-phenylacetate shows the highest activity of any 12-deoxy ester (Evans and Edwards, 1987). For more about the irritancy of other phorbol esters, see Schmidt and Evans (1980).

Despite a somewhat different three-dimensional appearance, the highly irritant ingenol esters (fig. 7.3) are still closely related to those of phorbol, the principal difference being the attachment of C-11 to C-10 rather than to C-9 and a conversion of the C-9 hydroxyl to a carbonyl (Schmidt, 1986a). Except for just a few instances, ingenol is esterified only on the 3-hydroxyl. The unusual orthoesters of the daphnane series (Schmidt, 1986a), such as the resiniferatoxins from *Euphorbia* (fig. 7.3), are notable for being the most irritant plant chemicals known. In irritant dermatitis, quantitative structure–activity relations (QSAR) for the skin corrosivity of 123 organic acids and bases (Barratt, 1995) and that for skin irritation by 52 neutral substances (Barratt, 1996) underline the key importance of physical and chemical properties such as acidity–basicity (pK_a) and K_{ow}.

Phototoxicity in coumarins is governed by the ability to absorb available radiation (such as sunlight) and to enter (intercalate) into and bind strands of DNA or RNA. A rigid planar structure is required, so simple or partially reduced coumarins are inactive. Alternatively or in addition, the absorbed energy may be transferred to oxygen to generate the very reactive singlet oxygen in situ, where it can do the most damage to cell constituents. Among furocoumarins, psoralen is the most phototoxic (relative activity 100; Musajo and Rodghiero, 1962); xanthotoxin is next at 38, followed by bergapten (28), angelicin (12), and isobergapten (10). Thus, the linear structures are far more phototoxic than are the angular ones (fig. 7.1), possibly because of their relative adaptability to intercalation.

9.9 Conclusions

Although all skin allergens and irritants are toxic to some degree, most show rather low toxicity via the mouth. Instead, they produce characteristic skin damage that may include redness (erythema), itching (pruritis), and eruptions that vary from rough skin (papules) to huge blisters (bullae). Symptoms can appear quickly, as is the case with irritation, or go through stages over a period of days as in ACD, but the end results are similar: The final stage always involves a release of mediators such as histamine from dermal or epidermal cells (or by direct injection from nettles), and it is they that do the actual damage.

The effects normally are temporary, although some forms of photodermtitis leave pigmentation that may last for years, and a few types of irritants such as phorbol esters and lyngbyatoxin A promote skin cancer. Although the relation of chemical structure to allergenicity and irritancy sometimes is obscure, the Michael addition reaction often is implicated. For phototoxicity, an ability to absorb solar radiation and slip between DNA strands or generate singlet oxygen remains important.

If, as the Vickery quotation states, "anything can make a rash," how is it that anyone escapes a continual case of dermatitis? First, with our increasingly urban and sedentary lives, many people never have an opportunity to be exposed to something like poison oak. Also, ACD and ICU require prior sensitization, so despite cross-reactions, it is possible to avoid the necessary second exposure. One's age, clothing, and environmental conditions also affect susceptibility, but skin rash of some kind indeed has become so commonplace that we may take little notice of it and certainly never associate it with plants.

TEN

"The long-standing effort to find an effective topical medication for acute poison ivy dermatitis is not one of the proud chapters in the history of medicine."
—*A. M. Kligman, 1958*

"The best prophylaxis for any type of allergic contact dermatitis is complete avoidance of the allergen."
—*Alexander A. Fisher, 1986*

10.1   Prevention and Treatment

This is the shortest chapter of the book, perhaps reflecting Kligman's view. However, there has been considerable progress since 1958: barrier lotions that minimize the contact of dermatotoxic substances with skin, measures to alleviate symptoms, and promising new treatments that could forestall the effects in the first place.

At this point, you should be able to recognize the principal plants and plant products that are toxic to skin, the routes of exposure to them, how they act, and what symptoms are to be expected. But how can those symptoms best be avoided? The ideal way is to avoid *any* exposure to the offending plants, contaminated tools, exposed pets, phototoxic foods, and so on. In reality, the sources are so diverse and widespread (tables 8.1 and 8.4) that even the best of intentions probably are doomed to failure. However, marked sensitivity to a particular type of plant usually can be detected through skin tests.

10.2   Patch Tests

If you have been hiking in poison ivy country and develop "reddness, itchinge, and blysters" a day or two later, you probably don't need a dermatologist to tell you that you have a toxicodendron allergy. However, the situation is seldom that simple—you could be mistaken and the symptoms are caused by something else—so skin tests are available to verify the type of dermatitis and perhaps the agent responsible. They include prick and scratch tests, scratch chamber tests, the RAST (radio-allergosorbent test), and several others, but by far the most common is the patch test. It is, of course, artificial in that it will not duplicate the original exposure conditions of temperature, dose, or duration, but it certainly is more reproducible, controllable, and scientific.

In the simplest test, the dermatologist or allergist tapes a small aluminum or plastic ring containing a highly diluted standard allergen to the upper back or arm, such that the substance is in contact with the skin. After two or three days, or a few minutes or hours for irritants, the "patch" is removed, the skin beneath it examined for a response, and the degree of response graded. Several subtances can be tested at the same time, but at least one nonallergic person, and perhaps several, should also receive the same allergen as a control.

Do not attempt this at home. Dosing and interpretation require professional experience. For example, a patch test for poison ivy is not advisable because of the danger of accidental sensitization of an unsensitized patient; after a few questions, the allergist may be able to diagnose this particular problem even without a test. One contemporary patch test kit is the TRUE (Thin-layer Rapid Use Epicutaneous) test, a convenient, off-the-shelf, standardized system that employs a film of allergen in a hydrophilic absorbent, which, on the skin, forms an allergen-releasing gel (Fischer and Maibach, 1989).

There are many standard allergens available for patch testing (Gebhardt et al., 2000), and there are kits representing groups of related allergens. Table 10.1 lists two such batteries of materials, one for people who regularly encounter plants (nurserymen, florists, gardeners, foresters) and the other for the general public who frequently react to the now nearly ubiquitous fragrance materials (section 8.3). Test allergens seldom cross-react, and they represent broad types the affected person might reasonably encounter. If no skin reaction is observed, other tests could be added or

Table 10.1 Standard Allergens for Patch Testing

Fragrances[a]	Plants[b]
2-Amylcinnamaldehyde, 1%	Arnica extract, 0.5%
Cinnamyl alcohol,* 1%	Chamomile extract, 2.5%
Cinnamaldehyde,* 1%	Dipentene (*dl*-limonene), 2%
Eugenol,* 1%	Feverfew flower extract, 1%
Geraniol,* 1%	Tansy extract, 1%
Hydroxycitronellal, 1%	Usnic acid, 0.1%
Isoeugenol,* 1%	Yarrow extract, 1%
Oak moss absolute,* 1%	

[a]Duus Johansen (2002). [b]Gebhardt et al. (2000). *Plant constituent.

higher test concentrations applied if it is considered safe to do so. Other examples include an STL mix, cosmetics mix, balsam of Peru, and a plant mix containing extracts of feverfew, chamomile, tansy, arnica, and yarrow (Gebhardt et al., 2000).

At times, application of actual plant material or product has been necessary when the standard allergen was unknown or unavailable. For example, leaflets of a suspect plant would be placed on the skin, or oleoresin extract from mature leaves, diluted with corn oil by 1:100 to 1:20,000, would be administered instead (Shelmire, 1941). Doing this may have significant adverse consequences: With poison oak, for example, a person who reacted to the equivalent of 500 μg of urushiol might be considered too sensitive to work in a forestry job (Epstein, 1990), or a fragrance allergy might require a change in one's favorite cosmetics. And does everyone react? In the case of poison ivy, about 61% of twenty-somethings did react and another 31% became eligible (sensitized), whereas a general survey of 24 common chemicals in over 30,000 Europeans showed that 10% of the subjects reacted to a fragrance mix, 7% to balsam of Peru, and 3% to colophony (Schnuch et al., 1997).

Patch tests are influenced by gender, age, and especially any history of previous exposures. For instance, a gardener long sensitive to poison oak could suddenly develop a rash after handling ladyslipper (*Cypripedium*) orchids, but a patch test might suggest only allergy to toxicodendrons unless the administering physician knew about the flowers. This is an example of a cross-reaction (section 8.6): Many allergens cross-react, including both natural and synthetic ones, so the exact source of allergenicity may be difficult and perhaps impossible to define (Benezra et al., 1985). Indeed, a person could respond to a plant he or she has never seen before, or several different allergies could be superimposed. Clearly, patch tests by themselves provide only general guidance in helping to avoid future allergic reactions.

10.3   Prevention

Even without the comfort of knowing to which specific allergens one is sensitive, it may be possible to ward off most skin damage with some form of general protection: a barrier, timely removal of the offending substance, immunization, or—most effective of all—avoidance of the cause. This subject was introduced in section 8.8 in relation to human exposure.

Reduced Contact

Complete avoidance of noxious plants is ideal but impractical for most people, so common sense must take its place. As one example, the ACD from primroses (*Primula* spp.) is caused simply by contact with trichomes on the flowers and stems and is largely preventable just by not stripping off dead blossoms with one's bare fingers. Alternatively, the chief culprit, a common *P. obconica* variety, could be replaced by newer nonallergenic forms such as 'Freedom,' 'Beauty,' or 'Libre' (Richards, 1993), or perhaps by another kind of plant entirely.

This careful choice of species actually allows one to have a low-allergen garden as described by Huntington (1998). The British Horticultural Trades Association (HTA) Code of Practice specifies safety labeling for plants grown for public sale, categorizes them according to the degree of hazard (table 10.2), and helps buyers avoid the most dangerous ones. The list is interesting both for what it includes (poison ivy) and what it does not (euphorbs, for example). In my experience as a gardener, California nurseries and florists have not yet taken up this laudable practice.

Table 10.2 Plants Listed as Allergenic or Irritant by the British Horticultural Trades Association

Category A. Sale should be discouraged[a]

Rhus radicans	Poison ivy
Rhus succedanea	Wax tree
Rhus verniciflua	Varnish tree

Category B. Warning required on plant and bed labels

Arum spp.	Black calla (example)
Daphne laureola	Spurge laurel
Daphne mesereum	February daphne
Dictamnus albus	Gas plant
Dieffenbachia spp.	Dumbcane
Primula obconica	Primrose
Ruta graveolens	Rue

Category C. Warning label required for less toxic plants

Alstroemeria spp.	Peruvian lily
Cupressocyparis leylandii	Leyland cypress
Dendranthema spp.[b]	Chrysanthemum
Echium spp.	Pride of Madeira
Fremontodendron spp.	Flannel bush
Hedera helix	English ivy
Hyacinthus varieties	Hyacinth
Lobelia tupa	Tupa
Narcissus varieties	Daffodil
Schefflera spp.	Umbrella plant
Tulipa varieties	Tulip

See Huntington (1998). [a]*Rhus* = *Toxicodendron*. [b]Called "chrysanthemum" in the United States.

Allergens seemingly are almost everywhere. There is even an account of a girl who contracted ACD on her bare legs merely from climbing a lichen-covered tree in her yard, proving the futility of complete avoidance. However, appropriate clothing, nonlatex gloves where warranted, washing hands and arms often, and especially learning to recognize the dangerous plants in your own surroundings will go a long way toward more comfort and safety.

Physical Barriers

This form of protection is moderately effective—and strongly advised—although it is far from foolproof. Long trousers, a long-sleeved shirt, and a hat or cap can provide at least an initial barrier. Experiments show that wool is the most effective fabric (it often reacts with and binds the allergen), but *any* clothing will probably be of some help. Of course, the clothes have to be washed and preferably treated with bleach after each exposure, and footware also should be washed or cleaned, especially shoe laces (which inevitably will be touched by hands).

Tools are best wiped down with dilute bleach, dried, and oiled; rinsing with rubbing alcohol is often suggested but still leaves a toxic residue unless a large volume is used, and disposal of the contaminated solvent then provides yet another means of exposure. The variety of exposure opportunities (tables 8.1–8.4) indicates why physical barriers are not uniformly successful.

A major source of exposure can be the sawdust formed during cutting or planing of various woods. Inhalation is easily remedied with a dust mask, and sawdust under one's ring or watch band is effectively avoided by wearing a long-sleeved shirt and removing any jewelry before working with the wood. Similar protection is called for when pruning or cutting silky oaks (*Grevillea robusta*), Christmasberry (*Schinus terebinthifolius*), or any other dermatotoxic woody species, when mowing a meadow or even a weedy lawn, or when pulling allergenic weeds in the garden. Lichens and liverworts, notably *Frullania* species, that adhere to tree bark cause woodcutter's eczema (lactone ACD), so it might be beneficial to wear gloves, long sleeves, and a hat even when cutting a Christmas tree.

Gloves do offer important protection, but they also provide hazards. For example, thin rubber (latex) gloves actually dissolve lactones and urushiols and conduct them directly to the skin beneath. Moderately heavy plastic gloves, the kind used for washing dishes, are better and can be rinsed with dilute bleach before removing them; leather work gloves are all right but hard to decontaminate; and even cotton gardening gloves are better than nothing if the hands first receive a barrier lotion and the gloves are bleached afterward. Contaminated gloves obviously should not be removed by unprotected hands or teeth, and the temptation to rub an itchy nose or wipe perspiration from one's brow with the gloved hands must be resisted.

It's also worth noting that many latex gloves are themselves allergenic, although efforts are being made to remove or deactivate the responsible proteins. A 1998 survey by Palosuo et al. (1998) showed that of 20 brands of surgical and examining gloves tested, over half had a low allergen content—Ansell and Baxter Ultraderm were among the best—whereas several others were on the high side.

Chemical Barriers

In recent years, several skin creams have become available that hinder an allergen's penetration. The subject has been reviewed briefly by Zhai and Maibach (2000), who provide examples of this kind of protection. For instance, preexposure treatment of the skin with polyamine salts of linoleic acid dimer afforded 70% protection in sensitive individuals, quaternary ammonium bentonite (clay) provided over 90% protection, and another organoclay preparation was 95% effective. Most proprietary protective lotions tested were less effective, although Hydropel, Stokogard, and Hollister Moisture Barrier reduced the incidence of toxicodendron dermatitis by about half (Grevelink et al., 1992).

In my experience, Ivy Block (Enviroderm Pharmaceuticals Inc., Louisville, KY) affords an effective barrier against poison oak and presently is the only one approved by the FDA. It contains bentonite clay to bind the allergens, whereas Oak-N-Ivy Armor (Tec Laboratories, Albany, OR) employs mineral oil and beeswax to dissolve and sequester them. The barrier must be washed off with cool water every few hours and then newly applied, but any sequestered allergen comes off with it. Another successful approach is to apply Tec-Nu (also from Tec Laboratories), a petroleum emulsion, *after* a possible exposure; it extracts the unabsorbed and uncombined allergen that is later washed away.

Immunization

ACD is an immune reaction, so protection of sensitive individuals by immunization theoretically should be possible. However, it has never become practical (Epstein, 1990). Some foresters and lacquer workers eventually become desensitized ("hardened") naturally, and Native Americans attempted desensitization by occasionally eating a small *Toxicodendron* leaf. However, many Caucasians also have tried the leaves, with either no result or, if enough were chewed, a serious case of internal poisoning (McNair, 1923). At one time, an extract of poison ivy allergen was available; it was to be swallowed daily in water, starting with a single drop and then regularly increasing the dose. Admittedly, 2 to 4 months of treatment were required for any benefit, and dosing had to be maintained to prevent a return of sensitivity (Epstein, 1990). With my hypersensitive son, a month of treatment resulted in a rash that covered most of his body.

Although protection against poison oak and poison ivy has received the most attention, the same products and principles apply equally well to most other plant allergens and irritants. Barrier lotions probably would not offer much protection against nettles, but clothes and the thicker kinds of gloves would.

10.4   Treatment: What Works, What Doesn't

Chapter 8 described the many ways in which one can become exposed to plant allergens and irritants. Avoidance or protection sometimes may be impractical, for example, when changing a tire on a weedy roadside, and an allergen-sensitive person's need to find something—*anything*—to alleviate the inevitable symptoms can be extreme. The most readily available help is also the least desirable: scratching. The intense itching is actually a sign that healing and the growth of new skin are already in progress, but even though abrasion may feel good at the time, it damages this tender skin, spreads any unabsorbed allergen, and opens the way for bacterial infection. The title of a popular booklet about poison oak treatment says it all: *Don't Scratch!* (Leite, 1982).

Washing contaminated skin with soap and water is of limited value unless it is done at once, because the skin absorbs up to half of many allergens within the first 10–20 minutes, and the spread of the rest of the allergens to nearby areas is a real danger. Therefore, although removal of excess allergen before it can do more damage is very desirable, the use of solvents such as alcohol or acetone still carries the danger that the poisons will spread—and who carries a bottle of solvent anyway? Still, even plain water may be better than no treatment at all, especially as first aid (Guin and Reynolds, 1980), and washing with a kerosene emulsion (Tec-Nu) literally extracts fat-soluble urushiols and other plant allergens off and out of the skin. This treatment has always benefited my wife and me, even hours after exposure.

Once a mild dermatitis has started, nonprescription hydrocortisone ointment to reduce the itching also works well for us, although a severe case would require the higher potency and professional judgment that only a physician can offer. A number of other over-the-counter products such as calamine lotion (primarily zinc oxide) sooth the itching, although *nothing actually cures the allergic reaction*. Local anesthetics such as benzocaine and topical (skin-applied) antihistamines must be used with caution, because they sometimes are sensitizers themselves (Fisher, 1986). Those that contain zirconium compounds may cause a form of tumor known as granuloma.

More serious cases of dermatitis, where blistering and swelling are severe, require the aid of a physician. Here, the goal is not only to make the victim as comfortable as possible but especially to avoid bacterial infection. Careful and sterile opening of blisters, cool boric acid compresses, antibiotics, and corticosteroid therapy for several weeks have been suggested (Fisher, 1986). The most serious cases may require a physician's administration of a steroid such as methylprednisolone (Medrol, for example), its acetate (Depo-Medrol), or a solution of its sodium succinate salt (Solu-Medrol); the ultimate step is hospitalization.

On the other hand, many traditional remedies such as poisonous wormwood (*Artemisia absinthium*), the irritant horsetails such as *Equisetum arvense*, camphor, baking soda, an ointment from castor oil and tobacco, or a paste of salt and vinegar once purported to cure the dermatitis (Horsfield, 1798). Combinations also were tried, for instance, a mixture of glycerine, tincture of iodine, carbolic acid (phenol), and morphine (DeWitt, 1874), but if they worked at all, which is doubtful, it was only because they themselves were powerful irritants. McNair (1923) lists over 300 supposed remedies (see table 10.3), many, such as mercury chloride, nitric acid, and *aqua regia* (nitric and sulfuric acids), that are truly frightening. Besides their immediately agonizing effects, some obviously produce long-term damage: For instance, the once-popular iron chloride binds to *Toxicodendron* catechols to form coordination complexes—and dark and long-lasting

Table 10.3   Some Traditional Remedies for Rhus Dermatitis

THESE TREATMENTS ARE NOT RECOMMENDED.

Ammonia water (ammonium hydroxide)	Monsel's solution (ferric sulfate in sulfuric acid)
Aqua regia (nitric and sulfuric acids)	
Baking soda (sodium bicarbonate)	Morphine sulfate
Bluestone (copper sulfate)	Nitric acid
Bromine in olive oil	Potassium chlorate
Butter	Potassium permanganate
Carbolic acid (phenol) in glycerine	Sal ammoniac (ammonium chloride)
Coffee	Silver nitrate
Corrosive sublimate (mercuric chloride)	Slaked lime (calcium hydroxide)
Cream and marshmallows	Sugar of lead (lead acetate)
Ferric chloride	Thornapple (*Datura stramonium*)
	Tincture of iodine
	White oak bark (*Quercus alba*)

Data from McNair (1923).

tatoos—whereas another old favorite, potassium permanganate, is toxic, irritating, and dyes the skin brown.

In her self-published booklet, Sandra Baker (1979) lists over 100 other folk remedies for poison oak and poison ivy, from alder bark and *Aloe vera* to yarrow and yerba santa. Hair spray, canned pineapple, and meat tenderizer are included "just for laughs," but several others have a long and distinguished history. Cornstarch and oatmeal help dry up fluid from broken blisters, alcohol or an extract of witch hazel (*Hamamelis virginiana*) feels cool on the rash, and a bath with Epsom salt (magnesium sulfate) likewise is soothing. If most of the others on her list may do little good, they also do little harm and might at least take your mind off your troubles.

Throughout history, treatments have been concocted from local wild plants. The leaves or juice of (mostly eastern U.S.) plants such as jimsonweed (*Datura stramonium*), bloodroot (*Sanguinaria canadensis*), goldenrod (*Salidago canadensis*), and jewel weed (*Impatiens biflora*) have all been prescribed at one time or another, and Native Americans in California painted on extracts of a sunflower (*Wyethia* spp.), manzanita (*Arctostaphylos* spp.), or gumplant (*Grindelia camporum* or *G. robusta*), as cited by Balls (1962). A popular current book on herbal medicine (Hobbs, 1998) recommends drinking an infusion of echinacea root (*E. purpurea*), or flowers of red clover (*Trifolium pratense*), elder (*Sambucus* spp.), or grindelia (*Grindelia* spp.) several times daily "to clear the blood." Although an aqueous extract of yerba santa (*Eriodictyon trichocalyx*) also is said to cure poison oak rash within a day or so, only jewel weed has received serious scientific attention (Guin and Reynolds, 1980). Unfortunately, it was shown to be ineffective.

A treatment recommended by Leite (1982) is known as the Miracle Method (after a park aide named Mike Miracle—no joke). It consists simply of taking a shower in water as hot as can be tolerated. (This is *not* recommended after blisters break and reveal tender new skin.) According to park ranger Leite, "the steaming spray completely satisfies the desire to scratch; the intensely hot water melts any remaining sap and carries it away before it can do further damage; and a forceful spray scrubs away dead skin while vigorously bringing healing oxygen to the area." It does seem to work, especially if some hydrocortisone ointment is applied soon afterward!

10.5 "Rational" Treatment

The term *rational* implies a scientific basis for the attempted cure (McNair, 1923). Most earlier treatments were based on, at best, a superficial understanding of the chemical properties of the allergens, the idea being to force a chemical modification that would provide nonallergenic products (chapters 5 and 6). For example, because catechols are readily nitrated or brominated, either nitric acid or a solution of bromine in olive oil were proposed as poison ivy treatments. Catechols also are easily oxidized, so potassium permanganate was a common treatment, and because phenolic hydroxyls combine with metals such as iron, bathing in a solution of iron chloride was particularly recommended by McNair (1923). These methods were actually used on real people, ignoring the serious damage to the rest of the skin, and they turned out to be very dangerous.

At the other extreme, topical (skin surface) application of corticosteroids such as hydrocortisone was introduced in the late 1950s and soon became the treatment of choice. According to Kligman and Kaidbey (1978), a prominent dermatologist at the University of California at San Francisco, Howard Maibach, suggested that the historical designation B.C. should stand for "before corticosteroids." Since that time, literally hundreds of these products have been tested and marketed in varying degrees of potency; Zhai et al. (2000) provide a brief evaluation. Used judiciously, corticosteroids safely relieve symptoms of ACD but of course do not cure it.

As the mechanism of ACD becomes clearer at the molecular level, opportunities have emerged for biological rather than chemical intervention in the process (Kalish, 1995). For example, if the biochemical oxidation of urushiols and laccols to their quinones could be inhibited, no antigen would be formed. Indeed, applied antioxidants do reduce urushiol ACD in mice (Schmidt et al., 1990), although the effect might also be due to inhibition of cytokine release from inflammatory cells or to interference with their accumulation (Ikeda et al., 1994). The blood-thinning drug pentoxiphylline (Trental) inhibits TNF-α formation and the elicitation phase of ACD, although it does not prevent initial sensitization (Schwarz et al., 1993).

Also, when applied to skin, several immunosupressant drugs inhibit the formation of interleukin-2 (IL-2) by activated T-cells (Duncan, 1994). Prevention of ACD in guinea pigs by injection of their own red blood cells externally treated with pentadecylcatechol has long been established (Watson et al., 1981). Although none of these treatments presently is approved for use against human ACD, feasible anti-ACD therapy finally may be on the horizon.

Topical treatment with corticosteroids inhibits both the induction (antigen formation and T-cell activation) and elicitation (degranulation and mediator release) of ACD (Burrows and Stoughton, 1976). The effect is due to reduction in the number of markers on Langerhans cell membranes and thus a decreased ability to present the antigens to T-cells. Treatment with UV-B radiation (290–320 nm) or PUVA (the photosensitizer psoralen under 320–400-nm UV irradiation) act in much the same way (Breathnach, 1986) and currently enjoy wide therapeutic use.

Of course, still another rational treatment may be no treatment at all. According to no less an authority than Captain John Smith, the redness, itching, and blisters "the which howsoever, after a while they passe awaye of themselves without further harme" (Smith, 1624). I find that removing the allergen, keeping the affected area clean and dry, applying something soothing to counteract the itch, and simply letting nature take its course is a very satisfactory procedure. However, *nothing beats staying away from the offending plants in the first place!*

10.6 Future Possibilities

During the half-million years or so since human beings lost most of their protective body hair, they have suffered from plant allergens and irritants and struggled to do something about it. For ages, natural materials were all they had (McNair, 1921c). As if in response to Kligman's indictment cited at the head of this chapter, the late 1950s ushered in the use of topical steroids, and now our growing knowledge of the immunological basis of contact dermatitis (Basketter et al., 1999) can lead to novel methods of protection and therapy.

Rather than only treating symptoms, some newer materials are showing promise for affecting early steps in the allergic reaction. The macrolide antibiotic tacrolimus inhibits ACD and ICD by limiting activation of the sensitized T-cells, at least in guinea pigs; the antiinflammatory ascomycin macrolactam pimecrolimus (STZ ASM-981) reduces formation of cytokines produced in the antigen-specific activation of T-cells; the fluorinated corticosteroid Kenalog (triamcinolone acetonide) is under examination for control of chronic contact dermatitis; and other semisynthetic steroids are being tested for suppression of the histamine release from mast cells (Rietschel and Fowler, 2001; Zhai et al., 2000).

Such potential treatments admittedly may produce serious side effects. For example, Azanin (azathioprine) is effective against *Parthenium* dermatitis but is considered a human carcinogen, and decades ago, Kligman and Kaidbey (1978) foresaw the dangers of corticosteroid overuse. Under any circumstances, altering the body's immune system is to be approached with caution, but the important thing is that this type of research and application actually seems to be progressing. However, as summarized in table 10.4, we still have a long way to go.

The discovery of such valuable medication requires bioassays, which until now were a time-consuming process using live guinea pigs and even human volunteers (Basketter et al., 1999). A recent innovation, the

Table 10.4 Present Status of Practical Treatments for ACD and ICD

Treatment	Allergens	Irritants
Compresses	Probably effective but little scientific evidence	Success based on scientific evidence
Topical corticoids	Requires high-potency corticoids, more study	Presumed effective but some evidence negative
Systemic corticoids	Probably effective but no controlled studies	No data

Courtesy of H. I. Maibach (personal communication, 2002).

LLNA (local lymph node assay), quickly measures the proliferation of mouse lymph node cells in vitro during skin sensitization in vivo. Its results correlate well with those from standard guinea pig and human tests and thus present possibilities for greatly expanded dermatologic risk assessment. This new assay might also allow more thorough examination of newly introduced plants to head off a future disaster like that caused by congress grass in India in the 1950s (section 1.2).

The principal interest of both government agencies and the medical community appears, perhaps rightly, to be the control of occupational dermatitis due principally to industrial chemicals. The future medical treatments just described generally would apply only to the most serious cases of dermatitis, especially those where the victims had not been responsible for their own exposure. On the other hand, the recent developments in barrier creams and other over-the-counter skin-protective products suggest that consumers have not been forgotten, and that even better protection will be forthcoming. This could eventually take the form of a barrier material so safe and persistent that it would be worn routinely by anyone who goes outdoors, just as sunscreens and insect repellents are now.

It is both easier and more effective to prevent plant dermatitis than to treat it afterward. The key lies in much more effective education. Of the students, plant scientists, and even health professionals interviewed during the preparation of this book, most were acquainted with poison oak or poison ivy, nettles, and sometimes other local dermatotoxic plants, but few had ever heard of toxic euphorbs or daisies, phototoxic figs or limes, secondary exposure, or Tec-Nu. In this country, at least, the information could be provided by the USDA Cooperative Extension Service, the U.S. Forest Service, nurserymen's associations (as it is in Great Britain), garden clubs, and horticultural societies—anyplace where people and plants are brought together. The time to start doing it is now.

10.7 Conclusions

The good news is that there are a number of fairly effective means for protection against ACD and irritants, including suitable clothing, gloves, washing, and barrier lotions, although immunization is questionable. If one does contract the malady, symptoms usually can be alleviated by simple means such as over-the-counter corticosteroids. Many home remedies range from ineffective to downright scary, but newer rational methods based on dermatotoxicity mechanisms already are being used. The bad news is that once you have ACD, there is still no *cure*. According to an old saying, "if you don't do anything [to treat poison ivy allergy], it lasts two weeks; if you treat it, it only lasts 14 days."

APPENDICES

Appendix A Urushiols in *Toxicodendron*

			% of Purified Extractives			
Structure, R =	Configuration	Name	*T. diversilobum*[a]	*T. radicans*[a]	*T. vernix*[a]	*T. vernicifluum*[b]
(15')		Urushiol I	3.4–22.3	0–7.6	15.3	3.1–4.3
(8', 15')	8'Z	Urushiol II	1.4–8.4	3.1–41.6	41.4	19.3–25.8
(8', 11')	8'Z, 11'Z	Urushiol III	0.2–2.7	17.9–83.1	32.7	2.5–14.5
(11')	8'Z, 11'E		0	0		1.0–1.6
(11', 13')	8'Z, 11'Z, 13'Z	Urushiol IV	0	0	—[c]	0.2–0.4
(11', 14')	8'Z, 11'E, 14'	Urushiol V	0–0.6	3.3–62.5	10.6	—
(11')	8'Z, 11'Z, 13'Z		0	0	—	51.3—67.0

[a] *T. diversilobum* (CA), *T. radicans* (NY and MD), and *T. vernix* (NJ), see Gross et al. (1975). [b] *T. vernicifluum* (Japan), see Du et al. (1984a). [c] Not reported.

Appendix B Laccols in *Toxicodendron*

Structure, R =	Configuration	Name	% of Purified Extractives		
			T. diversilobum[a]	*T. radicans*[a]	*T. Vernicifluum*[b]
17'		Laccol I	0–2.1	0–0.2	3.8
8' 17'	8'Z	Laccol II	5.7–10.7	0–2.1	9.6
8' 11'	8'Z, 11'Z	Laccol III	18.7–24.9	0–22	3.2
11' 14'	8'Z, 11'E, 14'E	Laccol V	35.1–62.5	0–4.2	—[c]
11'	8'Z, 11'E, 13'E		0	0	0.6
11' 14'	8'Z, 11'Z, 14'Z, 16		0–1.3	0	—
10'	10'Z		—	—	0.3–1.3
10' 13'	10'Z, 13'Z		—	—	0.3–0.7
13' 16'	10'Z, 13'Z, 16'		—	—	0.6–1.0

[a]*T. diversilobum* (CA), *T. radicans* (NY and MD); *T. vernix* (NJ) contained no laccols (Gross et al., 1975). [b]*T. vernicifluum* (Japan), see Du et al. (1984a). [c]Not reported.

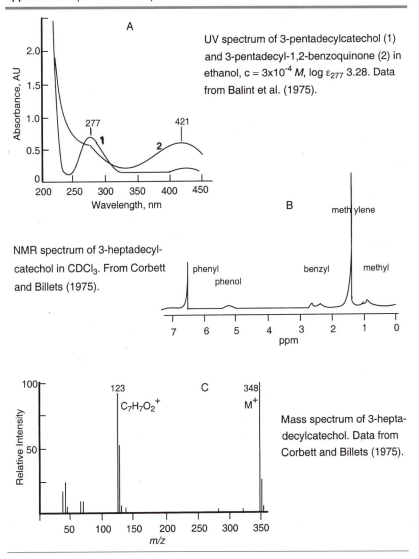

A UV spectrum of 3-pentadecylcatechol (1) and 3-pentadecyl-1,2-benzoquinone (2) in ethanol, c = 3×10^{-4} M, log ε_{277} 3.28. Data from Balint et al. (1975).

NMR spectrum of 3-heptadecyl-catechol in CDCl$_3$. From Corbett and Billets (1975).

Mass spectrum of 3-hepta-decylcatechol. Data from Corbett and Billets (1975).

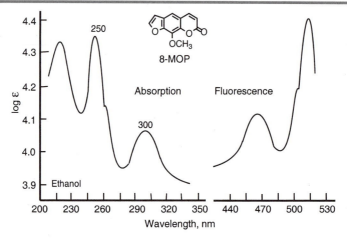

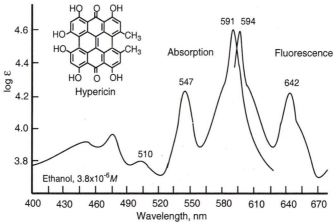

Appendix E Composition of Garlic Oils

Component	Structure	Oil A[a] %	Oil B[b] %
Diallyl disulfide	$(CH_2=CHCH_2)_2S_2$	26	4
Diallyl trisulfide	$(CH_2=CHCH_2)_2S_3$	19	8
Allyl methyl trisulfide	$CH_2=CHCH_2S_3CH_3$	15	7
Allyl methyl disulfide	$CH_2=CHCH_2S_2CH_3$	13	nd[c]
Diallyl trisulfide	$(CH_2=CHCH_2)_2S_4$	8	nd
Allyl methyl tetrasulfide	$CH_2=CHCH_2S_4CH_3$	6	nd
Dimethyl trisulfide	$CH_3S_3CH_3$	3	nd
Monosulfides	RSR'	3	nd
Pentasulfides	RS_5R'	4	nd
2-Vinyl-4H-1,3-dithiin	See display 7.6	nd	50
3-Vinyl-4H-1,2-dithiin	See display 7.6	nd	19
E- and Z-Ajoene	See display 7.6	nd	12
Total		97	100

Lawson et al. (1991). [a]Steam-distilled. [b]Oil-macerated. [c]None detected.

Appendix F Thiosulfinates in Seven *Allium* Species

Thiosulfinate[a]	MW	Yellow Onion[b]	Red Onion	Leek	Garlic	Indian Garlic	Elephant Garlic	Bear Garlic
AS-SOA	162.3	—[c]	—	—	2066	3140	162	954
AS-SOPn	162.3	—	—	—	37	59	3	—
ASO-SPn	162.3	—	—	—	123	178	11	31
ASO-SM	136.2	—	—	—	27	547	59	458
AS-SOM	136.2	—	—	—	57	1342	103	973
MSO-SM	110.2	5	0.7	0.5	—	161	26	463
MSO-SPr	138.2	0.5	8	1	—	—	—	—
MS-SOPr	138.2	0.5	6	1	—	—	—	—
MSO-SPn	136.2	12	1	6	—	50	6	20
MS-SOPn	136.2	11	1	3	27	547	—	—
PrSO-SPr	166.3	8	1	6	—	—	—	—
PrSO-SPn	164.3	6	4	4	—	—	—	—
PrS-SOPn	164.3	3	3	2	—	—	—	—
Bissulfine	178.1	1	4	0.8	—	—	—	—
Zwiebelanes[d]	162.3	6	8	3	—[e]	—[e]	—[e]	—[e]
Total		53	36.7	27.3	2337	6024	370	2899

Block et al. (1992a). [a]A, allyl; M, methyl; Pn, 1-propenyl; Pr, propyl. [b]In order across: *Allium cepa, A. cepa, A. porrum, A. sativum, A. sativum, A. ampeloprasum,* and *A. ursinum.* [c]Mg/kg wet wt; — means not detected. [d]Block et al. (1992b). [e]Not reported and not expected (Bayer et al., 1989).

General

Avalos, J., and H. I. Maibach (eds.). 2000. *Dermatologic Botany*. Boca Raton, FL: CRC Press.

Basketter, D., F. Gerberick, I. Kimber, and C. Willis. 1999. *Toxicology of Contact Dermatitis: Allergy, Irritancy, and Urticaria*. Chichester, UK: John Wiley and Sons.

Benezra, C., G. Ducombs, Y. Sell, and J. Foussereau. 1985. *Plant Contact Dermatitis*. Toronto: B.C. Decker Inc.

Kanerva, L., P. Elsner, J. E. Wahlberg, and H. I. Maibach, eds. 2000. *Handbook of Occupational Dermatitis*. Berlin: Springer Verlag.

Lovell, C. R. 1993. *Plants and the Skin*. Oxford: Blackwell Scientific Publications.

Mitchell, J. C., and A. Rook. 1979. *Botanical Dermatology*. Vancouver, BC: Greengrass Ltd.

Rietschel, R. L., and J. F. Fowler. 2001. *Fisher's Contact Dermatitis*, 5th ed. Philadelphia: Lippincott, Williams and Wilkins.

Plants

Avalos, J. 2000. Urticaceae, in *Dermatologic Botany* (J. Avalos and H. I. Maibach, eds.). Boca Raton, FL: CRC Press, pp. 237–50.

Bruneton, J. 1999. *Toxic Plants Dangerous to Humans*. Andover, U.K.: Intercept Ltd.

Burrows, G. E., and R. J. Tyrl. 2001. *Toxic Plants of North America*. Ames: Iowa State University Press.

Kingsbury, J. M. 1964. *Poisonous Plants of the United States and Canada*. Englewood Cliffs, NJ: Prentice-Hall.

Fuller, T. C., and E. McClintock. 1986. *Poisonous Plants of California*. Berkeley: University of California Press.

Gillis, W. T. 1971. The systematics and ecology of poison ivy and poison oaks (*Toxicodendron*, Anacardiaceae). *Rhodora*, 73: 72–159, 161–237, 370–443, 465–540.

Guin, J. D., and J. H. Beaman. 1986. Toxicodendrons of the United States. *Clin. Dermatol*. 4: 137–48.

Guin, J. D., J. H. Beaman, and H. Baer. 2000. Toxic Anacardiaceae, in *Dermatologic Botany* (J. Avalos and H. I. Maibach, eds.). Boca Raton, FL: CRC Press, pp. 85–142.

Hausen, B. M. 1981. *Woods Injurious to Human Health: A Manual*. Berlin: DeGruyter and Co.

Heywood, V. H., J. B. Harborne, and B. L. Turner. 1977. *The Biology and Chemistry of the Compositae*. vols. I and II. New York: Academic Press.

McNair, J. B. 1923. *Rhus Dermatitis (Poison Ivy): Its Pathology and Chemotherapy*. Chicago: University of Chicago Press.

Mitchell, J. D. 1990: The poisonous Anacardiaceae genera of the world. *Adv. Econ. Botany* 8: 103–29.

Mitchell, J. C., and A. Rook. 1979. *Botanical Dermatology.* Vancouver, BC: Greengrass Ltd. (For an update, see Schmidt, 2001.)

Morton, J. F. 1982. *Plants Poisonous to People in Florida and Other Warm Areas,* 2nd ed. Miami, FL: Julia F. Morton.

Seaman, F. C. 1982. Sesquiterpene lactones as taxonomic characters in the Asteracee. *Bot. Revs.* 48: 121–595.

Chemicals

Baer, H. 1986a. Chemistry and immunochemistry of poisonous Anacardiaceae, *Clin. Dermatol.* 4: 152–59.

Culberson, C. F. 1969. *Chemical and Botanical Guide to Lichen Products.* Chapel Hill, NC: University of North Carolina Press.

Evans, F. J. 1986a. *Naturally Occurring Phorbol Esters.* Boca Raton, FL: CRC Press.

Evans, F. J., and R. J. Schmidt. 1980. Plants and plant products that induce contact dermatitis. *Planta Med.* 38: 289–316.

Koch, H. P., and L. D. Lawson. 2000. *Garlic: The Science and Therapeutic Application of* Allium sativum *L. and Related Species,* 2nd ed. Baltimore, MD: Williams and Wilkins.

Murray, R. D. H. 1997. Naturally occurring plant coumarins. *Prog. Chem. Org. Nat. Products* 72: 1–120. A 1989–96 update of Murray's previous reviews of 1978, 1984, and 1991.

O'Neil, M. J. 2001. *The Merck Index,* 13th ed. Whitehouse Station, NJ: Merck and Co., Inc.

Seaman, F. C. 1982. Sesquiterpene lactones as taxonomic characters in the Asteracee. *Bot. Revs* 48: 121–595.

Thompson, R. H. 1987. *Naturally Occurring Quinones. III. Recent Advances.* London: Chapman and Hall.

Tyman, J. H. P. 1979. Non-isoprenoid long chain phenols. *Chem. Soc. Revs.* 8: 499–537.

Yoshioka, H., T. J. Mabry, and B. N. Timmermann. 1973. *Sesquiterpene Lactones: Chemistry, NMR, and Plant Distribution.* Tokyo: University of Tokyo Press.

Exposure

de Groot, A. C., and P. J. Frosch. 1997. Adverse reactions to fragrances, *Contact Dermat.* 36: 57–86.

Guin, J. D. 2000. Occupational contact dermatitis to plants, in *Handbook of Occupational Dermatitis* (L. Kanerva, P. Elsner, J. E. Wahlberg, and H. I. Maibach, eds.). Berlin: Springer Verlag, pp. 730–66.

Huntington, L. 1998. *Creating a Low-Allergen Garden.* San Diego, CA: Laurel Glen Publishing.

Kanerva, L., P. Elsner, J. E. Wahlberg, and H. I. Maibach, eds. 2000. *Handbook of Occupational Dermatitis.* Berlin: Springer Verlag.

Effects

Benezra, C., G. Ducombs, Y. Sell, and J. Foussereau. 1985. *Plant Contact Dermatitis*. Toronto: B.C. Decker Inc.

Kligman, A.M. 1958. Poison ivy (*Rhus*) dermatitis: an experimental study. *Arch. Dermat.* 77: 149–80.

McNair, J. B. 1923. *Rhus Dermatitis (Poison Ivy): Its Pathology and Chemotherapy*. Chicago: University of Chicago Press.

Mechanisms

Basketter, D., F. Gerberick. I. Kimber, and C. Willis. 1999. *Toxicology of Contact Dermatitis: Allergy, Irritancy, and Urticaria*. Chichester, UK: John Wiley and Sons.

Kalish, R. S. 1995. Poison ivy dermatitis: Pathogenesis of allergic contact dermatitis to urushiol. *Prog. Dermatol.* 29: 1–12.

Prevention and Treatment

Epstein, W. L. 1990. Poison oak and poison ivy dermatitis, in *Occupational Skin Disease* (R. M. Adams, ed.), 2nd ed. Philadelphia: W. B. Saunders Co., pp. 536–42.

Zhai, H., A. Anigbogu, and H. I. Maibach. 2000. Treatment and protection, in *Handbook of Occupational Dermatitis* (L. Kanerva, P. Elsner, J. E. Wahlberg, and H. I. Maibach, eds.). Berlin: Springer Verlag, pp. 402–11.

REFERENCES

For a list of key references, see appendix G.

Abell, C., and J. Staunton. 1984. Biosynthesis of 6-methylsalicylic acid; the combined use of mono- and trideuterated acetate precursors to investigate the degree of stereocontrol in the aromatization sequence. *Chem. Commun.* 1984: 1005–7.

Abraham, M. H., H. S. Chadha, and R. C. Mitchell. 1995. The factors that influence skin penetration of solutes. *J. Pharm. Pharmacol.* 47: 8–16.

Adams, R. M. 1990. Job descriptions with their irritants and allergens, in *Occupational Skin Disease* (R. M. Adams, ed.), 2nd ed. Philadelphia: W. B. Saunders Co., pp. 578–691.

———, and T. Fischer. 1990. Diagnostic patch testing, in *Occupational Skin Disease* (R. M. Adams, ed.), 2nd ed. Philadelphia: W. B. Saunders Co., pp. 223–53.

Adolf, W., and E. Hecker. 1984. Irritant phorbol derivatives from four jatropha species. *Phytochem.* 23: 129–32.

———, B. Sorg, M. Hergenhahn, and E. Hecker. 1982. Structure-activity relations of polyfunctional diterpenes of the daphnane type. 1. Revised structure for resiniferatoxin and structure-activity relations of resiniferol and some of its esters. *J. Nat. Prod.* 45: 347–54.

Aitken, A. 1986. The biochemical mechanism of action of phorbol esters, in *Naturally Occurring Phorbol Esters* (F. J. Evans, ed.). Boca Raton, FL: CRC Press, pp. 272–88.

Alanko, K. 2000. Aromatherapists, in *Handbook of Occupational Dermatitis* (L. Kanerva, P. Elsner, J. E. Wahlberg, and H. I. Maibach, eds.). Berlin: Springer Verlag, pp. 811–13.

Alber, J. I., and D. M. Alber.1993. *Baby-safe Houseplants and Cut Flowers*. Pownal, VT: Storey Communications, Inc.

Ale, S. I., F. Feneira, G. Gonzales, and W. Epstein. 1997. Allergic contact dermatitis caused by *Lithrea mollioides* and *Lithrea brasiliensis*: Identification and characteristics of the responsible allergens. *Amer. J. Contact Dermat.* 8: 144–49.

Ali, H., S. B. Christensen, J. C. Foreman, F. L. Pearce, W. Piotrowski, and O. Thastrup. 1985. The ability of thapsigargin and thapsigargicin to activate cells involved in the inflammation response. *Brit. J. Pharmacol.* 85: 705–12.

Ando, M. 1992. Studies on the synthesis of biologically active sesquiterpene lactones. *Yuki Gosei Kagaku Kyokaishi* 50: 858–74.

Apostolou, A., R. E. Williams, and C. R. Comerski. 1979. Acute toxicity of micronized 8-methoxypsoralen in rodents. *Drug Chem. Toxicol.* 2: 309–13.

Arditti, J., and E. Rodriguez. 1982. Dieffenbachia: Uses, abuses, and toxic constituents. A review. *J. Ethnopharmacol.* 5: 293–302.

Aregullin, M., and E. Rodriguez. 2000. Hydrophyllaceae, in *Dermatologic Botany* (J. Avalos and H. I. Maibach, eds.). Boca Raton, FL: CRC Press, pp. 187–99.

Arnold, H. L. 1968. *Poisonous Plants of Hawaii.* Rutland, VT: Charles E. Tuttle Co.

Asahina, Y., and S. Shibata. 1954. *Chemistry of Lichen Substances.* Tokyo: Japan Society for the Promotion of Science.

Avalos, J. 2000. Urticaceae, in *Dermatologic Botany* (J. Avalos and H. I. Maibach, eds.). Boca Raton, FL: CRC Press, pp. 237–50.

———, and H. I. Maibach, eds. 2000. *Dermatologic Botany.* Boca Raton, FL: CRC Press.

Baer, H. 1986. Chemistry and immunochemistry of poisonous Anacardiaceae, *Clin. Dermatol.* 4: 152–59.

———, R. C. Watkins, A. P. Kurtz, J. S. Byck, and C. R. Dawson. 1967. Delayed contact sensitivity to catechols. II. Cutaneous toxicity of catechols chemically related to the active principles of poison ivy. *J. Immunol.* 99: 365–69.

———, M. Hooten, H. Fales, A. Wu, and F. Schaub. 1980. Catecholic and other constituents of the leaves of *Toxicodendron radicans* and variation of urushiol concentrations within one plant. *Phytochem.* 19: 799–802.

Baker, S. J. 1979. *Poison Oak and Poison Ivy: Why it Itches, What to Do.* Soquel, CA: Sandra Baker.

Bakker, J., F. J. Gommers, I. Nieuwenhuis, and H. Wynberg. 1979. Photoactivation of the nematicidal compound α-terthienyl from roots of marigolds (*Tagetes* species). A possible singlet oxygen role. *J. Biol. Chem.* 254: 1841–44.

Balint, A. V., J. H. Dawson, and C. R. Dawson. 1975. A spectroscopic and chromatographic investigation of the behavior of 3-pentadecylcatechol (PDC) in various solvents under aerobic conditions. *Anal. Biochem.* 66: 340–52.

Balls, E. K. 1962. *Early Uses of California Plants.* Berkeley: University of California Press.

Bandyopadhyay, C., A. S. Gholap, and V. R. Mamdapur. 1985. Characterization of alkylresorcinol in mango (*Mangifera indica* L.) latex. *J. Agric. Food Chem.* 33: 377–79.

Barbier, P., and C. Benezra. 1982. Stereospecificity of allergic contact dermatitis (ACD) induced by two natural enantiomers, (+)- and (−)-frullanolides, in guinea pigs. *Naturwiss.* 69: 296–97.

Barkley, F. A., and E. D. Barkley. 1938. A short history of Rhus to the time of Linnaeus. *Amer. Midland Nat.* 19: 265–333.

Barley, G. C., E. R. H. Jones, and V. Thaller. 1988. Crepenynate as a precursor of falcarinol in carrot tissue culture. *Bioact. Molec.* 7: 85–91.

Barratt, M. D. 1995. Quantitative structure activity relationships for skin corrosivity of organic acids, bases, and phenols. *Toxicol. Lett.* 75: 169–76.

———. 1996. Quantitative structure activity relationships for skin irritation and corrosivity of neutral and electrophilic chemicals. *Toxicol. in Vitro* 10: 247–56.

Barton, D. H. R., A. M. Deflorin, and O. E. Edwards. 1956. The synthesis of usnic acid. *J. Chem. Soc.* 1956: 530–34.

Baruah, R. N., F. Bohlmann, and R. M. King. 1985. Novel sesquiterpene lactones from *Anthemis cotula. Planta Med.* 1985: 531–32.

Basketter, D., F. Gerberick. I. Kimber, and C. Willis. 1999. *Toxicology of Contact Dermatitis: Allergy, Irritancy, and Urticaria.* Chichester, UK: John Wiley and Sons.

Bayer, T., H. Wagner, E. Block, S. Grisoni, S. Zhao, and A. Neszmelyi. 1989. Zwiebelanes: Novel biologically-active 2,3-dimethyl-5,6-dithiabicyclo [2.1.1]hexane-5-oxides from onion. *J. Amer. Chem. Soc.* 111: 3085–86.

Beaman, J. H. 1986. Allergenic Asian Anacardiaceae. *Clin. Dermatol.* 4: 191–203.

Beckmann, B., and H. Ippen. 1998. Teebaum-Öl. *Dermatosen* 46: 120–24.

Beier, R. C., G. W. Ivie, and E. H. Oertli. 1983. Psoralens as phytoalexins in food plants of the family Umbelliferae, in *Xenobiotics in Food and Feed* (J. W. Finley and D. E. Schwass, eds.). *Advan. in Chem. Series* 234: 295–310.

Benezra, C., and H. I. Maibach. 1984. True cross-sensitization, false cross-sensitization and otherwise. *Contact Dermat.* 11: 65–69.

———, G. Ducombs, Y. Sell, and J. Foussereau. 1985. *Plant Contact Dermatitis.* Toronto, Canada: B.C. Decker Inc.

Bentley, R. K., and V. Thaller. 1969. The structure of carotatoxin, a natural toxicant from the carrot. *Chem. Commun.* 1967: 439–40.

Berry, D. L., M. R. Lieber, S. M. Fischer, and T. J. Slaga. 1977. Qualitative and quantitative separation of a series of phorbol-ester tumor-promoters by high-pressure liquid chromatography. *Cancer Letters* 3: 128–32.

Bestmann, H.-J., B. Classen, U. Kobold, O. Vostrowsky, F. Klingauf, and U. Stein. 1988. Steam volatile constituents from leaves of *Rhus typhina. Phytochem.* 27: 85–90.

Birmingham, D. J., M. M. Key, and G. E. Tublich. 1961. Phototoxic bullae among celery harvesters. *Arch. Dermat.* 83: 73–87.

Björkman, B. 1976. Properties and function of plant myrosinases, in *The Biology and Chemistry of the Cruciferae* (J. G. Vaughn, A. J. Macleod, and B. M. G. Jones, eds.). New York: Academic Press, pp. 191–205.

Bleumink, E., J. C. Mitchell, and J. P. Nater. 1973. ACD from wood (*Thuja plicata*). *Brit. J. Derm.* 88: 499–504.

———, H. M. G. Doeglas, A. H. Klokke, and J. P. Nater. 1972. ACD due to garlic. *Brit. J. Dermatol.* 87: 6–9.

Block, E., and T. Bayer. 1990. (Z,Z)-d,l-2,3-Dimethyl-1,4-butanedithial 1,4-dioxide: A novel biologically active organosulfur compound from onion. *J. Amer. Chem. Soc.* 112: 4584–85.

————, and E. M. Calvey. 1994. Facts and artifacts in *Allium* chemistry, in *Sulfur Compounds in Foods* (C. J. Mussinan and M. E. Keelan, eds.). *ACS Sympos. Series* 564: 63–79.

————, D. Putnam, and S.-H. Zhao. 1992a. *Allium* Chemistry: GC-MS analysis of thiosulfinates and related compounds from onion, leek, scallion, shallot, chive, and Chinese chive. *J. Agric. Food Chem.* 40: 2431–38.

————, S. Naganathan, D. Putnam, and S.-H. Zhao. 1992b. *Allium* chemistry: HPLC analysis of thiosulfinates from onion, garlic, wild garlic (ramsoms), leek, scallion, shallot, elephant (great-headed) garlic, chive, and Chinese chive. Uniquely high allyl to methyl ratios in some garlic samples. *J. Agric. Food Chem.* 40: 2418–30.

————, L. K. Revelle and A.A. Bazzi. 1980. Chemistry of sulfides. 5. The lachrymatory factor of the onion: An NMR study. *Tetrahed. Lett.* 21: 1277–80.

Blohm, H. 1962. *Poisonous Plants of Venezuela*. Cambridge, MA: Harvard University Press.

Blumstein, G. I. 1935. Buckwheat sensitivity. *J. Allergy Clin. Immunol.* 7: 74–79.

Bohlmann, F., and C. Zdero. 1985. Naturally occurring thiophenes, in *Thiophene and Its Derivatives, Part I* (S. Gronowitz, ed.). New York: John Wiley and Sons, pp. 261–323.

————, F. Burkhardt, and C. Zdero. 1973. *Naturally Occurring Acetylenes*. London: Academic Press.

Bolkart, K. H., and M. H. Zenk. 1968. Zur Biosynthese methoxylierter Phenole in höheren Pflanzen. *Z. Pflanzenphysiol.* 59: 439–44.

————. 1969. The homogentisate pathway in the biosynthesis of 2,7-dimethyl-1,4-naphthoquinone. *Z. Pflanzenphysiol.* 61: 356–59.

Boll, P. M., and L. Hansen. 1987. On the presence of falcarinol in the Aralaceae, *Phytochem.* 26: 2955–56.

Bos, J. D., and M. L. Kapsenberg. 1986. The skin immune system: Its cellular constituents and their interactions. *Immunol. Today* 7: 235–40.

Bosland, P. W., and E. J. Votava. 1999. *Peppers: Vegetable and Spice Capsicums*. Wallingford, UK: CABI Publishing Co.

Brandle, I., A. Boujnah-Khouadja, and J. Foussereau. 1983. Allergy to castor oil. *Contact Dermat.* 9: 424–25.

Breathnach, S. M. 1991. Origin, cell lineage, ontogeny, tissue distribution, and kinetics of Langerhans cells, in *Epidermal Langerhans Cells* (G. Schuler, ed.). Boca Raton, FL: CRC Press, pp. 23–49.

Breathnach, S. M. 1986. Immunologic aspects of contact dermatitis. *Clin. Dermat.* 4: 5–71.

Bremer, K. 1994. *Asteraceae: Cladistics and Classification*. Portland, OR: Timber Press.

Briggs, D. E. 1974. Hydrocarbons, phenols, and sterols of the testa and pigment strand in the grain of *Hordeum distichon*. *Phytochem.* 13: 987–96.

Brockmann, H. 1957. Photodynamisch wirksame Pflanzenfarbstoffe. *Prog. Chem. Org. Nat. Products* 14: 141–85.

————, and H. Lackner. 1979. Zur Konstitution des Fagopyrins. *Tetrahed. Lett.* 1979: 1575–78.

Brockmöller, J., T. Reum, S. Bauer, R. Kerb, W.-D. Hübner, and I. Roots. 1997. Hypericin and pseudohypericin: Pharmacokinetics and effects on photosensitivity in humans. *Pharmacopsychiatry* 30 (Supp. 2): 94–101.

Bronaugh, R. L., M. E. K. Kraeling, J. L. Yourick, and H. L. Hood. 1999. Cutaneous metabolism during *in vitro* percutaneous absorption, in *Percutaneous Absorption: Drugs-Cosmetics-Mechanisms-Methodology* (R. L. Bronaugh and H. I. Maibach, eds.). New York: Marcel Dekker, pp. 57–64.

Brooks, G. 1934. *Laque d'Indochine*, Rhus succedanea: *La Laccase et le Laccol.* Paris: Herman et Cie.

Brophy, J. J., N. W. Davies, I. A. Southwell, I. A. Stiff, and L. R. Williams. 1989. Gas chromatographic quality control for oil of *Melaleuca* terpinen-4-ol (Australian tea tree). *J. Agric. Food Chem.* 37: 1330–35.

Brown, N. J., and L. J. Roberts. 2001. Histamine, bradykinin, and their antagonists, in *Goodman and Gilman's The Pharmacological Basis of Therapeutics* (J. G. Hardman and L. E. Limbird, eds.), 10th ed. New York: McGraw-Hill, pp. 645–67.

Bruneton, J. 1999. *Toxic Plants Dangerous to Humans.* Andover, UK: Intercept Ltd.

Burgess, J. F. 1952. Occupational dermatitis due to onion and garlic. *Can. Med. Assoc. J.* 66: 275.

Burrows, G. E., and R. J. Tyrl. 2001. *Toxic Plants of North America.* Ames: Iowa State University Press.

Burrows, W. M., and R. B. Stoughton. 1976. Inhibition of induction of human contact sensitization by topical glucocorticosteroids. *Arch. Dermat.* 112: 175–78.

Burry, J. N., J. C. Reid, and J. Kirk. 1975. Australian bush dermatitis. *Contact Dermat.* 1: 263–64.

Bussy, A. 1840. Untersuchungen über die bildung des ätherischen Senföls. *Liebig's Ann.* 34: 223–30.

Byck, J. S., and C. R. Dawson. 1968. Assay of protein-quinone coupling involving compounds structurally related to the active principle of poison ivy. *Anal. Biochem.* 25: 123–35.

Cai, X. J., E. Block, P. C. Uden, B. D. Quimby, and J. J. Sullivan. 1995. Allium chemistry: Identification of natural abundance of organoselenium compounds in human breath after ingestion of garlic using gas chromatography with atomic emission detection. *J. Agric. Food Chem.* 43: 1751–53.

Camarasa, J. G. 2000. Algae, in *Dermatologic Botany* (J. Avalos and H. I. Maibach, eds.). Boca Raton, FL: CRC Press, pp. 261–71.

Camm, E., H. W. L. Buck, and J. C. Mitchell. 1976. Phytophotodermatitis from *Heracleum mantegazzianum. Contact Dermat.* 2: 68–72.

Camp, B. J., C. H. Bridges, D. W. Hill, and B. Patamalai. 1988. Isolation of a steroidal sapogenin from the bile of a sheep fed *Agave lecheguilla. Vet. Human Toxicol.* 30: 533–35.

Carson, C. F., and T. V. Riley. 2001. Safety, efficacy, and provenance of tea tree (*Melaleuca alternifolia*) oil. *Contact. Dermat.* 45: 65–67.

Casal, U. A. 1961. *Japanese Art Lacquers*. Tokyo: Sophia University.

Catalano, P. N. 1984. Mango sap and poison ivy. *J. Amer. Acad. Dermatol.* 10: 522.

Chan-Yeung, M. 1994. Mechanism of occupational asthma due to western red cedar (*Thuja plicata*). *Amer. J. Indust. Med.* 25: 13–18.

Chaudhary, S., O. Ceska, P. J. Warrington, and M. J. Ashwood-Smith. 1985. Increased furocoumarin content of celery during storage, *J. Agric. Food Chem.* 33: 1153–57.

Cheminat, A., J. L. Stampf, and C. Benezra. 1984. ACD to laurel *Laurus nobilis* L.: Isolation and identification of haptens. *Arch. Dermatol. Res.* 276: 178–81.

Chen, C.-L., H.-M. Chang, and T. K. Kirk. 1977. Betulachrysoquinone hemiketal: A benzoquinone hemiketal macrocyclic compound produced by *Phanerochaete chrysosporum*. *Phytochem.* 16: 1983–85.

Chew, A.-L., and H. I. Maibach. 2000. Botanical photoallergy, in *Dermatologic Botany* (J. Avalos and H. I. Maibach, eds.). Boca Raton, FL: CRC Press, pp. 77–81.

Chopra, R. N., R. L. Badhawar, and S. Ghosh. 1965. *Poisonous Plants of India*, vol. 1. 2nd ed. New Delhi: Indian Council of Agricultural Research.

Christensen, L. P. 1999. Direct release of the allergen tulipalin A from Alstroemeria cut flowers: A possible source of airborne contact dermatitis? *Contact Dermat.* 41: 320–24.

———, 2000. Primulaceae, in *Dermatologic Botany* (J. Avalos and H. I. Maibach, eds.). Boca Raton, FL: CRC Press, pp. 201–35.

———, and E. Larsen. 2000. Direct emission of the allergen primin from intact *Primula obconica* plants. *Contact Dermat.* 42: 149–53.

———, K. Kristiansen, and M. Ørgaard. 2000. Alstroemeriaceae, in *Dermatologic Botany* (J. Avalos and H. I. Maibach, eds.). Boca Raton, FL: CRC Press, pp. 273–310.

———, H. B. Jakobsen, E. Paulsen, L. Hodal, and K. E. Andersen. 1999. Airborne Compositae dermatitis. Monoterpenes and no parthenolide are released from flowering *Tanacetum parthenium* (feverfew) plants. *Arch. Dermatol. Res.* 291: 425–31.

Christensen, S. B., A. Andersen, and U. W. Smitt. 1997. Sesquiterpenoids from *Thapsia* species and medicinal chemistry of the thapsigargins. *Prog. Chem. Org. Nat. Products* 71: 129–67.

———, I. Kjoller-Larsen, U. Rasmussen, and C. Christoperssen. 1982. Thapsigargin and thapsigargicin, two histamine-liberating sesquiterpene lactones from *Thapsia garganica*. X-ray analysis of the 7,11-epoxide of thapsigargin. *J. Org. Chem.* 47: 649–52.

Cirigottis, K. A., L. Cleaver, J. E. T. Corrie, R. G. Grasby, G. H. Green, J. Mock, S. Nimgirawath, R. W. Read, E. Ritchie, W. C. Taylor, A. Vadasz, and W. R. G. Webb. 1974. Chemical studies of the Proteaceae. VII. An

examination of the woods of 17 species for resorcinol derivatives.
Austral. J. Chem. 27: 345–55.

Cleland, J. B. 1914. Plants, including fungi, poisonous or otherwise injurious to man
in Australia. *Austral. Med Gaz.* 35: 569.

Collins, F. W., and J. C. Mitchell. 1975. Aroma chemicals: Reference sources for
perfume and flavour ingredients, with special reference to cinnamic aldehyde.
Contact Dermat. 1: 43–47.

Connolly, J. D., and I. M. S. Thornton. 1973. Sesquiterpenoid lactones from the
liverwort *Frullania tamarsci. Phytochem.* 12: 631–32.

Connor, H. F. 1951. *The Poisonous Plants of New Zealand.* Wellington, NZ:
DSIRO, Bulletin 99.

Corbett, M. D., and S. Billets. 1975. Characterization of poison oak urushiol.
J. Pharm. Sci. 64: 1715–18.

Cordiero, R. S. B., J. B. Aragao, and L. Morhy. 1983. The presence of histamine in
Cnidoscolus oligandrus. An. Acad. Bras. Cienc. 55: 123–28. *Chem. Abstr.* 98:
212904^{w} (1983).

Cornell University. 1976. *Hortus Third.* New York: Macmillan Publishing Co.

Corner, E. J. H. 1952. *Wayside Trees of Malaya.* Singapore: Government Printing
Office, 2 vols.

Cornut, J. P. 1635. *Canadensium Plantarum Aliarumque Nondum Editarum
Historia.* Paris: Simon LeMayne.

Crombie, L. M., M. L. Games, and D. J. Pinter. 1968. Chemistry and structure of
phorbol, the diterpene parent of the cocarcinogens of *Croton* oil. *J. Chem.
Soc.* 1968C: 1347–62.

Cronin, E., and C. D. Calnan. 1978. Allergy to hydroabietyl alcohol in adhesive
tape. *Contact Dermat.* 4: 57.

Crosby, D. G., and N. Aharonson. 1967. The structure of carotatoxin, a natural
toxicant from the carrot. *Tetrahedron* 23: 465–72.

Culberson, C. F. 1969. *Chemical and Botanical Guide to Lichen Products.* Chapel
Hill: University of North Carolina Press.

Culpeper, N. 1653. *The Complete Herbal.* London: Thomas Kelly & Co. Reprinted
in 1869.

Czarnetzki, B. M. 1986. *Urticaria.* Berlin: Springer Verlag.

———, T. Thiele, and T. Rosenbach. 1990. Immunoreactive leukotrienes in nettle
plants (*Urtica urens*). *Intern. Arch. Allergy Appl. Immunol.* 91: 43–46.

D'Arcy, W. G. 1974. Severe CD from Poinsettia. *Arch. Dermat.* 109: 909–10.

Dahlquist, I., and S. Fregert. 1980. Contact allergy to atranorin in lichens and
perfumes. *Contact Dermat.* 6: 111–19.

Dawson, C. R., and G. P. Ng. 1978. An improved synthesis of 3-n-pentadecylca-
techol (3-PDC). *Org. Prep. Proced. Int.* 10: 167–72.

de Groot, A. C. 2000. Fragrances, in *Handbook of Occupational Dermatitis*
(L. Kanerva, P. Elsner, J. E., Wahlberg, and H. I. Maibach, eds.). Berlin:
Springer Verlag, pp. 497–508.

———, and P. J. Frosch. 1997. Adverse reactions to fragrances, *Contact Dermat.* 36:
57–86.

De Kraker, J.-W., M. C. R. Franssen, A. de Groot, W. A. König, and H. J. Bouwmeester. 1998. (+)-Germacrene A biosynthesis. *Plant Physiol.* 117: 1381–92.

DeLeo, V. A. 1992. Photocontact dermatitis, in *Photosensitivity* (V. A. DeLeo, ed.). New York: Igaku-Shoin Medical Publishers, pp. 84–99.

———, S. C. Taylor, D. V. Belsito, J. F. Fowler, A. F. Fransway, H. I. Maibach, J. G. Marks, C. G. T. Mathias, J. R. Nethercott, M. D. Pratt, R. R. Reitschel, E. F. Sherertz, F. J. Storrs, and J. S. Taylor. 2002. The effect of race and ethnicity on patch test results. *J. Amer. Acad. Dermatol.* 46: S107–112.

DeNapoli, F. 1917. Simulation of skin disease by soldiers. *Brit. Med. J.*, 3 March: 9.

Deuel, P. G., and T. A. Geissman. 1957. Xanthinin. II. The structures of xanthanin and xanthatin. *J. Amer. Chem. Soc.* 79: 3778–83.

De Wit, R. J. G. M., and E. Kodde. 1981. Induction of polyacetylenic phytoalexins in *Lycopersicon esculentum* after inoculation with *Cladosporium fulvum* (syn. *Fulvia fulva*). *Physiol. Plant Pathol.* 18: 143–48.

DeWitt, W. H. 1874. Poisoning by *Rhus Toxicodendron*. *Amer. J. Med. Sci.* 67: 116–18.

Diawara, M. M., J. T. Trumble, C. F. Quiros, and R. Hansen. 1995. Implications of distribution of linear furocoumarins within celery. *J. Agric. Food Chem.* 43: 723–27.

DiTomaso, J. M., and W. T. Lanini. 1996. *Poison Oak*. Davis, CA: UC Statewide IPM Project, University of California, Pest Notes No. 32.

Dooms-Goossens, A. 1993. Cosmetics as causes of allergic contact dermatitis. *Cutis* 52: 316–20.

Dooms-Goossens, J. M., and H. Deleu. 1991. Airborne contact dermatitis: An update. *Contact Dermat.* 25: 211–17.

———, A., R. Dubelloy, and H. Degreef. 1990. Contact and systemic contact-type dermatitis to spices. *Dermatol. Clin.* 8: 89–93.

Du, Y. 1990. Chemical composition of essential oil from the sap of the Rhus lac tree. *Gaodeng Xuexiao Huaxue Xuebao* 11: 605–10; *Chem. Abstr.* 114: 88400^m.

———, R. Oshima, and J. Kumanotani. 1984a. Reversed-phase liquid chromatographic separation and identification of constituents of urushiol in the sap of the lac tree, *Rhus vernicifera*. *J. Chromatog.* 284: 463–73.

———, R. Oshima, and H. Iwatsuki. 1984b. High-resolution gas-liquid chromatographic analysis of urushiol from the lac tree, *Rhus vernicifera*, without derivatization. *J. Chromatog.* 295: 179–86.

———, R. Oshima, Y. Yamauchi, J. Kumanotani, and T. Miyakoshi. 1986. Long chain phenols from the Burmese lac tree, *Melanorrhoea usitata*. *Phytochem.* 25: 2211–18.

Ducombs, G. 1978. Allergy to colophony. *Contact Dermat.* 4: 118–19.

Duncan, J. 1994. Differential inhibition of cutaneous T-cell mediated reactions and epidermal cell proliferation by cyclosporin, FK506, and rapamycin. *J. Invest. Dermatol.* 102: 84–88.

Dunn, I. S., J. C. Mitchell, and G. H. N. Towers. 1974. Reactions of alantolactone, an allergenic sesquiterpene lactone, with some amino acids, *Can. J. Biochem.* 52: 575–81.

———, D. J. Liberato, N. Castagnoli, and V. S. Byers. 1982. Contact sensitivity to urushiol: Role of covalent bond formation. *Cell. Immunol.* 74: 220–33.

Dupuis, G., J. C. Mitchell, and G. H. N. Towers. 1974. Reaction of alantolactone, an allergenic sesquiterpene lactone, with some amino acids. Resultant loss of immunologic activity. *Can. J. Biochem.* 52: 575–81.

Duus Johansen, J. 2002. Contact allergy to fragrances: Clinical and experimental investigations of the fragrance mix and its ingredients. *Contact Dermat.* 46 (Suppl. 3): 1–31.

Elias, P. 1992. Role of lipids in barrier function of the skin, in *Pharmacology of the Skin* (H. Mukhtar, ed.). Boca Raton, FL: CRC Press.

ElSohly, M. A., P. D. Adawadkar, D. A. Benigni, E. S. Watson, and T. L. Little. 1986. Analogues of poison ivy urushiol. Synthesis and biological activity of disubstituted *n*-alkylbenzenes. *J. Med. Chem.* 29: 606–11.

EPA. 1993. *Reregistration Eligibility Decision (RED): Glyphosate.* Washington, DC: U.S. Environmental Protection Agency, EPA 738-R-93-015.

———. 1998. *Reregistration Eligibility Decision (RED): Triclopyr.* Washington, DC: U.S. Environmental Protection Agency, EPA 738-F-98-007.

Epstein, J. H. 1991. Photocontact allergy in humans, in *Dermatotoxicology* (F. N. Marzulli and H. I. Maibach, eds.). New York: Hemisphere Publishing Corp., pp. 607–21.

———, A. Ormsby, and R. M. Adams. 1990. *Occupational Skin Cancer*, 2nd ed. Philadelphia: W. B. Saunders Co.

Epstein, W. L. 1990. Poison oak and poison ivy dermatitis, in *Occupational Skin Disease* (R. M. Adams, ed.), 2nd ed. Philadelphia: W. B. Saunders Co., pp. 536–42.

———. 1994. Occupational poison ivy and oak dermatitis. *Dermatol. Clin.* 12: 511–16.

———, V. S. Byers, and W. Franklin. 1982. Induction of antigen specific hyposensitization to poison oak in sensitized adults. *Arch Dermatol.* 118: 630–33.

Erman, E. 1985. Chemistry of the Monoterpenes. Parts A and B. New York: Marcel Dekker, Inc.

Estlander, T., R. Jolanki, K. Alanko, and L. Kanerva. 2001. Occupational allergic contact dermatitis caused by wood dusts. *Contact Dermat.* 44: 213–17.

Etzstorfer, C., H. Falk, and M. Oberreiter. 1993. On the tautomerism of hypericin: The 1,6-dioxo tautomer. *Monatsh. Chem.* 124: 923–29.

Evans, F. J. 1986a. *Naturally Occurring Phorbol Esters.* Boca Raton, FL: CRC Press.

———. 1986b. Phorbol: Its esters and derivatives, in *Naturally Occurring Phorbol Esters* (F. J. Evans, ed.). Boca Raton, FL: CRC Press, pp. 171–215.

———, and M. C. Edwards. 1987. Activity correlations in the phorbol ester series, in *The Euphorbiales: Chemistry, Taxonomy, and Economic Botany* (S. L. Jury, T. Reynolds, D. F. Cutler, and F. J. Evans, eds.). Orlando,

FL: Academic Press Inc., pp. 231–46. Reprinted from *Bot. J. Linn. Soc.* 94(1,2).

———, and A. D. Kinghorn. 1977. A comparative phytochemical study of the diterpenes of some species of the genera *Euphorbia* and *Elaeophorbia* (Euphorbiaceae). *Bot. J. Linn. Soc.* 74: 23–35.

———, and R. J. Schmidt. 1980. Plants and plant products that induce contact dermatitis. *Planta Med.* 38: 289–316.

———, R. J. Schmidt, and A. D. Kinghorn 1975. A microtechnique for the identification of diterpene inflammatory toxins. *Biomed. Mass Spectrom.* 2: 126–30.

———, and S. E. Taylor. 1983. Pro-inflammatory, tumor-promoting and antitumor diterpenes of the plant families Euphorbiaceae and Thymelaeaceae. *Prog. Chem. Org. Nat. Products* 44: 1–99.

Falk, H. and W. Schmitzberger. 1992. On the nature of "soluble" hypericin in *Hypericum* species. *Monatsh. Chem.* 123: 731–39.

———, J. Meyer, and M. Oberreiter. 1992. Deprotonation and protonation of hydroxyphenanthroperylenes. *Monatsh. Chem.* 123: 277–84.

Farracane, J. 2001. Conquering the mango. *Island Scene* (3): 23–26.

Feldmann, R. J., and H. I. Maibach. 1970. Absorption of some organic compounds through the skin in man. *J. Invest. Dermatol.* 54: 399–404.

Findlay, G. H., D. A. Whiting, S. H. Eggers, and R. P. Ellis. 1974. Smodingium (African "poison ivy") dermatitis. History, comparative plant chemistry and anatomy, clinical and histological features, *Brit. J. Dermatol.* 90: 535–41.

Finley, K. T. 1988. Quinones as synthones, in *The Chemistry of Quinonoid Compounds* (S. Patai and Z. Rappoport, eds.), vol. 2, part 1. Chichester: John Wiley and Sons, pp. 1–878.

Fischer, T., and H. I. Maibach. 1989. Easier patch testing with TRUE Test. *J. Amer. Acad. Dermatol.* 20: 447–53.

Fisher, A. A. 1986. *Contact Dermatitis*, 3rd ed. Philadelphia: Lea and Febiger.

Fisher, A. A., and A. Dooms-Goossens. 1976. The effect of perfume "ageing" on the allergenicity of individual perfume ingredients. *Contact. Dermat.* 2: 155–59.

———, and J. C. Mitchell. 1986. Dermatitis due to plants and spices, in *Contact Dermatitis* (A. A. Fisher, ed.), 4th ed. Philadelphia: Lea and Febiger, pp. 418–53.

Fochtman, F. W., J. E. Manno, C. L. Winek, and J. A. Cooper. 1969. Toxicity of the genus *Dieffenbachia*. *Toxicol. Appl. Pharmacol.* 15: 38–45.

Foussereau, C. Benezra, and H. I. Maibach. 1982. *Occupational Contact Dermatitis: Clinical and Chemical Aspects.* Copenhagen: Munksgaard Publishers.

Fraginals, R., M. Schaeffer, J.-L. Stampf, and C. Benezra. 1991. Perfluorinated analogues of poison ivy allergens. Synthesis and skin tolerogenic activity in mice. *J. Med Chem.* 34: 1024–27.

Frankel, E. 1991. *Poison Ivy, Poison Oak, Poison Sumac, and Their Relatives.* Pacific Grove, CA: Boxwood Press.

Freeman, S. 1990. Fragrance and nickel: Old allergies in new guises. *Amer. J. Contact Dermat.* 1: 47–52.

Fregert, J., and H. Möller. 1963. Contact allergy to balsam of Peru. *Brit. J. Dermatol.* 75: 218–20.

———, and H. Horsman. 1963. Hypersensitivity to balsams of pine and spruce. *Arch. Dermat.* 87: 693–95.

Frey-Wyssling, A. 1981. Crystallography of the two hydrates of crystalline calcium oxalate in plants. *Amer. J. Bot.* 68: 130–41.

Frohne, D., and H. Pfänder. 1984. *A Color Atlas of Poisonous Plants.* London: Wolfe Publications.

Fronczek, F. R., D. Vargas, N. H. Fischer, G. Chiari, F. Balza, and G. H. N. Towers. 1989. Structures of three pseudoguaianolides: Parthenin, hymenolin (11β,13-dihydroparthenin), and bipinnatin. *Acta Cryst.* 45C: 2006–10.

Fujiki, H., M. Suganuma, H. Suguri, S. Yoshizawa, K. Kakagi, M. Nakayasu, M. Ojika, K. Yamada, T. Yasumoto, R. E. Moore, and T. Sugimura. 1990. New tumor promoters from marine natural products, in *Marine Toxins: Origin, Structure, and Molecular Pharmacology* (S. Hall and G. Strichartz, eds.). *ACS Sympos. Ser.* 418: 87–106.

Fujiwara, M., M. Yoshimura, and S. Tsuno. 1955. "Allithiamine," a newly found derivative of vitamin B1. III. On the allicin homologues in the plants of the allium species. *J. Biochem. (Japan)* 42: 591–601; *Chem. Abstr.* 50: 1132.

Fuller, T. C., and E. McClintock. 1986. *Poisonous Plants of California.* Berkeley, CA: University of California Press.

Gäfvert, E., U. Nilsson, and A.-T. Karlberg. 1992. Rosin allergy: Identification of dehydroabietic acid peroxide with allergenic properties. *Arch. Dermatol. Res.* 284: 409–13.

Gambaro, V., M. C. Chamy, E. von Brand, and J. A. Garbarino. 1986. 3-(Pentadec-10-enyl)catechol, a new allergenic compound from *Lithrea caustica* (Anacardiaceae). *Planta Med.* 1986: 20–22.

Gebhardt, M., P. Elsner, and J. G. Marks. 2000. *Handbook of Contact Dermatitis.* London: Martin Dunitz, Ltd.

Gillis, W. T. 1971a. The systematics and ecology of poison ivy and poison oaks (*Toxicodendron,* Anacardiaceae). *Rhodora,* 73: 72–159.

———. 1971b. The systematics and ecology of poison ivy and poison oaks (*Toxicodendron,* Anacardiaceae). *Rhodora* 73: 161–237.

———. 1971c. The systematics and ecology of poison ivy and poison oaks (*Toxicodendron,* Anacardiaceae). *Rhodora* 73: 370–443.

———. 1971d. The systematics and ecology of poison ivy and poison oaks (*Toxicodendron,* Anacardiaceae). *Rhodora* 73: 465–540.

Gochfeld, M., and J. Burger. 1983. Sexual transmission of nickel and poison oak contact dermatitis. *The Lancet* 1(8324): 589.

Gommers, F. J. 1972. Increase of the nematocidal activity of α-terthienyl and related compounds by light. *Nematologica* 18: 458–62.

Gonçalo, S., F. Cabral, and M. Gonçalo. 1988. Contact sensitivity to oak moss. *Contact Dermat.* 19: 355–57.

Good, R. 1953. *The Geography of Flowering Plants*, 2nd. ed. London: Longman Green and Co.

Goodman, I., J. R. Foutes, E. Bresnick, R. Menegas, and G. H. Hitchings. 1959. A mammalian thioglycosidase. *Science* 130: 450–51.

Gottlieb, P., H. Gall, and R. U. Peter. 2000. Allergic contact dermatitis from natural rubber latex. *Contact Dermat.* 42: 240.

Granroth, B., and A. I. Virtanen. 1967. *S*-(2-Carboxypropyl)-cysteine and its sulfoxide as precursors in the biosynthesis of cycloalliin. *Acta Chem. Scand.* 21: 1654–56.

Grevelink, S. A., D. F. Murrell, and E. A. Olsen. 1992. Effectiveness of various barrier preparations in preventing and/or ameliorating experimentally produced *Toxicodendron* dermatitis, *J. Amer. Acad. Dermatol.* 27: 182–88.

Gross, M., H. Baer, and H. M. Fales. 1975. Urushiols of poisonous Anacardiaceae. *Phytochem.* 14: 2263–66.

Guenther, E. 1975. *The Essential Oils.* Huntington, NY: R. E. Krieger Publishing Co.

Guin, J. D. 1980. The black spot test for recognizing poison ivy and related species. *J. Amer. Acad. Dermatol.* 2: 332–33.

———. 2000. Occupational contact dermatitis to plants, in *Handbook of Occupational Dermatitis* (L. Kanerva, P. Elsner, J. E. Wahlberg, and H. I. Maibach, eds.). Berlin: Springer Verlag, pp. 730–66.

———, and J. H. Beaman. 1986. Toxicodendrons of the United States. *Clin. Dermatol.* 4: 137–48.

———, and R. Reynolds. 1980. Jewelweed treatment of poison ivy dermatitis. *Contact. Dermat.* 6: 287–88.

———, J. H. Beaman, and H. Baer. 2000. Toxic Anacardiaceae, in *Dermatologic Botany* (J. Avalos and H. I. Maibach, eds.). Boca Raton, FL: CRC Press, pp. 85–142.

———, M. Lelong, and R. Karl. 1981. Recognition of eastern poison oak with emphasis on plants in Alabama. *J. South. Med Assoc.* 74: 435–43.

Gunther, R. T. 1959. *The Greek Herbal of Dioscorides.* London: Hafner Publishing Company.

Hansch, C., A. Leo, and D. Hoekman. 1995. *Exploring QSAR: Hydrophobic, Electronic, and Steric Constants.* Washington, DC: The American Chemical Society.

Hansen, L., and P. M. Boll. 1986. Polyacetylenes in Araliaceae: Their chemistry, biosynthesis, and biological significance. *Phytochem.* 25: 285–93.

Hartwell, J. L., and A. W. Schrecker. 1958. The chemistry of podophyllum. *Prog. Chem. Org. Nat. Products* 15: 83–166.

Hausen, B. M. 1978a. On the occurrence of the contact allergen primin and other quinoid compounds in species of the family Primulaceae. *Arch. Dermatol. Res.* 261: 311–21.

———. 1978b. Sensitizing capacity of naturally occurring quinones. V. 2,6-Dimethoxy-*p*-benzoquinone: Occurrence and significance as a contact allergen. *Contact Dermat.* 4: 204–13.

————. 1980. Allergic contact dermatitis to quinones in *Paphiopedilum haynaldianum* (Orchidaceae). *Arch. Dermat.* 116: 327–28.

————. 1981. *Woods Injurious to Human Health: A Manual.* Berlin: DeGruyter and Co.

————. 1991. A simple method of isolating parthenolide from *Tanacetum* and other sensitising plants. *Contact Dermat.* 24: 153–55.

———— 2000a. Allergenic hardwoods, in *Dermatologic Botany* (J. Avalos and H. I. Maibach, eds.). Boca Raton, FL: CRC Press, pp. 389–408.

————. 2000b. Aralaceae, in *Dermatologic Botany* (J. Avalos and H. I. Maibach, eds.). Boca Raton, FL: CRC Press, pp. 143–49.

————, and R. M. Adams. 1990. Woods, in *Occupational Skin Disease* (R. M. Adams, ed.), 2nd ed. Philadelphia: W. B. Saunders Co., pp. 524–36.

————, and O. Helmke. 1995. Butenylbithiophene, alpha-terthienyl, and hydroxytremetone as contact allergens in cultvars of marigold (*Tagetes* sp.). *Contact Dermat.* 33: 33–37.

————, and K. H. Schulz. 1976. Chrysanthemum allergy. III. Identification of the allergens. *Arch. Dermatol. Res.* 255: 111–21.

————. 1977. Occupational contact dermatitis due to Croton (*Codiaeum variegatum* L.) A. Juss var. *pictum* (Lodd.) Muell. Arg. *Contact Dermat.* 3: 289–92.

————, and O. Spring. 1989. Sunflower allergy: On the constituents of the trichomes of *Helianthus annuus* L. (Compositae). *Contact Dermat.* 20: 326–34.

————, and C. Wolf. 1996. 1,2,3-Trithiane-5-carboxylic acid, a first contact allergen from *Asparagus officinalis* (Liliaceae). *Amer. J. Contact Dermat.* 7: 41–46.

————, E. G. Devries, and J. M. C. Geuns. 1988. Sensitizing potency of coleon O in *Coleus* sp. (Lamiaceae). *Contact Dermat.* 19: 217–18.

————, H. R. Herrmann, and G. Willuhn. 1978. The sensitizing capacity of Compositae plants. I. ACD from *Arnica longifolia* Eaton. *Contact Dermat.* 4: 3–10.

————, A. Shoji, and O. Jarchow. 1984. Orchid allergy. *Arch. Dermat.* 120: 1206–8.

————, H. W. Schmalle, D. Marshall, and R. H. Thomson. 1983. 5,8-Dihydroxyflavone (primetin), the contact sensitizer of *Primula mistassinica* Michaux. *Arch. Dermatol. Res.* 275: 365–70.

————, P. Evers, H.-T. Stüwe, W. A. König, and E. Wollenweber. 1992. Propolis allergy (IV). Studies with further sensitizers from propolis and constituents common to propolis, poplar buds, and balsam of Peru. *Contact. Dermat.* 26: 34–44.

————, J. Bröhan, W. A, König, H. Faasch, H. Hahn, and G. Bruhn. 1987. Allergic and irritant contact dermatitis from falcarinol and didehydrofalcarinol in common ivy (*Hedera helix* L.). *Contact Dermat.* 17: 1–9.

————, H. Heitsch, B. Borrmann, D. Koch, R. Rathmann, B. Richter, and W. A. Koenig. 1995. Structure-activity relationships in allergic contact dermatitis. (I). Studies on the influence of side-chain length with derivatives of primin. *Contact Dermat.* 33: 12–16.

Hauser, S. C. 1996. *Nature's Revenge: The Secrets of Poison Ivy, Poison Oak, Poison Sumac, and Their Remedies*. New York: Lyons and Burford.

Hecker, E. 1981. Co-carcinogens and tumor promoters of the diterpene ester type as possible carcinogenic risk factors. *J. Cancer Res. Clin. Oncol.* 99: 103–24.

Hellerström, S., N. Thyresson, and G. Widmark. 1957. Chemical aspects of turpentine eczema. *Dermatologica* 115: 277–86.

Herz, W. 1977. Sesquiterpene lactones, in *The Biology and Chemistry of the Compositae*, Vol. 1 (V. H. Heywood, J. B. Harborne, and B. L. Turner, eds). New York: Academic Press, pp. 337–57.

Heskel, N. S., R. B. Amon, F. J. Storrs, and C. R. White. 1983. Phytophotodermatitis due to *Ruta graveolens*. *Contact Dermat.* 9: 278–80.

Hickman, J. C. 1993. *The Jepson Manual: Higher Plants of California*. Berkeley, CA: University of California Press.

Hill, G. A., V. Mattacotti, and W. D. Graham. 1934. The toxic principle of the poison ivy. *J. Amer. Chem. Soc.* 56: 2736–38.

Hjorth, N. 1982. Allergy to balsams. *Clin. Exp. Dermatol.* 7: 1–9.

———, and D. S. Wilkinson. 1968. Contact dermatitis. IV. Tulip fingers, hyacinth itch, and lily rash. *Brit. J. Dermatol.* 80: 696–98.

Hobbs, C. 1998. *Herbal Remedies of Dummies*. Foster City, CA: IDG Books Worldwide, Inc.

Holzer, P. 1991. Capsaicin: Cellular targets, mechanisms of action, and selectivity for thin sensory neurons. *Pharm. Rev.* 43: 143–201.

Hooker, W. J., and G. A. W. Arnott. 1832. *The Botany of Captain Beechy's Voyage*, Part III. London: Henry G. Bohn, p. 137. Reprinted by S. Cramer, Weinheim, Germany, in 1965.

Hoppe, W., K. Zechmeister, M. Röhrl, F. Brandl, E. Hecker, G. Kreibach, and H. Bartsch. 1969. The structure determination of a solvate of phorbol, the diterpene parent of the tumor promoters from *Croton* oil. *Tetrahed. Lett.* 1969: 667–70.

Horper, W., and F.-J. Marner. 1995. Phenols and quinones from leaves of *Primula obconica*. *Nat. Prod. Lett.* 41: 163–170.

———. 1996. Biosynthesis of primin and miconidin and its derivatives. *Phytochem.* 41: 451–56.

Horsfield, T. 1798. *An Inaugural Dissertation on Rhus vernix, R. radicans, and R. glabrum, Commonly Known in Pennsylvania as Poison Oak, Poison Vine, and Common Sumac*. Philadelphia, PA.

Howard, P. H., and W. M. Meylan. 1997. *Physical Properties of Organic Chemicals*. Boca Raton, FL: CRC Press.

Huffaker, C. B., and C. E. Kennett. 1959. A ten-year study of vegetational changes associated with biological control of Klamath weed. *J. Range Mgmt.* 12: 69–82.

Huneck, S. 1981. The absolute configuration of (+)-usnic and (+)-isousnic acids. X-ray analysis of the (−)-α-phenylethylamine derivative of (+)-usnic acid and of (−)-pseudoplacodiolic acid, a new dibenzofuran from the lichen *Rhizoplaca chrysoleuca*. *Tetrahed. Lett.* 22: 351–52.

Huntington, L. 1998. *Creating a Low-Allergen Garden*. San Diego: Laurel Glen Publishing.

Hurtado, I. 1986. Poisonous Anacardiaceae of South America. *Clin. Dermatol.* 4: 183–90.

Hurwitz, R. M., H. P. Rivera, and J. D. Guin. 1984. Black spot poison ivy dermatitis. An acute irritant contact dermatitis superimposed upon allergic contact dermatitis. *Amer. J. Dermatopathol.* 4: 319–22.

Hutchinson, C. R., and E. Leete. 1970. Biosynthesis of α-methylene-γ-butyrolactone, the cyclized aglycone of tuliposide A. *Chem. Commun.* 1970: 1189–90.

Huygens, S., and A. Goossens. 2000. An update on airborne contact dermatitis. *Contact Dermat.* 44: 1–6.

IARC. 1986. Some naturally occurring and synthetic food components, furocoumarins, and ultraviolet radiation. Vol. 40. *IARC Monographs on the Evaluation of the Carcinogenic Risk of Chemicals to Humans*. Geneva: World Health Organization, pp. 327–47.

———. 1993. Some naturally occurring substances: Food items and constituents, heterocyclic aromatic amines and mycotoxins. Vol. 56. *IARC Monographs on the Evaluation of the Carcinogenic Risk of Chemicals to Humans*. Geneva: World Health Organization, pp. 135–62.

Ikeda, M., K. K. Schroeder, L. B. Mosher, C. W. Woods, and A. L. Akeson. 1994. Suppressive effects of antioxidants on intracellular adhesion molecule-1 (ICAM-1) expression in human epidermal keratinocytes. *J. Invest. Dermatol.* 103: 791–96.

Imamoto, T., Y. Tsuno, and Y. Tukawa. 1971. Hofmann rearrangement. I. Kinetic substituent effects of *ortho-*, *meta-*, and *para*-substituted *N*-bromobenzamides. *Bull. Chem. Soc. Japan* 44: 1632–38.

International Union of Biochemistry. 1979. *Enzyme Nomenclature: Recommendations (1978) of the Committee on Nomenclature and Classification of Enzymes of the International Union of Biochemistry*. New York: Academic Press.

Itokawa, H., N. Totsuka, K. Nakahara, K. Takeya, J.-P. Lepoittevin, and Y, Asakawa. 1987. Antitumor principles from *Ginkgo biloba* L. *Chem. Pharm. Bull.* 35: 3016–20.

———, M. Maezuru, K. Takeya, M. Kondo, M. Inamatsu, and H. Morita. 1989. A quantitative structure-activity relationship for antitumor activity of long-chain phenols from *Ginkgo biloba* L. *Chem. Pharm. Bull.* 37: 1619–21.

Ivie, G. W., R. C. Beier, and D. L. Holt. 1982. Analysis of the garden carrot (*Daucus carota* L.) for linear furocoumarins (Psoralens) at the sub parts per million level. *J. Agric. Food Chem.* 30: 413–16.

Jakupovic, J., T. Morgenstern, M. Bittner, and M. Silva. 1998. Diterpenes from *Euphorbia peplus*. *Phytochem.* 47: 1601–1809.

Jansen, H., B. Müller, and K. Knobloch. 1989. Characterization of an alliin lyase preparation from garlic (*Allium sativum*). *Planta Med.* 55: 434–39.

Jardon, P., N. Lazortchak, and R. Gautron. 1987. Formation of singlet oxygen $^1\Delta g$ photosensitized by hypericin. *J. Chim. Phys., Phys.-Chim. Biol.* 84: 1141–45.

Jenner, P. M., E. C. Hagen, J. M. Taylor, E. C. Cook, and O. G. Fitzhugh. 1964. Food flavourings and compounds of related structure. I. Acute oral toxicity. *Food Cosmet. Tox.* 2: 327–43.

Johnson, R. A., H. Baer, C. H. Kirkpatrick, C. R. Dawson, and R. G. Khurana. 1972. Comparison of the contact allergenicity of the four pentadecylcatechols derived from poison ivy urushiol in human subjects. *J. Allerg. Clin Immun.* 49: 27–35.

Jones, H. E., C. W. Lewis, and S. L. McMarlin. 1973. Allergic contact sensitivity in atopic dermatitis. *Arch. Dermat.* 107: 217–22.

Jones, S. T., J. K. Wipff, and P. N. Montgomery. 1997. *Vascular Plants of Texas.* Austin: University of Texas Press.

Josephy, P. D. 1997. *Molecular Toxicology.* New York: Oxford University Press.

Kagan, J. 1991. Naturally occurring di- and trithiophenes. *Prog. Chem. Org. Nat. Products* 56: 87–169.

Kalish, R. S. 1995. Poison ivy dermatitis: Pathogenesis of allergic contact dermatitis to urushiol. *Prog. Dermatol.* 29: 1–12.

Kanerva, L., T. Estlander, and R. Jolanki. 1995. Occupational allergic contact dermatitis caused by ylang-ylang oil. *Contact Dermat.* 33: 198–99.

Kanerva, L., P. Elsner, J. E. Wahlberg, and H. I. Maibach, eds. 2000. *Handbook of Occupational Dermatitis.* Berlin: Springer Verlag.

Kanerva, L., T. Estlander, and R. Jolanki. 1995. Occupational allergic contact dermatitis caused by ylang-ylang oil. *Contact Dermat.* 33: 198–99.

Kao, J., and M. P. Carver. 1991. Skin metabolism, in *Dermatotoxicology* (F. N. Marzuli and H. I. Maibach, eds.), 4th ed. New York: Hemisphere Publishing Corp., pp. 143–200.

Karlberg, A.-T. 2000. Colophony, in *Handbook of Occupational Dermatitis* (L. Kanerva, P. Elsner, J. E. Wahlberg, and H. I. Maibach, eds.). Berlin: Springer Verlag, pp. 509–16.

———, K. Bohlinder, and A. Bohman. 1988. Identification of 15-hydroperoxy-abietic acid as a contact allergen in Portuguese colophony. *J. Pharm. Pharmacol.* 40: 42–47.

———, K. Magnusson, and U. Nilsson. 1992. Air oxidation of *d*-limonene (the citrus solvent) creates potent allergens. *Contact Dermat.* 26: 332–40.

Kavli, G., G. Volden, K. Midelfart, S. Haugsbø, and J. O. Prytz. 1983. Phototoxicity of *Heracleum laciniatum. Contact Dermat.* 9: 27–32.

Keil, H., D. Wasserman, and C. R. Dawson. 1944. The relation of chemical structure in catechol compounds and derivatives to poison ivy hypersensitiveness in man as shown by the patch test. *J. Exp. Med.* 80: 275–87.

Keith, I., W. Rerich, and I. M. Bush. 1969. Toilet paper dermatitis. *J. Amer. Med. Assoc.* 209: 269.

Kerner, J., J. Mitchell, and H. I. Maibach. 1973. Irritant contact dermatitis from *Agave americana* L. Incorrect use of sap as "hair restorer." *Arch. Dermat.* 108: 102–3.

Khan, S. R. 1995. *Calcium Oxalate in Biological Systems*. Boca Raton, FL: CRC Press.

Kimber, I., and R. J. Dearman. 2002. Allergic contact dermatitis: The cellular effectors. *Contact Dermat.* 46: 1–5.

King, L. J. 1957. A unique reported use for the fruit of *Semicarpus anacardium* L. f. (Anacardiaceae) in ancient Arabian and Indian medicine. *Economic Bot.* 11: 263–66.

Kinghorn, A. D., and F. J. Evans. 1975. A biological screen of selected species of the genus *Euphorbia* for skin irritant effects. *Planta Medica* 28: 325–35.

Kingsbury, J. M. 1964. *Poisonous Plants of the United States and Canada.* Englewood Cliffs, NJ: Prentice-Hall.

Kinsella, A. R. 1986. Multistage carcinogenesis and the biological effects of tumor promoters, in *Naturally Occurring Phorbol Esters* (F. J. Evans, ed.). Boca Raton, FL: CRC Press, pp. 33–61.

Kjaer, A. 1960. Naturally derived isothiocyanates (mustard oils) and their parent glucosides. *Prog. Chem. Org. Nat. Products* 18: 122–76.

———. 1976. Glucosinolates in the Cruciferae, in *The Biology and Chemistry of the Cruciferae* (J. G. Vaughn, A. J. Macleod, and B. M. Jones, eds.). New York: Academic Press, pp. 207–19.

Klaassen, C. D., M. O. Amdur, and J. Doull. 1996. *Casarett and Doull's Toxicology: The Basic Science of Poisons*, 5th ed. New York: McGraw-Hill.

Klauder, J. V., and J. M. Kimmich. 1956. Sensitization dermatitis to carrots: Report of cross-sensitization phenomenon and remarks on phytophotodermatitis. *Arch. Dermat.* 74: 149–58.

Kligman, A. M. 1958. Poison ivy (*Rhus*) dermatitis: An experimental study. *Arch. Dermat.* 77: 149–80.

———, and K. H. Kaidbey. 1978. Hydrocortisone revisited. *Cutis* 22: 232–44.

Knight, T. E. 1991. *Philodendron*-induced dermatitis: Report of cases and review of the literature. *Cutis* 48: 375–78.

———, and B. M. Hausen. 1994. Melaleuca oil (tea tree oil) dermatitis. *J. Amer. Acad. Dermatol.* 30: 423–27.

Koch, H. P., and L. D. Lawson. 2000. *Garlic: The Science and Therapeutic Application of Allium sativum L. and Related Species*, 2nd ed. Baltimore: Williams and Wilkins.

Kolis, S. J., T. H. Williams, E. J. Postma, G. J. Sasso, P. N. Confalone, and M. A. Schwartz. 1979. The metabolism of ^{14}C-methoxalen by the dog. *Drug Metab. Dispos.* 7: 220–25.

Kornhauser, A., W. G. Wamer, and L. A. Lambert. 1996. Cellular and molecular events following ultraviolet irradiation of skin, in *Dermatotoxicology* (F. N. Marzulli and H. I. Maibach, eds.), 5th ed. Washington, DC: Taylor and Francis, pp. 189–230.

Kouakou, B. 1991. *Fate of Urushiol (Poison Oak Toxicant) When Consumed by Dairy Goats.* Ph.D. dissertation, University of California, Davis, CA.

Kozubek, A. 1984. Thin-layer chromatographic mapping of 5-*n*-alk(en)ylresorcinol homologues from cereal grains. *J. Chromatog.* 295: 304–7.

————, W. S. M. Geurts Van Kessel, and R. A. Demel. 1979. Separation of 5-n-alkylresorcinols by reversed-phase high-performance liquid chromatography. *J. Chromatog.* 169: 422–25.

Krajewska, A., and J. J. Powers. 1988. Sensory properties of naturally occurring capsaicinoids. *J. Food Sci.* 53: 902–5.

Krenzelok, E. P., T. D. Jacobsen, and J. M. Aronis. 1996. A review of 96,659 *Dieffenbachia* and *Philodendron* exposures. *J. Toxicol. Clin. Toxicol.* 34: 601.

Kumanotani, J. 1983. Japanese lacquer: A super durable coating, in *Polymer Applications of Renewable-Resource Materials* (C. E. Carraher and L. H. Sperling, eds.). New York: Plenum Press, pp. 225–48.

Kurtz, A. P., and C. R. Dawson. 1971a. Synthesis of compounds structurally related to poison ivy urushiol. 3. 3-n-Pentadecylcatechol and 3-n-alkylcatechols of varying side-chain length. *J. Med. Chem.* 14: 729–32.

————. 1971b. Synthesis of compounds structurally related to poison ivy urushiol. 4. 3-(1-Alkylalkylcatechols of varying sidechain shape and flexibility. *J. Med. Chem.* 14: 733–37.

Kwangsukstith, C., and H. I. Maibach. 1995. Effect of age and sex on the induction and elicitation of allergic contact dermatitis. *Contact Dermat.* 33: 289–98.

Laakso, I., T. Seppänen, R. Hiltunin, B. Müller, H. Jansen, and K. Knobloch. 1989. Volatile garlic odor components: Gas phases and adsorbed exhaled air analyzed by headspace gas chromatography-mass spectrometry. *Planta Med.* 55: 257–61.

Lahti, A. 1986. Contact urticaria to plants. *Dermatol. Clin.* 4: 127–36.

————, and M. Hannuksela. 1978. Hypersensitivity to apple and carrot can be reliably detected with fresh material. *Allergy* 33: 143–46.

Lammintausta, K., and H. I. Maibach. 1990. Contact dermatitis due to irritation, in *Occupational Skin Disease* (R. M. Adams, ed.). Philadelphia: W. B. Saunders, pp. 1–15.

Lampe, K. F. 1986. Dermatitis-producing Anacardiaceae of the Caribbean area. *Clin. Dermatol.* 4: 171–82.

Lange, G. L., and M. Lee. 1987. Synthesis of four sesquiterpenoid lactone skeletons, germacranolide, elemanolide, cadinanolide, and guaianolide, from a single photoadduct. *J. Org. Chem.* 52: 325–31.

Lawson, L. D. 1996. The composition and chemistry of garlic cloves and processed garlic, in *Garlic: The Science and Therapeutic Application of* Allium sativum *L. and Related Species* (H. P. Koch and L. D. Lawson, eds.), 2nd ed. Baltimore: Williams and Wilkins, pp. 37–107.

————, and B. G. Hughes. 1992. Characterization of the formation of allicin and other thiosulfinates from garlic. *Planta Med.* 58: 345–50.

————, and Z. J. Wang. 1993. Prehepatic fate of the organosulfur compounds derived from garlic (*Allium sativum*). *Planta Med.* 59: A688.

————, and B. G. Hughes. 1991. Identification and HPLC quantitation of the sulfides and dialk(en)yl thiosulfinates in commercial garlic products. *Planta Med.* 57: 363–70.

Lee, J., and B. C. Uff. 1967. Organic reactions involving electrophilic oxygen. *Quart. Rev. Chem. Soc.* 21: 429–57.

Lee, K.-H., I. H. Hall, E.-C. Mar, C. O. Starnes, S. A. ElGebaly, T. G. Waddell, R. I. Hadgraft, C. G. Ruffner, and I. Weidner. 1977. Sesquiterpene antitumor agents: Inhibitors of cellular metabolism. *Science* 196: 533–36.

Leite, D. 1982. *Don't Scratch!* Walnut Creek, CA: Weathervane Books.

Lejman, E., T. Stoudemayer, G. Grove, and A. M. Kligman. 1984. Age differences in poison ivy dermatitis. *Contact Dermat.* 11: 163–67.

Leung, T.-W. C., D. H. Williams, J. C. J. Baarna, S. Foti, and P. B. Oelrichs. 1986. Structural studies on the peptide moroidin from *Laportea moroides. Tetrahed.* 42: 3333–48.

Lewis, W. H., and M. P. F. Elvin-Lewis. 1977. *Medical Botany.* New York: John Wiley and Sons.

Leyden, J. L., and A. M. Kligman. 1977. Allergic contact dermatitis: Sex differences. *Contact Dermat.* 3: 333–36.

Liberato, D. J., V. S. Byers, R. G. Dennick, and N. Castagnoli. 1981. Regiospecific attack of nitrogen and sulfur nucleophiles on quinones derived from poison oak/ivy catechols (urushiols) and analogues as models for urushiol-protein conjugate formation. *J. Med. Chem.* 24: 28–33.

Lookadoo, S. E., and A. J. Pollard. 1991. Chemical contents of stinging trichomes of *Cnidoscolus texanus. J. Chem. Ecol.* 17: 1909–16.

Lovell, C. R. 2000a. Florists, in *Handbook of Occupational Dermatitis* (L. Kanerva, P. Elsner, J. E. Wahlberg, and H. I. Maibach, eds.). Berlin: Springer Verlag, pp. 935–37.

———. 2000b. Phytophotodermatoses, in *Dermatologic Botany* (J. Avalos and H. I. Maibach, eds.). Boca Raton, FL: CRC Press, pp. 201–235.

Lund, E. D., and J. H. Bruemmer. 1991. Acetylenic compounds in stored packaged carrots. *J. Sci. Food Agric.* 54: 287–94.

Lunggren, B. 1977. Psoralen photoallergy caused by plant contact. *Contact Dermat.* 3: 85–90.

Lyman, W. J., R. F. Reehl, and D. H. Rosenblatt. 1990. *Handbook of Chemical Property Estimation Methods.* Washington, DC: The American Chemical Society.

Lyon, C. C. 2000. Confectionery and candy makers, in *Handbook of Occupational Dermatitis* (L. Kanerva, P. Elsner, J. E. Wahlberg, and H. I. Maibach, eds.). Berlin: Springer Verlag, pp. 863–67.

Mackoff, S., and A. G. Dahl. 1951. A botanical consideration of the weed oleoresin problem. *Minnesota Medicine* 34: 1169.

Majima, R. 1909. Über den Hauptbestandteil des Japanlacks. I. Mitteilung. Über Urushiol und Urushiol-dimethyl Äther. *Ber.* 42: 1418–23.

———. 1912. Über den Hauptbestandteil des Japanlacks. III. Mitteilung. Die katalytische Reduktion von Urushiol. *Ber.* 45: 2727–30.

———. 1915. Über den Hauptbestandteil des Japanlacks. V. Mitteilung. Über die Konstitution von Hydro-urushiol. *Ber.* 48: 1593–97.

———. 1922a. Über den Hauptbestandteil des Japan-Lacks. VIII. Mitteilung. Stellung der Doppelbindungen in der Seitenkette des Urushiols und Beweisführring, dass das Urushiol eine Mischung ist. *Ber.* 55B: 172–77.

———. 1922b. Über den Hauptbestandteil des Japan-Lacks. IX Mitteilung. Chemische Untersuchung der verschiedenen natürlichen Lackarten, die dem Japan-Lack nahe verwandt sind. *Ber.* 55B: 191–214.

———, and I. Nakamura. 1913. Über den Hauptbestandteil des Japanlacks. IV. Mitteilung. Einige Derivate des Hydrourushiols. *Ber.* 46: 4080–88.

———, and J. Tahara. 1915. Über den Hauptbestandteil des Japanlacks. VI. Mitteilung. Über die Synthese des Hydro-urushiols. *Ber.* 48: 1607–11.

March, J. 1992. *Advanced Organic Chemistry: Reactions, Mechanisms, and Structure,* 4th ed. New York: John Wiley and Sons.

Markiewitz, K. H., and C. R. Dawson. 1965. On the isolation of the allergenically active components of the toxic principle of poison ivy. *J. Org. Chem.* 30: 1610–13.

Marks, J. G., T. Demelfi, and M. A. McCarthy. 1984. Dermatitis from cashew nuts. *J. Amer. Acad. Dermatol.* 10: 627–31.

Marley, K. A., R. A. Larson, and R. Davenport. 1995. Alternative mechanisms of psoralen photoxicity, in *Light-Activated Pest Control* (J. R. Heitz and K. R. Downum, eds.). *ACS Sympos. Series* 616: 179–88.

Marner, F.-J., and W. Horper. 1992. Phenols and quinones from seeds of different *Iris* species. *Helv. Chim. Acta* 75: 1557–62.

Martínez, M. 1979. *Catálogo de Nombres Vulgares y Científicos de Plantas Mexicanas.* Mexico City: Fondo de Cultura Económica.

Marzulli, F. N., and H. I. Maibach. 1991. *Dermatotoxicology,* 4th ed. New York: Hemisphere Publishing Corp.

Mason, H. S. 1945a. The allergenic principles of poison ivy. V. The synthesis of 3-n-pentadecyl-catechol (hydrourushiol). *J. Amer. Chem. Soc.* 67: 1538–40.

———. 1945b. The toxic principles of poison ivy. III. The structure of bhilawanol. *J. Amer. Chem. Soc.* 67: 418–20.

May, S. B. 1960. Dermatitis due to *Grevillea robusta* (Australian Silky Oak). *Arch. Dermat.* 82: 1006.

McDonald, C. J. 1973. Dermatological problems in black skin. *Prog. Dermatol.* 7(4): 15–19.

McDougal, J. N., G. W. Jepson, and H. J. Clewell. 1990. Dermal absorption of organic chemical vapors in rats and humans. *Fundam Appl. Tox.* 14: 229–308.

McNair, J. B. 1916. The poisonous principle of poison oak. *J. Amer. Chem. Soc.* 38: 1417–21.

———. 1921a. Lobinol—A dermatitant from *Rhus diversiloba* (poison oak). *J. Amer. Chem. Soc.* 53: 159–64.

———. 1921b. A study of *Rhus diversiloba* with special reference to its toxicity. *Amer. J. Botany* 8: 127–46.

———. 1921c. Remedies for Rhus dermatitis. *Arch. Dermat.* 4: 217–34.

———. 1923. *Rhus Dermatitis (Poison Ivy): Its Pathology and Chemotherapy.* Chicago: University of Chicago Press.

Mennella, J. A., and G. K. Beauchamp. 1991. Maternal diet alters the sensory qualities of human milk and the nursling's behavior. *Pediatrics* 88: 737–44.

———. 1993. The effects of repeated exposure to garlic-flavored milk on the nursling's behavior. *Pediatr. Res.* 34: 805–8.

Menz, J., and R. K. Winkelmann. 1987. Sensitivity to wild vegetation. *Contact Dermat.* 16: 179–73.

Metcalfe, D. D., H. A. Samson, and R. A. Simon. 1997. *Food Allergy: Adverse Reactions to Foods and Food Additives*, 2nd ed. Cambridge, UK: Blackwell Science.

Milne, J. A. 1972. *Introduction to the Diagnostic Histopathology of the Skin.* Baltimore: The Williams and Wilkins Co.

Mitchell, J. C. 1974. Contact dermatitis from plants of the caper family, Capparidaceae. *Brit. J. Dermatol.* 71: 13–20.

———. 1981a. Parthenium pollen—Parthenium dermatitis. *Contact Dermat.* 7: 212–13.

———. 1981b. Industrial aspects of 112 cases of allergic contact dermatitis from *Frullania* in British Columbia during a 10-year period. *Contact Dermat.* 7: 268–69.

———. 1986. Frullania (Liverwort) phytodermatitis (woodcutter's eczema). *Clin. Dermat.* 4: 62–64.

———, and G. Dupuis. 1971. Allergic contact dermatitis from sesquiterpenoids of the Compositae family of plants. *Brit. J. Dermatol.* 84: 139–150.

———, and W. P. Jordan. 1974. Allergic contact dermatitis from the radish, *Raphanus sativus. Brit. J. Dermatol.* 91: 183–89.

———, and H. I. Maibach. 2000. Diagnosis and patch testing of plant dermatitis, in *Dermatologic Botany* (J. Avalos and H. I. Maibach, eds.). Boca Raton, FL: CRC Press, pp. 39–44.

———, and A. Rook. 1979. *Botanical Dermatology.* Vancouver, BC: Greengrass Ltd. (For an update, see Schmidt, 2001.)

———, and S. Shibata. 1969. Immunological activity of some substances derived from lichenized fungi. *J. Invest. Dermat.* 52: 517–20.

———, G. Dupuis, and T. A. Geissman. 1972. Allergic contact dermatitis from sesquiterpenoids in plants, *Brit. J. Dermatol.* 87: 235–40.

———, H. I. Maibach, and J. Guin. 1981. Leaves of *Ginkgo biloba* not allergenic for *Toxicodendron*-sensitive subjects. *Contact Dermat.* 7: 47–8.

———, B. Fritig, B. Singh, and G. H. N. Towers. 1970. Allergic contact dermatitis from *Frullania* and Compositae: The role of sesquiterpene lactones. *J. Invest. Dermatol.* 54: 233–39.

———. A. K. Roy, G. Dupuis, and N. Towers. 1971. Allergic contact dermatitis from ragweed (*Ambrosia* species). The role of sesquiterpene lactones. *Arch. Dermat.* 104: 73–76.

Mitchell, J. D. 1990. The poisonous Anacardiaceae genera of the world. *Adv. Econ. Botany* 8: 103–29.

———, and S. A. Mori. 1987. The cashew and its relatives (*Anacardium*: Anacardiaceae). *Mem. N.Y. Bot. Garden* 42: 1–76.

Miyakoshi, T., and H. Togashi. 1990. Synthesis of 3-alkylcatechols via intramolecular cyclization. *Synthesis* 1990: 407–10.

———, H. Kobuchi, N. Niimura, and Y. Yoshihiro. 1991. Synthesis of urushiols with pentadecatrienyl side chain, two constituents of the sap of the lac tree, *Rhus vernicifera. Bull. Chem. Soc. Japan* 64: 2569–72.

Monsereenusorn, Y., S. Kongsamut, and P. D. Pezalla. 1982. Capsaicin: A literature survey. *Crit. Rev. Toxicol.* 10: 321–39.

Morren, M.-A., R. Rodrigues, and A. Dooms-Goossens. 1992. Connubial contact dermatitis: A review. *Europ. J. Dermatol.* 2: 219–23.

Morton, J. F. 1982. *Plants Poisonous to People in Florida and Other Warm Areas,* 2nd ed. Miami: Julia F. Morton.

Muenscher, W. C., and B. I. Brown. 1944. Dermatitis and photosensitization produced by *Ptelea angustifolia. Madroña* 7: 184.

Mukhtar, H. 1992. *Pharmacology of the Skin.* Boca Raton, FL: CRC Press.

Murdoch, S. R., and J. Dempster. 2000. Allergic contact dermatitis from carrot. *Contact. Dermat.* 42: 236.

Murphy, J. C., E. S. Watson, and E. C. Harland. 1983. Toxicological evaluation of poison oak urushiol and its esterified derivative. *Toxicology* 26: 135–42.

Murray, R. D. H. 1997. Naturally occurring plant coumarins. *Prog. Chem. Org. Nat. Products* 72: 1–120. (A 1989–96 update of Murray's previous reviews of 1978, 1984, and 1991.)

———, J. Mendez, and S. A. Brown. 1982. *The Natural Coumarins: Occurrence, Chemistry and Biochemistry.* New York: John Wiley & Sons.

Musajo, L., and G. Rodigheiro. 1962. The skin-photosensitizing furocoumarins. *Experientia* 18: 153–200.

Nahrstedt, A., and V. Butterweck. 1997. Biologically active and other chemical constituents of the herb of *Hypericum perforatum* L. *Pharmacopsychiatry* 30 (Suppl. 2): 129–34.

Nakano, T., J. D. Medina, and I. Hurtado. 1970. The chemistry of *Rhus striata* ("Manzanillo"). *Planta Med.* 18: 260–65.

Naves, Y. R., and G. Mazuyer. 1947. *Natural Perfume Materials: A Study of Concretes, Resinoids, Floral Oils, and Pomades.* New York: Reinhold Publishing Corp.

Neal, M. C. 1965. *In Gardens of Hawaii.* Honolulu: Bishop Museum Press.

Neering, H., B. E. J. Vitanyi, K. E. Malten, W. G. Van Ketel, and E. Van Djik. 1975. Allergens in sesame oil. *Acta Dermat.* 55: 31–34.

Nielsen, B. E. 1971. Coumarin patterns in the Umbelliferae, in *The Biology and Chemistry of the Umbelliferae* (V. H. Heywood, ed.). London: Academic Press, pp. 325–36.

Oakes, A. J., and J. O. Butcher. 1962. *Poisonous and Injurious Plants of the U.S. Virgin Islands.* Washington, DC: U.S. Department of Agriculture, Miscellaneous Publication 882.

Occolowitz, J. L. 1964. Mass spectrometry of naturally-occurring alkenylphenols and their derivatives. *Anal. Chem.* 36: 2177–81.

O'Malley, M. A., and R. Barba. 1990. Bullous dermatitis in field workers associated with exposure to mayweed. *Amer. J. Contact Dermat.* 1: 34–42.

———, and C. G. T. Mathias. 1988. Distribution of lost-work-time claims for skin disease in California Agriculture: 1978–1983. *Amer. J. Indust. Med.* 14: 715–20.

O'Neill, M. J. 2001. *The Merck Index*, 13th ed. Whitehouse Station, NJ: Merck and Co., Inc.

Opdyke, D. L. J. 1973. Monographs on fragrance raw materials. *Food Cosmet. Tox.* 11: 1011–81.

———. 1975a. Rue Oil. *Food Cosmet. Tox.* 13: 455–56.

———. 1975b. Monographs on fragrance raw materials. *Food Cosmet. Tox.* 13: 681–923.

Osawa, T., A. Suzuki, and S. Tamura. 1971. Isolation of chrysartemins A and B as rooting cofactors in *Chrysanthemum morifolium. Agr. Biol. Chem.* 35: 1966–72.

Pace, N. 1942. The etiology of hypericism, a photosensitivity produced by St. Johnwort. *Amer. J. Physiol.* 136: 650–56.

Palosuo, T., S. Mäkinen-Kiljunen, H. Alenius, T. Reunala, E. Yip, and K. Turjanmaa. 1998. Measurement of natural rubber latex allergen levels in medical gloves by allergen-specific IgE-ELISA inhibition, RAST inhibition, and skin prick test. *Allergy* 53: 59–67.

Pangilinan, N. C., G. W. Ivie, B. A. Clement, R. C. Beier, and M. Uwayjan. 1992. Fate of [^{14}C]xanthotoxin (8-methoxypsoralen) in laying hens and lactating goat. *J. Chem. Ecol.* 18: 253–70.

Papageorgiou, C., J.-L. Stampf, and C. Benezra. 1988. Allergic contact dermatitis to tulips: An example of enantiospecificity. *Arch. Dermatol. Res.* 280: 5–7.

———, J. P. Corbet, F. M. Brandão, M. Pecequeiro, and C. Benezra. 1983. Allergic contact dermatitis due to garlic (*Allium sativum* L.). Identification of the allergens: The role of mono-, di-, and trisulfide present in garlic. A comparative study in man and animal (guinea pig). *Arch. Dermatol. Res.* 275: 229–34.

Parke, D. V. 1968. *The Biochemistry of Foreign Compounds*. Oxford: Pergamon Press.

Parker, P. J., S. Stabel, and M. D. Waterfield. 1984. Purification to homogeneity of protein kinase C from bovine brain; identity with phorbol ester receptor. *EMBO J.*, 3: 953–59.

Parsons, W. T., and E. G. Cuthbertson. 1992. *Noxious Weeds of Australia*. Melbourne: Inkata Press.

Pathak, M. A. 1974. Phytophotodermatitis, in *Sunlight and Man* (T. B. Fitzpatrick, M. A. Pathak, L. C. Harber, M. Seiji, and A. Fukita, eds.). Tokyo: University of Tokyo Press, p. 502.

———, F. Daniels, T. B. Fitzpatrick. 1962. The presently known distribution of furocoumarins (psoralens) in plants. *J. Invest. Dermatol.* 39: 225–39.

Paulsen, E. 1992. Compositae dermatitis: A survey. *Contact Dermat.* 26: 76–86.

————, K. E. Anderson, and B. M. Hausen. 2001. Sensitization and cross-reaction patterns in Danish Compositae-allergic patients. *Contact Dermat.* 45: 197–204.

————, L. P. Christensen, and K. E. Andersen. 2002. Do monoterpenes released from feverfew (*Tanacetum parthenium*) plants cause airborne Compositae dermatitis? *Contact Dermat.* 47: 14–18.

Pax, F., and H. Hoffman. 1931. Euphorbiaceae, in *Die Natürlichen Pflanzenfamilien* section 19C (A. Engler and K. Prantl, eds.), 2nd ed. Leipzig: Engleman, p. 208.

Pecequeiro, M., and F. M. Brandão. 1985. Airborne contact dermatitis to plants. *Contact. Dermat.* 13: 277–79.

Peekel, P. G. 1984. *Flora of the Bismarck Archipelago for Naturalists.* Lae (Papua New Guinea): Office of Forests.

Perold, G. W., J. C. Muller, and G. Ourisson. 1972. Structure d'un lactone allergisante: Le Frullanolide. *Tetrahedron* 28: 5797.

Pfaff, F. 1897. On the active principle of *Rhus toxicodendron. J. Exper. Med.* 2: 181–96.

Phillips, F. S., M. B. Chenowith, and C. C. Hunt. 1948. Studies on the toxicology of podophyllotoxin and related substances. *Fed. Proc.* 7: 249.

Picman, A. K., and G. H. N. Towers. 1982. Sesquiterpene lactones in various populations of *Parthenium hysterophorus. Biochem. System. Ecol.* 10: 145–55.

————, J. Pickman, and G. H. N. Towers. 1982. Cross-reactivity between sesquiterpene lactones related to parthenin in parthenin-sensitized guinea pigs. *Contact Dermat.* 8: 2294–301.

Pirilä, V., O. Kilpi, A. Olkonnen, L. Pirilä, and E. Siltanen. 1969. On the chemical nature of the eczematogens in oil of turpentine. *Dermatologica* 139: 183–94.

Potts, R. O., D. B. Bommannan, and R. H. Guy. 1992. Percutaneous absorption, in *Pharmacology of the Skin* (H. Mukhtar, ed.). Boca Raton, FL: CRC Press.

Powell, S. M., and D. K. Barrett. 1986. An outbreak of contact dermatitis from *Rhus verniciflua* (*Toxicodendron vernicifluum*). *Contact Dermat.* 14: 288–89.

Prodi, R., P. DeCastro, and G. A. Malorgio. 1994. *The World Cashew Economy.* Bologna, Italy: Oltremare SpA.

Pugh, W. J. 1999. Relationship between H-bonding of penetrants to stratum corneum lipids and diffusion, in *Percutaneous Absorption: Drugs— Cosmetics—Mechanisms—Methodology* (R. L. Bronaugh and H. I. Maibach, eds.), 3rd ed. New York: Marcel Decker, Inc.

Quattrone, A. J. 1977. Nonenzymic spectrophotometric determination of potential poison ivy cross-reactors. *Clin. Chem.* 23: 571–75.

Quirce, S., A. I. Tabar, M. D. Muro, and J. M. Olaguibel. 1994. Airborne contact dermatitis from *Frullania. Contact Dermat.* 30: 73–6.

Radcliffe-Smith, A. 1986. A review of the family Euphorbiaceae, in *Naturally Occurring Phorbol Esters* (F. J. Evans, ed.). Boca Raton, FL: CRC Press.

Rademacher, M. 2000. Lichens, in *Dermatologic Botany* (J. Avalos and H. I. Maibach, eds.). Boca Raton, FL: CRC Press, pp. 365–74.

Rastogi, S. C., S. Heydorn, J. D. Johansen, and D. A. Basketter. 2001. Fragrance chemicals in domestic and occupational products. *Contact Dermat.* 45: 221–25.

———. 1986. Dermatotoxic phenolics from trichomes of *Phacelia companularia* and *P. pedicellata*. *Phytochem.* 25: 1617–19.

Reynolds, G. W., and E. Rodriguez. 1989. Contact allergens of an urban shrub *Wigandia caracasana*. *Contact Dermat.* 21: 65–9.

Reynolds, N. J., J. L. Burton, and J. W. B. Bradfield. 1991. Weed whacker dermatitis. *Arch. Derm.* 127: 1419–20.

Richards, J. 1993. *Primula*. London: Batsford, Ltd.

Ridley, D. D., E. Ritchie, and W. C. Watson. 1968. Chemical studies of the Proteaceae. II. Some further constituents of *Grevillea robusta* A. Cunn.: Experiments on the synthesis of 5-n-tridecylresorcinol (grevillol) and related substances. *Austral. J. Chem.* 21: 2979–88.

Rietschel, R. L., and J. F. Fowler. 2001. *Fisher's Contact Dermatitis*, 5th ed. Philadelphia: Lippincott, Williams and Wilkins.

Ritchie, E., W. C. Taylor, and S. T. K. Vautin. 1965. Chemical studies of the Proteaceae. I. *Grevillea robusta* A. Conn and *Orites excelsa* R. Br. *Austral. J. Chem.* 18: 2015–20

Rivero-Cruz, J. F., D. Chavez, B. Hernandez Bautista, A. L. Anaya, and R. Mata. 1997. Separation and characterization of *Metopium brownei* urushiol components. *Phytochem.* 45: 1003–8.

Rizk, A. M., F. M. Hammouda, M. M. El-Missiry, H. M. Radwan, and F. J. Evans. 1984. Constituents of Egyptian Euphorbiaceae. XIII. Biologically active diterpene esters from *Euphorbia peplus*. *Phytochem.* 24: 1605–6.

Roberts, D. W., and C. Benezra. 1993. Quantitative structure-activity relationships for skin sensitization potential of urushiol analogues. *Contact Dermat.* 29: 78–83.

Roberts, M. S., R. A. Anderson, and J. Swarbrick. 1977. Permeability of human epidermis to phenolic compounds. *J. Pharm. Pharmacol.* 29: 677–83.

Roberts, S. G. 1989. Mexico's killer tree "chechén" (*Rhus radicans*) (sic). *American Woodturner* 4(2): 24.

Robinson, D. R., and C. A. West. 1970. Biosynthesis of cyclic diterpenes in extracts of seedlings of *Ricinus communis* L. I. Identification of diterpene hydrocarbons formed from mevalonate. *Biochemistry* 9: 70–9.

Robles, M., J. West, E. Rodriguez, and M. Heinrich. 2000. Asteraceae, in *Dermatologic Botany* (J. Avalos and H. I. Maibach, eds.). Boca Raton, FL: CRC Press, pp. 151–68.

Rodriguez, E., M. O. Dillon, T. J. Mabry, J. C. Mitchell, and G. H. N. Towers. 1976a. Dermatologically active sesquiterpene lactones in trichomes of *Parthenium hysterophorus* L. (Compositae). *Experentia* 32: 236–38.

———, G. H. N. Towers, and J. C. Mitchell. 1976b. Biological activities of sesquiterpene lactones. *Phytochem.* 15: 1573–80.

Rodriguez, E., P. L. Healey, and I. Mehta. 1984. *Biology and Chemistry of Plant Trichomes*. New York: Plenum Press.

Rogers, T. H. 1974. Natural rubber, in *Chemical and Process Technology Encyclopedia* (D. M. Considine, ed.). New York: McGraw-Hill, p. 984.

Ross, C. M. 1959. Poison ivy dermatitis: The first South African cases. *S. Afr. Med. J.* 33: 657–60.

Ross, W. C. J. 1962. *Biological Alkylating Agents*. London: Butterworth.

Rougier, A., C. Lotte, and H. I. Maibach. 1989. In vivo relationship between percutaneous absorption and transdermal water loss, in *Percutaneous Absorption*, 2nd ed. (R. L. Bronaugh and H. I. Maibach, eds.). New York: Marcel Dekker, pp. 175–90.

————, D. Dupuis, C. Lotte, R. Roguet, and H. Schaefer. 1983. *In vivo* correlation between stratum corneum reservoir function and percutaneous absorption. *J. Invest. Dermatol.* 81: 275–78.

Roy, A. B. 1987. Sulfatases from *Helix pomatia. Methods in Enzymol.* 143: 361–66.

Rudzki, E., and Z. Dajek. 1975. Dermatitis caused by buttercups (Ranunculus). *Contact Dermat.* 1: 322.

————. Z. Grzywa, and W. S. Bruo. 1976. Sensitivity to 35 essential oils. *Contact Dermat.* 2: 196–200.

Rytand, D. A. 1948. Fatal anuria, the nephrotic syndrome, and glomular nephritis as sequels of the dermatitis of poison oak. *Am. J. Med.* 5: 548–60.

Sahasrabudhe, S. R., D. Lala, and V. V. Modi. 1986. Degradation of orcinol by *Aspergillus niger, Can. J. Microbiol.* 32: 535–38.

Salinas, M. L., T. Ogura, amd L. Soffchi. 2001. Irritant contact dermatitis caused by needle-like calcium oxalate crystals, raphides, in *Agave tequilana* among workers in tequila distilleries and agave plantations. *Contact Dermat.* 44: 94–6.

Salo, H., M. Hannuksela, and B. M. Hausen. 1981. Lichen picker's dermatitis (*Cladonia alpestris* (L.) Rab). *Contact Dermat.* 7: 9–13.

Sams, W. M. 1941. Photodynamic action of lime oil (*Citrus aurantifolia*). *Arch. Dermat.* 44: 571–87.

Samson, A. W., and K. W. Parker. 1930. St. Johnswort on range lands in California. *Calif. Agric. Exper. Station Bull.* 503.

Santesson, J. 1973. Identification and isolation of lichen substances, in *The Lichens* (V. Ahmadjian and M. E. Hale, eds.). New York: Academic Press, pp. 633–52.

Santucci, B., M. Picardo, and A. Cristaudo. 1985. Contact dermatitis from *Euphorbia pulcherrima. Contact Dermat.* 12: 285–86.

Sargent, C. S. 1916. *Plantae Wilsonianae: An Enumeration of the Woody Plants Collected in Western China for the Arnold Arboretum of Harvard University During the Years 1907, 1908, and 1910 by E. H. Wilson.* Cambridge: Cambridge Univ. Press. (Reprinted in 1988 by Dioscorides Press, Portland).

Saxena, D. B., P. Dureja, B. Kumar, D. Rani, and R. K. Kohli. 1991. Modification of parthenin. *Indian J. Chem.* 30B: 849–58.

Scaiano, J. C., R. W. Redmond, B. Mwhta, and J. T. Arnason. 1990. Efficiency of the photoprocesses leading to singlet oxygen ($^1\Delta_g$) generation by α-terthienyl:

Optical absorption, optoacoustic calorimetry, and infrared luminescence studies. *Photochem. Photobiol.* 52: 655–59.

Schaeffer, M., P. Talaga, J.-L. Stampf, and C. Benezra. 1990. Cross-reaction in allergic contact dermatitis from α-methylene-γ-butyrolactones: Importance of the *cis* or *trans* ring junction. *Contact Dermat.* 22: 32–36.

Scheel, L. D., V. B. Perone, R. L. Larkin, and R. E. Kupel. 1963. The isolation and characterization of two toxic furanocoumarins (psoralens) from diseased celery. *Biochemistry* 2: 1127–31.

Scheinman, P. 1996. Allergic contact dermatitis to fragrance: A review. *Am. J. Contact Dermat.* 7: 65–76.

Schmidt, R. J. 1985. When is a chrysanthemum dermatitis not a *Chrysanthemum* dermatitis? *Contact Dermat.* 13: 115–19.

———. 1986a. The ingenane polyol esters, in *Naturally Occurring Phorbol Esters* (F. J. Evans, ed.). Boca Raton, FL: CRC Press, pp. 245–69.

———. 1986b. Biosynthetic and chemosystematic aspects of the Euphorbiaceae and Thymelaeaceae, in *Naturally Occurring Phorbol Esters* (F. J. Evans, ed.). Boca Raton, FL: CRC Press, pp. 87–106.

———. 1996. Allergic contact dermatitis to liverworts, lichens, and mosses, *Semin. Dermatol.* 15: 95–102.

———. 2001. The *Botanical Dermatitis* database. *Amer. J. Contact Dermat.* 12: 40–42.

———, and F. J. Evans. 1979. Investigations into the skin-irritant properties of resiniferonol orthoesters. *Inflammation* 3: 273–80.

———. 1980. The skin irritant effects of phorbol and related polyols. *Arch. Toxicol.* 44: 279–89.

———, L. Khan, and L. Y. Chung. 1990. Are free radicals and not quinones the haptenic species derived from urushiol and other contact allergenic mono- and dihydric alkylbenzenes? The significance of NADH, glutathione, and redox cycling in the skin. *Arch. Dermatol. Res.* 282: 56–64.

Schnuch, A., J. Geier, W. Uter, P. J. Frosch, W. Lehmacher, W. Aberer, M. Agathos, R. Arnold, T. Fuchs, B. Laubstein, G. Lischka, P. M. Pietrzyk, J. Rakoski, G. Richter, and F. Rueff. 1997. National rates and regional differences in sensitization to allergens of the standard series. *Contact Dermat.* 37: 200–9.

Schuler, G. 1991. *Epidermal Langerhans Cells.* Boca Raton, FL: CRC Press.

Schulte, K. E., G. Henke, G. Rücker, and S. Foerster. 1968. Beitrag zur Biogenese des α-Terthienyls. *Tetrahedron* 24: 1899–1903.

Schwartz, I., L. Tulipan, and D. J. Birmingham. 1957. *Occupational Diseases of the Skin,* 2nd ed. Philadelphia: Lea and Febiger.

Schwarz, A., C. Krone, F. Trautinger, Y. Aragane, P. Neuner, T. A. Luger, and T. Schwarz. 1993. Pentoxifylline suppresses irritant and contact hypersensitivity reactions. *J. Invest. Dermatol.* 101: 549–52.

Scott, F. M., and K. C. Baker. 1947. Anatomy of Washington navel orange rind in relation to water spot. *Bot. Gaz.* 108: 459–75.

Seaman, F. C. 1982. Sesquiterpene lactones as taxonomic characters in the Asteracee. *Bot. Revs.* 48: 121–595.

Seip, H., H. H. Ott, and E. Hecker. 1983. Skin irritant and tumor promoting diterpene esters of the tigliane type from the Chinese tallow tree (*Sapium sebiferum*). *Planta Med.* 49: 199–203.

Seligman, P. J., C. G. Mathias, and M. A. O'Malley. 1987. Phytophotodermtitis from celery among grocery store workers. *Arch. Dermat.* 123: 1478–82.

SGCAFS. 1996. *Inherent Natural Toxicants in Food*, Steering Group on Chemical Aspects of Food Surveillance. London: Ministry of Agriculture, Fisheries, and Food (UK), Food Surveillance Paper No. 51.

Shelmire, B. 1941. The poison ivy and its oleoresin. *J. Invest. Derm.* 4: 337–48.

Shin, Y. G., G. A. Cordell, Y. Dong, and J. M. Pazzuto. 1999. Rapid identification of cytotoxic alkenyl catechols in *Semecarpus anacardium* using bioassay-linked high-performance liquid chromatography-electrospray/mass spectrometric analysis. *Phytochem. Anal.* 10: 208–12.

Slater, J. E. 1994. Latex allergy. *J. Allerg. Clin. Immunol.* 94: 139–49.

Smith, J. 1624. *The Generall Historie of Virginia, New England, and the Summer Isles with the names of the Adventurers, Planters, and Governours from their first beginning An: 1584 to this present 1624*. Printed by J. D. and I. H. for Michael Sparkes, 1624. Reprinted 1966, Ann Arbor: University Microfilms, Inc., p. 170.

Smith, J. G., R. G. Crounce, and D. Spence. 1970. The effects of capsaicin on human skin, liver, and epidermal liposomes. *J. Invest. Dermatol.* 54: 170–3.

Smitt, U. W. 1995. A chemotaxonomic investigation of *Thapsia villosa* L. Apiaceae (Umbelliferae). *Bot. J. Linn. Soc.* 119: 367–77.

Southwell, I. A., and M. H. Campbell. 1991. Hypericin content variation in *Hypericum perforatum* in Australia. *Phytochem.* 30: 475–8.

Spurlock, G. M., R. E. Plaister, W. L. Graves, T. E. Adams, Jr., and R. B. Bushnell. 1980. *Goats for California Brush Control*. Richmond, CA: Division of Agricultural Sciences, University of California, Leaflet 21044.

Srinivas, S. R. 1986. *Atlas of Essential Oils*. New York: Anadams Consultant Service.

Stafford, R. G., M. Mehta, and B. W. Kemppainen. 1992. Comparison of the partition coefficient and skin penetration of a marine algal toxin (lyngbyatoxin A). *Food Cosmet Tox.* 30: 795–801.

Stahl, E., K. Keller, and C. Blinn. 1983. Cardanol, a skin irritant in pink pepper. *Planta Med.* 48: 5–9.

Stampf, J.-L., G. Schlewer, G. Ducombs, J. Foussereau, and C. Benezra. 1978. Allergic contact dermatitis due to sesquiterpene lactones. *Brit. J. Dermatol.* 99: 163–69.

Standley, P. C. 1923. Trees and shrubs of Mexico, *Contribs. U.S. National Herbarium* 23 (Part 3): 517–848.

Stauffer, J. 1972. *An Investigation of Hydrourushiol (PDC)-Protein Interactions. Formation and Properties of Various PDQ-Protein and Related Conjugates.* Ph.D. dissertation, Columbia University, New York, *Diss. Abstr. Internat. B* 33: 96–7.

Stevenson, R. L. 1883. *The Silverado Squatters*, chapter 4. London: Chatto & Windus.

Stoll, A., and E. Seebeck. 1947. Über alliin, die genuine Muttersubstanz des Knoblauchöls. *Experientia* 3: 114–15.

Straus, M. W. 1931. Artificial sensitization of infants to poison ivy. *J. Allergy* 2: 137–44.

Sunthankar, S. V., and C. R. Dawson. 1954. The structural identification of the olefinic components of Japanese lac urushiol. *J. Amer. Chem. Soc.* 76: 5070–74.

Suzuki, Y., Y. Esumi, H. Hyakutake, Y. Kono, and A. Sakurai. 1996. Isolation of 5-(8′Z- heptadecenyl)resorcinol from etiolated rice seedlings as an antifungal agent. *Phytochem.* 41: 1485–89.

Swan, R. J., W. Klyne, and H. MacLean. 1967. Optical rotatory dispersion studies. XLI. The absolute configuration of plicatic acid. *Can. J. Chem.* 45: 319–24.

Sweet, D. V. 1987. *Registry of Toxic Effects of Chemical Substances*, vol. 3A. Washington, DC: U.S. Public Health Service.

Symes, W. F., and C. R. Dawson. 1954. Poison Ivy "urushiol." *J. Amer. Chem. Soc.* 76: 2959–63.

Thompson, R. H. 1971. *Naturally Occurring Quinones*, 2nd ed. London: Academic Press.

———. 1987. *Naturally Occurring Quinones. III. Recent Advances*. London: Chapman and Hall.

Thurston, E. L. 1974. Morphology, fine structure, and ontogeny of the stinging emergence of *Urtica dioica*. *Am. J. Bot.* 61: 809–17.

———. 1976. Morphology, fine structure, and ontogeny of the stinging emergences of *Tragia ramosa* and *T. saxicola* (Euphorbiaceae). *Amer. J. Bot.* 63: 710–18.

Torrey, J., and A. Gray. 1840. *A Flora of North America*, vol. 1. New York: Wiley and Putnam. Reprinted by Hafner Publishing Co., New York, in 1969.

Towers, G. H. N., and J. C. Mitchell. 1983. The current status of the weed *Parthenium hysterophorus* L. as a cause of allergic contact dermatitis. *Contact Dermat.* 9: 465–69.

Toyama, I. 1918. Rhus dermatitis. *J. Cutan. Disease* 36: 157.

Tschesche, R., F.-J. Kämmerer, and G. Wulff. 1969. Über die Strukter der antibiotsch aktiven Substanzen der Tulpe (*Tulipa gesneriana* L.). *Chem. Ber.* 102: 2057–71.

Turjanmaa, K., H. Alenius, S. Mäkinen-Kiljunen, T. Reunala, and T. Palosuo. 2000. Natural rubber-latex allergy, in *Handbook of Occupational Dermatitis* (L. Kanerva, P. Elsner, J. E. Wahlberg, and H. I. Maibach, eds.). Berlin: Springer Verlag, pp. 719–29.

Turner, B. L. 1977. Fossil history and geography, in *The Biology and Chemistry of the Compositae*, vol. 1. (V. H. Heywood, J. B. Harborne, and B. L. Turner, eds). New York: Academic Press, pp. 21–39.

Turner, N. J., and A. F. Szczawinski. 1991. *Common Poisonous Plants and Mushrooms of North America*. Portland, OR: Timber Press.

Turner, R. J., and E. Wasson. 1997. *Botanica*. Milson's Point, New South Wales: Random House Australia.

Tyman, J. H. P. 1973. Long-chain phenols. Part III. Identification of the components of a novel phenolic fraction in *Anacardium occidentale* (Cashew Nut-Shell Liquid) and synthesis of the saturated member. *J. Chem. Soc. Perkin 1* 1973: 1639–47.

———. 1979. Non-isoprenoid long chain phenols. *Chem. Soc. Revs.* 8: 499–537.

———, and S. K. Lam. 1978. The conversion of anacardic acid to urushiol in vitro and in vivo, vol. 2, in *11th. International Symposium on the Chemistry of Natural Products, IUPAC* (N. Marekov, I. Ognyanov, and A. Orahovats, eds.). Sofia, Bulgaria: Izd. BAN, pp. 190–92.

———, and A. J. Mathews. 1982. Long-chain phenols. XXII. Compositional studies on Japanese lac (*Rhus vernicifera*) by chromatography and mass spectrometry. *J. Chromatog.* 235: 149–64.

———, V. Tychopoulos, and P. Chan. 1984. Long-chain phenols. XXV. Quantitative analysis of natural cashew nut-shell liquid (*Anacardium occidentale*) by high-performance liquid chromatography. *J. Chromatog.* 303: 137–50.

Tzeng, C.-C. 1993. *Effect of 24-, 48-, or 72-Hour In Vitro Rumen Fluid Incubation and Pepsin-HCl Treatment on Poison Oak Urushiol*. Ph.D. dissertation, University of California, Davis, CA.

Urbach, F. 1991. Photocarcinogenesis, in *Dermatotoxicology* (F. N. Marzulli and H. I. Maibach, eds.). New York: Hemisphere Publishing Corp., pp. 633–46.

USDA. 1970. *Selected Weeds of the United States*. Washington, DC: U.S. Dept. of Agriculture. Reprinted by Dover Publications Inc. in 1971 as *Common Weeds of the United States*.

Van Dijk, E., and L. Berrens. 1941. Plants as an etiological factor in dermatitis venenata due to plants. *Dermatologica* 129: 321–28.

VanEtten, C. H. 1969. Goitrogens, in *Toxic Constituents of Plant Foodstuffs* (I. E. Liener, ed.). New York: Academic Press, pp. 103–142.

———, M. E. Daxenbichler, and I. A. Wolff. 1969. Natural glucosinolates (thioglucosides) in foods and feeds. *J. Agr. Food Chem.* 17: 483–91.

Van Mons, J. B. 1797. Mémoire sur le *Rhus radicans*. *Act. Soc. Méd. Chir. Pharm.* 1(2): 136–67.

Verspyck Mijnssen, G. A. W. 1969. Pathogenesis and causative agent of "Tulip Finger," *Brit. J. Dermatol.* 81: 737–45.

Vickers, H. R. 1941. The carrot as a cause of dermatitis. *Brit. J. Dermatol.* 53: 52–7.

Walker, F. B. 1967. Genetic factors in human allergic contact dermatitis. *Internat. Arch. Allergy Appl. Immun.* 32: 453.

Watson, E. S., J. C. Murphy, and P. W. Wirth. 1981. Immunologic studies of poisonous Anacardiaceae. I. Production of tolerance and desensitization to poison ivy and oak urushiols using esterified urushiol derivatives in guinea pigs. *J. Invest. Dermatol.* 76: 164–70.

Weber, L. F. 1937. External causes of dermatitis: A list of irritants. *Arch. Dermat.* 35: 129–79.

Webster, G. L. 1975. Conspectus of a new classification of the Euphorbiaceae. *Taxon* 24: 593–601.

Weissman, G., L. Azaroff, S. Davidson, and P. Dunham. 1986. Synergy between phorbol esters, 1-oleyl-2-acetylglycerol, urushiol, and calcium ionophore in eliciting aggregation of marine sponge cells. *Proc. Nat. Acad. Sci. USA* 83: 2914–18.

Wender, P. A., K. D. Rice, and M. E. Schnute, 1997a. The first formal asymmetric synthesis of phorbol. *J. Amer. Chem. Soc.* 119: 7897–98.

———, C. D. Jesudason, H. Nakahira, N. Tamura, A. L. Tebbe, and Y. Ueno. 1997b. The first synthesis of a daphnane diterpene: The enantiocontrolled total synthesis of (+)-resiniferatoxin. *J. Amer. Chem. Soc.* 119: 12976–77.

Werker, E., and J. G. Vaughn. 1976. Ontogeny and distribution of myrosin cells in the shoot of *Sinapis alba* L. A light- and electron-microscope study. *Israel J. Bot.* 25: 140–51.

White, J. C. 1887. *Dermatitis Venenata: An Account of External Irritants Upon the Skin.* Boston: Cupples and Hurd.

Whiting, D. A. 1986. Smodingium: Allergenic Anacardiaceae in South Africa. *Clin. Dermatol.* 4: 204–7.

Wilks, W. 1914. *Journal Kept by David Douglas During His Travels in North America, 1823–1827.* London: The Royal Horticultural Society.

Williams, R. T. 1959. *Detoxication Mechanisms,* 2nd ed. New York: John Wiley.

Winek, C. L., J. Butala, S. P. Shanor, and F. W. Fochtman. 1978. Toxicology of Poinsettia. *Clin. Toxicol.* 13: 27–45.

Winkler, J. D., M. B. Rouse, M. F. Greaney, S. J. Harrison, and Y. T. Jeon. 2002. The first total synthesis of (±)-ingenol. *J. Amer. Chem. Soc.* 124: 9726–28.

Witzel, D. A., G. W. Ivie, and J. W. Dollahite. 1976. Mammalian toxicity of helenalin, the toxic principle of *Helenium microcephalum* DC (Smallhead Sneezeweed). *Amer. J. Vet. Res.* 37: 859–61.

Woods, B., and C. D. Calnan. 1976. Toxic Woods. *Brit. J. Dermatol.* 94 (Suppl. 13): 1–97.

Wrigley, J. W., and M. Fagg. 1988. *Australian Native Plants,* 3rd ed. Sydney: Collins Publishers Australia.

Wynn, J. L., and T. M. Cotton. 1995. Spectroscopic properties of hypericin in solution and at surfaces. *J. Phys. Chem.* 99: 4317–23.

Yamazaki, M., M. Matsuo, and S. Shibata. 1965. Biosynthesis of lichen depsides, lecanoric acid, and atranorin. *Chem. Pherm. Bull.* 13: 1015–17.

Yates, S. G., R. E. England, and W. F. Kwolek. 1983. Analysis of carrot constituents: Myristicin, falcarinol, and falcarindiol, in *Xenobiotics in Foods and Feeds* (eds.), *ACS Sympos. Ser.* 234: 333–44.

Yoshida, H. 1883. Chemistry of lacquer (Urushi). Part I. *J. Chem. Soc.* 43: 472–86.

Yoshioka, H., T. J. Mabry, and B. N. Timmermann. 1973. *Sesquiterpene Lactones: Chemistry, NMR, and Plant Distribution.* Tokyo: University of Tokyo Press.

Zajdela, E., and E. Bisagni. 1981. 5-Methoxypsoralen, the malanogenic additive in suntan preparations, is tumorigenic in mice exposed to 365 nm u.v. radiation. *Carcinog.* 2: 121–27.

Zarnowska, E. D., R. Zarnowski, and A. Kozubek. 2000. Alkylresorcinols in fruit pulp and leaves of *Ginkgo biloba* L. *Z. Naturforsch.* 55C: 881–85.

Zarnowski, R., Y. Suzuki, Y. Esumi, and S. J. Pietr. 2000. 5-*n*-Alkylreaorcinols from the green microalga *Apatococcus constipatus. Phytochem.* 55: 975–77.

Zechmeister, L., and J. W. Sease. 1947. A blue-fluorescing compound, terthienyl, isolated from marigolds. *J. Amer. Chem. Soc.* 69: 273–75.

Zhai, H., and H. L. Maibach. 2000. Prevention of allergic contact dermatitis to plants, in *Dermatologic Botany* (J. Avalos and H. I. Maibach eds.). Boca Raton, FL: CRC Press, pp. 45–50.

——, H., A. Anigbogu, and H. I. Maibach. 2000. Treatment and protection, in *Handbook of Occupational Dermatitis* (L. Kanerva, P. Elsner, J. E. Wahlberg, and H. I. Maibach, eds.). Berlin: Springer Verlag, pp. 402–11.

Zhan, D., Y. Du, and B. Qian. 1990. Oxidation of urushiol and its analogs catalyzed by *Rhus vernicifera* laccase in aqueous solution of ethanol. *Gaofenzi Xuebao* 1990: 327–31; *Chem. Abstr.* 114: 104405[z].

Zheng, G., W. Lu, H. A. Aisa, and J. Cai. 1999. Absolute configuration of falcarinol, a potent antitumor agent commonly occurring in plants. *Tetrahed. Lett.* 40: 2181–82.

Zubay, G. 1986. *Biochemistry.* Reading, MA: Addison-Wesley Publishing Co.

Zug, K. A., and J. G. Marks. 1999. Plants and woods, in *Occupational Skin Disease,* (R. M. Adams, ed.), 3rd ed. Philadelphia: W. B. Saunders Company, pp. 567–96.

GLOSSARY

Acuminate. Tapering to a sharp point.

Allergen. A chemical substance, sometimes generated metabolically, that causes an allergic reaction.

Antiinflammatory. An agent that reduces inflammation.

Asthma. An allergy of the respiratory tract.

Axil. The angle where a stem or petiole meets a main stalk.

Bioavailability. Here, the availability of a substance to be absorbed by the skin.

Bullae. Large blisters.

Cocarcinogen. A substance that does not initiate tumors but enhances the carcinogen's effect.

Conjugate (n.). A metabolite in which a reactive chemical group has been deactivated by combination with a natural reagent, for example, a glucose ester of a carboxylic acid.

Corticoid. Abbreviation for corticosteroid.

Corticosteroid. A steroid (hormone) of the adrenal cortex, such as hydrocortisone, used for treatment of dermatitis.

Coumarin. Benzo-2-pyrone, a common type of natural plant lactone.

Cross-reaction. An allergic reaction to a substance chemically related to the original sensitizer.

Cytokine. A low–molecular-weight messenger substance secreted by T-cells in response to an antigen.

Dendritic cell. A cell with many branches—in this context, of the epidermis—for example, a Langerhans cell.

Dermatotoxic. Toxic to skin.

Dermis. The skin layer beneath the epidermis, composed primarily of collagen, in which capillaries, nerve cells, and hair follicles are embedded.

Detoxication. Removal or reduction of toxicity, most often via metabolic processes.

Dicot. Abbreviation for dicotyledon; a broadleaf plant that produces two initial leaves from the sprouting seed. A majority of familiar flowering plants are dicots.

Dioecious. A plant that produces male and female structures on separate individuals.

Diterpene. A substance based on a 20-carbon skeleton composed of four isoprene units.

Drupe. A fruit with a hard exterior and a fleshy interior surrounding the single seed.

Eczema. The general term for a skin condition that produces inflammation (redness), itching, and/or oozing lesions.

Epidermis. The outer living layer of skin, beneath the stratum corneum, in which allergy is initiated.

Epoxide. A three-member cyclic structure containing two carbons and one oxygen; an oxirane.

Essential oil. A natural plant-derived extractive that produces an aroma or essence.

Euphorb. An abbreviation indicating a member of the family Euphorbiaceae.

Glabrous. Without hair, generally used to describe a plant.

Glucosinolate. A mustard oil glycoside, the sugar derivative of a thiohydroxamic acid sulfate, which forms an isothiocyanate upon hydrolysis; a thioglucoside.

Hapten. A low–molecular-weight substance that combines with protein to provide an antigen.

Hispid. Covered with stiff hairs or small spines.

HPLC. An abbreviation for the method of chemical separations known as high-performance liquid chromatography.

Hypoallergenic. Reduced ability to cause allergy.

Immunoglobulin. A class of immunologically active globe-shaped proteins.

Involucre. A whorl of bracts located below and close to a flower or fruit.

K_{ow}. Abbreviation for the octanol–water partition coefficient, the ratio of the concentration of a substance in an upper octyl alcohol phase of an aqueous mixture compared to that in the water below.

Laccol. Common name for an allergenic catechol containing a 17-carbon side chain.

Lachrymator. A substance that produces tears in the eyes of an exposed individual.

Lactone. A cyclic ester, that is, where the acid and alcohol groups are on the same molecule.

Latex. The milky sap (emulsion) produced by some plants, including those of the mango and spurge families.

Laticifer. The latex-carrying duct within a plant.

Lichen. A symbiotic combination of an alga and an Ascomycete fungus.

Lipophilic. Attracted to or soluble in fat (lipid).

Liverwort. A lower plant (bryophyte) of the class Hepaticae, related to mosses but possessing lobed leaves.

Lymph. The fluid, analogous to blood, that transports and disposes of foreign material in the body. It contains white cells (lymphocytes) but no red cells.

Lymph node. Locations in the body where lymph ducts meet.

Lymphocyte. A leukocyte (white cell) that mediates the immune reactions of the body, for example, Langerhans cells and T-cells.

Mast cell. A large dermal cell that contains numerous mediator-carrying granules.

Mediator. In this text, a substance, such as histamine, responsible for the swelling, itching, and blisters of allergy or irritation.

Metabolism. In this text, the biodegradative processes of living organisms.

Michael reaction. Addition of a nucleophile such as an amine across a carbon–carbon double bond that is adjacent to an electron-attracting group such as a carbonyl.

Monocot. Abbreviation for monocotyledon; a narrow-leafed plant with parallel veins that produces only one initial leaf from the sprouting seed; typically a grass.

Mustard oil. An old name for a natural isothiocyanate.

Nucleophile. An electron-rich chemical species that seeks electropositive centers in a chemical reaction. Amines and mercaptans are typical nucleophiles.

Oxidase. An enzyme that catalyzes biochemical oxidation (oxygenation) reactions.

Palmate. Resembling a hand with spread fingers; shaped like the silhouette of a palm tree.

Panicle. Flowers set in the form of a loose pyramid.

Partition coefficient. A constant representing the ratio of the concentration of a substance in one phase (such as fat) to that in an adjacent phase (usually liquid water).

Peduncle. The stem that connects a flower with a main stalk.

Petiole. The stem that connects a leaf with a main stalk.

Phenol. A benzene ring containing one or more hydroxyl groups; specifically, hydroxybenzene.

Photodermatitis. A skin condition resembling ACD brought on by a combination of certain chemicals and light.

Photodynamic. Inducing a toxic reaction to light and oxygen.

Pilose. Bearing soft, straight hairs.

Pinnate. Resembling a feather, with similar parts arranged opposite each other along a central axis.

Polyketide. A chemical structure composed of repeating acetyl (CH_3CO—) units.

Promoter. In this text, a cocarcinogen that promotes the carcinogenicity (tumor formation) of an initiator.

Pruritis. Itching.

Puberulent. Covered with fine hairs normally visible only under magnification.

Pubescent. Downy.

PUV. A form of allergy treatment involving simultaneous exposure to the phototoxic furocoumarin psoralen and ultraviolet radiation at 320–400 nm.

Raceme. Flowers borne on short stems set at intervals along a main stem.

Raphide. A cellular bundle of calcium oxalate crystals that may be forcibly ejected upon contact.

Rubefacient. A medication that reddens the skin, generally by bringing blood closer to the surface.

Sensitization. In this text, the initial reaction to an antigen that sets the stage for symptoms of allergy upon the next encounter.

Sesquiterpene. A substance based on a 15-carbon skeleton of three isoprene units.

Singlet oxygen. A reactive form of molecular oxygen in which the two oxygen atoms are connected by a double bond rather than the oxygen being a diradical.

Stratum corneum. The thin surface layer of skin, consisting of dead cells (the protein keratin), fat, and other chemicals.

Ternate. Arranged in threes.

Terpene. A type of natural chemical based on isoprene (2-methyl-1, 3-butadiene).

TLC. Abbreviation for thin-layer chromatography, where a solvent rises up a plate covered with a thin layer of adsorbent on which a mixture to be separated has been placed.

Trichome. An emergence or epidermal hair on a plant surface.

Trifoliate. Having three leaves.

Ultraviolet. The region of the electromagnetic spectrum with wavelengths between 180 and 400 nm. Solar ultraviolet spans 280–400 nm.

Umbel. A flower structure in which the stems (peduncles) appear to start from a common point, like spokes on an umbrella. Typical of the carrot family (Umbelliferae, now termed the Apiaceae).

Urticaria. Contact urticaria. An transient allergic or irritant skin reaction, such as that caused by a nettle (*Urtica*), whose symptoms often may be similar to those of allergic contact dermatitis.

Urushioid. A substance that is chemically and immunologically similar to urushiol, the allergen of toxicodendons.

UV. Abbreviation for ultraviolet (radiation). The UV-A region covers 320–400 nm and UV-B 290–320 nm.

Vapor pressure. The pressure exerted by vapor of a substance when in equilibrium with the liquid or solid form; a measure of volatility.

Vesicant. An agent that causes blisters.

Vitiligo. A skin condition characterized by smooth white patches.

Xenobiotic. A chemical that is foreign to an organism; not a natural substance.

INDEXES
INDEX OF PLANT NAMES

Numbers in italics indicate tables or figures, bold type indicates key information.

Bergamot orange. *See Citrus bergamia*
Betula spp., 50
Bishop's weed. *See Ammi* spp.
Bitter orange. *See Citrus aurantium*
Black mustard. *See Brassica nigra*
Blister plant. *See Ranunculus* spp.
Blue spurge. *See Euphorbia*
    coerulescens
Bowdichia nitida, 51, 110
Brassica hirta. See Sinapis alba
Brassica nigra, 78, 79, 140, 141
Brassica spp., 78, 79, 140, *140*, *141*,
    142
Brassicaceae, 6, **77**, 78, 140
Brazilian pepper tree. *See Schinus*
    terebinthifolius
Broccoli. *See Brassica* spp.
Buckwheat. *See Fagopyrum*
    esculentum
Burmese lac. *See Melanorrhoea usitata*
Buttercups. *See Ranunculus* spp.

Cabbage. *See Brassica* spp.
Cajeput. *See Melaleuca* spp.
California pepper tree. *See Schinus*
    molle
Calla lily. *See Zantedeschia aethiopica*
Calocedrus decurrens, 49, 110
Caltha palustris, 83
Campnosperma auriculata, **44**, 89
Canadian balsam. *See Abies balsamea*
Cananga odorata, 59
Canary Island spurge. *See Euphorbia*
    spp.
Candelabra cactus. *See Euphorbia* spp.
Candlenut. *See Aleurites moluccana*
Candytuft. *See Iberis* spp.
Capeweed. *See Arctotheca* spp.
Capsicum annuum, 6, 83, **84**
Cardwellia sublimis, 90
Carica papaya, 78, 141
Carrot. *See Daucus carota*
Cashew. *See Anacardium occidentale*
Castor bean. *See Ricinus communis*
Cauliflower. *See Brassica* spp.
Cedar. *See Calocedrus decurrens* (see
    also *Juniperus virginiana*)
Cedrella mexicana, 50
Celery. *See Apium graveolens*

Century plant. *See Agave* spp.
Chamaemelum nobile, 40, 56, 59, 114
Chamaesyce maculata, 74
Chamomile, German. *See Matricaria*
    chamomilla (= *Chamomilla*
    recutita)
Chamomile, Roman. *See*
    Chamaemelum nobile
    (= *Anthemis nobilis*)
Chicory. *See Chicorium* spp.
Chicorium spp., 53, 114, 158
Chili pepper. *See Capsicum annuum*
Chinese primrose. *See Primula* spp.
Chinese tallow tree. *See Sapium*
    sebiferum
Christmasberry. *See Schinus*
    terebinthifolius
Chrysanthemums, 54, 155, 156, *159*,
    (see also *Dendranthema*)
Chrysanthemum cinerariaefolium, 53,
    114
Chrysanthemum morifolium. See
    Dendranthema × *grandiflorum*
Cinnamomum spp., 40, **60**, 109, 121,
    163
Cinnamon. *See Cinnamomum* spp.
Citronella. *See Cymbopogon nardus*
Citrus aurantifolia (lime), 6, 67, 67–8
Citrus spp., 6, 59, **60**, 67–8, *67*, 121,
    163
Cladonia spp., 63
Clematis vitalba, 83
Cleome hassleriana, 141
Cloves. *See Syzygium aromaticum*
Cnidoscolus spp., 74, **82**, 147, 148
Cockleburr. *See Xanthium*
    pennsylvanicum
Cocobolo. *See Dalbergia obtusa*
    (*retusa*)
Cochleara officinalis, 141
Codiaeum variegatum, 19, 5, 74, 75
Coleus blumeii, 110, 113
Common rue. *See Ruta graveolens*
Comocladia spp., 44
Compositae. *See Asteraceae*
Congress grass. *See Parthenium*
    hysterophorus
Cooper's spurge. *See Euphorbia*
    cooperi

Cordia. *See Cordia goeldiana*
Cordia goeldiana, 51, *110*
Costus. *See Saussurea costus*
Cow parsnip. *See Heracleum lanatum*
Cowslip. *See Primula veris*
Creeping buttercup. *See Ranunculus
    repens*
Creosote bush. *See Larrea tridentata*
Croton spp., 75, 136
Croton, varigated. *See Codiaeum
    variegatum*
Crowfoot. *See Ranunculus* spp.
Crown-of-thorns. *See Euphorbia milii*
Cruciferaceae. *See* Brassicaceae
Cymbidium cultivars, 49, *110*
Cymbopogon citratus, 59
Cymbopogon nardus, 59
Cynara spp., *40*, 53, 114, 156
Cyperus dietrichae, *110*
Cypress spurge. *See Euphorbia
    cyparissias*
Cypripedium calceolus, 49, *110*

Daffodil. *See Narcissus* spp.
Dalbergia latifolia, 50, *51*
Dalbergia obtusa (retusa), 50, *51*,
    110, 113
Dalbergia spp., 50, *51*, *110*, 159
Dandelion. *See Taraxacum officinale*
Daphne spp., **77**, 136, 190, *196*
Daucus carota, 69, 119–120, 156
Dendranthema spp., 54, 114, *159*
Dendranthema × *grandiflorum*, *40*,
    54, 109, 158, plate 14
Dendrocnide spp., 81, 82, 147, 184
Desert bluebells. *See Phacelia* spp.
Desert heliotrope. *See Phacelia* spp.
Dictamnus albus, 67, 69, *196*
Dieffenbachia spp., 83, 84, **85–6**,
    149, 184, *196*
Dill. *See Anethum graveolens*
Diospyros celebica, 51, 109, *110*
Distemonanthus benthamianus, *110*
Dittrichia graveolens, 156
Dog fennel. *See Anthemis cotula*
Dumbcane. *See Dieffenbachia* spp.

Eastern poison oak. *See Toxicodendron
    diversilobum* ssp. *pubescens*

East Indian rosewood. *See Dalbergia
    latifolia*
Echinops exaltus, 67
Elecampane. *See Inula helenium*
Elephant garlic. *See Allium
    ampeloprasum*
El litre. *See Lithrea caustica*
English ivy. *See Hedera helix*
Erigeron strigosus, 55, 56, 158
Erysimum cheiri, 78, 141
Eucalyptus spp., 163
Eugenia caryophyllata. *See
    Syzygium aromaticum*
Euphorbiaceae, 6, 7, 8, **73**, 74, 178,
    179
Euphorbia characias wulfenii, 76,
    138, *179*; plates 19, 24
Euphorbia milii, 76, 137, 178, 179
Euphorbia spp., *6*, *19*, 74, 76, 77,
    138, 178, 179, 190
Euphorbia pulcherrima (poincettia),
    76
Euphorbia resinifera, 76, 137, 179
Euphorbia tirucalli, 75, 178, 179,
    plate 18
Euphorbium. *See Euphorbia resinifera*
Euphorbia wulfenii. *See Euphorbia
    characias wulfenii*
Eutrema wasabi, 78, 79
Evergreen candytuft. *See Iberis* spp.
Evernia prunastri, 64, 121

Fagopyrum esculentum, 67, 72, 134
Fatshedra. *See Fatshedra lizei*
Fatshedra lizei, 58
Fennel. *See Foeniculum vulgare*
Feverfew. *See Tanacetum parthenium*
Ficus spp., 6, 67, 71, 180
Fig. *See Ficus* spp.
Fleabane. *See Erigeron strigosus*
Florida holly. *See Schinus
    terebinthifolius*
Florist's chrysanthemum. *See
    Dendranthema* × *grandiflorum*
Foeniculum vulgare, 70
French marigold. *See Tagetes patula*
Fraxinella. *See Dictamnus albus*
Frullania dilatata, 63, 114, *155*,
    156

Lime. *See Citrus aurantifolia*
Lithrea caustica, 40, 51, 89
Lithrea spp., 44, 51, 89
Litre. *See Lithrea caustica*
Liverworts. *See* Hepaticae
Longleaf Pine. *See Pinus* spp.
Lyngbya majuscula, 64, 84

Macassar ebony. *See Diospyros
    celebica*
Machaerium scleroxylon, 51, 110
Mala mujer, 3
Manchineel. *See Hippomane
    mancinella*
Mandrake. *See Podophyllum peltatum*
Mango. *See Mangifera indica*
Mangifera indica, 40, **41–2**, 89, 158,
    160
Mansonia. *See Mansonia altissima*
Mansonia altissima, 50, 51, 109, 110
Manzanillo de Cerra. *See
    Toxicodendron striatum*
Marguerite. *See Argyanthemum
    frutescens*
Marigold. *See Tagetes* spp.
Marking nut. *See Semecarpus* spp.
Marsh marigold. *See Caltha palustris*
Matricaria chamomilla, 56, 114, 158,
    163
Mattiola incana, 78
Mayapple. *See Podophyllum peltatum*
Mayweed. *See Anthemis cotula*
Mecha. *See Phagnalon purpurescens*
Melaleuca alternifolia (tea tree), **60**,
    124, 163
Melaleuca spp., **60**, 124, 163
Melanochyla spp., 43
Melanorrhoea spp., 43, 51, 89
Melanorrhoea usitata (Burmese lac),
    51, 89
Mentha spp., 59, 121, 163
Menzies peppergrass. *See Lepidium*
    spp.
Metopium spp., 6, 40, 43, 89, 168
Mexican cedar. *See Cedrella mexicana*
Mignonette. *See Reseda odorata*
Milo. *See Thespesia populnea*
Mint. *See Mentha* spp.
Mokihana. *See Pelea anisata*

Mole plant. *See Euphorbia* spp.
Monarda spp., 121
Monstera deliciosa, 45
Moraceae, **71**
Mountain rockcress. *See Arabis alpina*
Mountain tobacco. *See Arnica
    montana*
Mustards. *See* Brassicaceae
Myristica fragrans, 60
Myroxylon balsamum, 62
Myroxylon toluiferum, 62

Narcissus spp., 55, 83
Nasturtium. *See Tropaeolum majus*
Nasturtium officinale, 78, 141
Nettle. *See Urtica* spp. (*see also
    Hespericnide tenella, Laportea*
    spp.)
Nicotiana tabacum, 159
Noseburn. *See Tragia ramosa*
Nutmeg. *See Myristica fragrans*

Oakmoss. *See Evernia prunastri*
Old man's beard. *See Clematis vitalba*
Onion. *See Allium cepa*
Opisthiolepis heterophylla, 90
Orange. *See Citrus* spp.
Oryza sativa (rice), 40, 45, 89
Oxlip. *See Primula* spp.

Panax ginseng, 58
Pao ferra. *See Machaerium scleroxylon*
Papaya. *See Carica papaya*
Papyrus. *See Cyperus dietrichae*
Pará rubber tree. *See Hevea
    brasiliensis*
Paratecoma peroba, 51
Parsley. *See Petroselinum sativum*
Parsnip. *See Pastinaca sativa*
Parthenium hysterophorus, 6, 7, 40,
    55, **56**, 114, 156, 158, 159
Pasque-flower. *See Pulsatilla vulgaris*
Pastinaca sativa, 67, 70, 132, 156
Pelargonium graveolens, 121
Pelea anisata, 69
Pencil bush. *See Euphorbia tirucalli*
Pentaspadon motleyi, 97
Pentaspadon officinalis, 89
Pepper. *See Capsicum annuum*

Peppermint. *See Mentha* spp.
Peppergrass. *See Lepidium* spp.
Pepper tree. *See Schinus molle*
Peroba do Campos. *See Tecoma peroba, Paratecoma peroba*
Persian lime. *See Citrus aurantifolia*
Persian ranunculus. *See Ranunculus* spp.
Persoonia eliptica, 90
Persoona linearis, 90
Petrophila shirleyae, 90
Petroselinum sativum, 70, 132
Phacelia spp., *48, 110*, plate 13
Phagnalon purpurescens, 110
Phebalium spp., 68
Philodendron spp., *40, 45, 86, 89*, plate 10
Physic nut. *See Jatropha curcas*
Pimpinella anisum, 59, 67
Pine. *See Pinus* spp.
Pinus spp., *62, 121*
Pistacia spp., *45*
Plumbago spp., *110*
Poaceae, *45, 89*
Podophyllum peltatum, 83, 84, 139
Poinsettia. *See Euphorbia pulcherrima*
Poison ivy. *See Toxicodendron radicans*
Poison oak, eastern. *See Toxicodendron diversilobum* ssp. *pubescens*
Poison oak., western. *See Toxicodendron diversilobum*
Poisonwood. *See Metopium* spp.
Prairie sage. *See Artemesia* spp.
Prima vera. *See Tabebuia donnell-smithii*
Primrose. *See Primula* spp.
Primula obconica, 6, 109, 109, 110–1, 196, plate 12
Primula × polyantha, 47
Primula spp., *47, 48, 48, 110, 152, 159, 195–6*
Primula veris (cowslip), *48*
Psoralea spp., *67, 73*
Pulsatilla vulgaris, 83
Pyrethrum daisy. *See Chrysanthemum cinerariaefolium*

Queen Anne's lace. *See Daucus carota*

Radish. *See Raphanus sativus*
Ragweed. *See Ambrosia* spp.
Ramp. *See Allium* spp.
Ranunculus bulbosa, 83
Ranunculus repens 83, plate 21
Ranunculus spp., *6, 19, 83, 114, 155, 156, 187*
Rape. *See Brassica* spp.
Raphanus sativus, 78
Red cedar. *See Thuja plicata*
Red onion. *See Allium cepa*
Rengas tree. *See Gluta rengas*
Reseda odorata, 78
Rhus, 5, 23, 24, 35
    toxicodendron, see Toxicodendron radicans
    typhina, 46
Rice. *See Oryza sativa*
Ricinus communis, 74, **77**
Rockcress. *See Arabis* spp.
Rocket candytuft. *See Iberis* spp.
Roman camomile. *See Chamaemelum nobile*
Rosa spp., *59, 121*
Rose. *See Rosa* spp.
Rosmarinus officinalis, 61
Rosemary. *See Rosmarinus officinalis*
Rosewoods. *See Dalbergia* spp.
Rutabaga. *See Brassica* spp.
Rutaceae, **67**, *68*
Ruta graveolens, 67, 68, 180, 196
Rye. *See Secale cereale*

Sage. *See Artemesia* spp. (*see also Salvia officinalis*)
Sagebrush. *See Artemesia* spp.
St. John's wort. *See Hypericum* spp.
Salvia officinalis, 59
Sandalwood. *See Santalum album*
Sandbox tree. *See Hura crepitans*
Santalum album, 61, 121
Sapium sebiferum, 74
Saussurea costus, 114
Schefflera spp., *58*
Schinus molle, 43
Schinus terebinthifolius, 6, 40, **42–43**, *58, 97, 154–5, 158, 168*, plate 9
Scurf pea. *See Psoralea corylifolia*
Scurvygrass. *See Cochleara officinalis*

INDEX OF CHEMICAL COMMON NAMES

Numbers in italics indicate tables or figures, bold type indicates key information.

Dihydrocapsaicin, 147
Dimethoxybenzoquinone (DMB),
    50, *51*, 108, *110, 111*
    reactions, **112**
    sources, *110*
Dimethoxydalbergione, *110, 111*
Dithiins, 145

Eugenol, 59, 121, 122, *122*, 123, *166, 175*
Euphorbium, 137
Evernic acid, 64, 125

Fagopyrin, *67*, 72, 133
Falcarindiol, 119
Falcarinol, 58, 109, 119–20
Falcarinone, 119
Farnesylhydroquinone, 109, *110, 111*
Ficusin, *129, 130*
Frullanolide, 63, *114, 115*, 189
Furocoumarins. *See the general index*

Geraniol, *59*, 121, *121*, 122, 161
2-Geranylhydroquinone, *110, 111*
2-Geranylquinone, *110, 111*
Gingerol, 59, *122*
Ginkgoic acid, *97*
Ginkgol, *97*
Ginkgolinic acid, *97*
Gluconapin and relatives. *See*
    glucosinolates
Glucosinolates, 79, *140*, 141–2, *141*
    (*see also* sinalbin, sinigrin)
Grevillol, *51, 93*

Helenalin, *11, 114, 115, 175*
Heraclenin, *129, 130*
Heraclenol, *129, 130*
Hevein, 126
Histamine, *139*, 147, 148, *148*, 149,
    180, 184
Huratoxin, *137*
Hydroginkgol, *97*
Hydroxycitronellal, *121*
Hypericin, *67*, 71, 133, 185
    uv absorption and fluorescence, *210*

Imperatorin, *129, 130*, 133
Ingenol and ingenol esters, 136,
    137, *138*

Irisquinone, *110, 111*
Isabelin, 57, *114, 115*
Isoalantolactone, 190
Isoalliin, *145*, 146
Isobergapten, *129, 130*, 132, 133
Isoimperatorin, *129, 130*, 132, 133
Isopimpinellin, *129, 130*, 132

Jasmone, *83*

Khellin, 130, *130*

Laccols, 9, 20, *51*, 87
    physical properties, *98*
    sources, *88, 208*
    spectra, *209*
    structures, *208*
Lachrymatory factor (LF), *144*,
    146
Lactones. *See the general index*
Lactucin, 53, *114, 115*
Lactucopicrin, *40*, 53, 109, *114, 115*
Lanatin, *129, 130*, 133
Lapachenol, *51, 110, 111*
Lapachol, *51, 110, 111*
Lapachonone, *110*
Laurenobiolide, 55, *114, 115*
Leucotrienes, *148*
Limonenes, *11*, 59, 109, 121, *121*,
    122, 124, *166*
Linalool, *11*, 121, 122, 161
Linalyl acetate, 59
Lobinol, 10
Ludovicin A, *114, 115*
Lyngbyatoxin A, 84, *139*, 148, 178

Macassar II, *51, 110, 111*
Mancinellin, *137*
Mansonone A, *51*, 109, *110–1*
Mansonone X, 109, *110, 111*, 113
Melacacidin, *110, 111*
l-Menthol, *59*, 109, 121, *122*, 162
Methiin, 144, *145, 211*
4-Methoxydalbergione, *110, 111*
γ-Methylionone, *121*
Miconidin, 113
Miliamine A, *137*
8-MOP. *See* Xanthotoxin
Moroidin, 147, *148*

GENERAL INDEX

Numbers in italics indicate tables or figures, bold type indicates key information.

Resin ducts. *See* laticifers
Resorcinols, 45–46, 64, 96, 102, **105–6**, 126, 188
  biosynthesis, 103–5, *103*
  sources, *89–90*
  structures, 93
Rosin. *See* colophony
Rubber, 126, 165

Sap, 8, 61, 62, 70, 80, 133, **151**
  from *Euphorbia*, 73, 178
  from *Mangifera* and *Semecarpus*, 44, 58, 158
  from *Toxicodendron*, 26, 28, 90, 163–4, 167, 201
Sawdust, 49, 156, 159, 197
Scoville scale, 84
Sensitization, **17–8**, 165, 166, 167, 183, 187, 189, 190
Sesquiterpene lactones. *See* lactones
Singlet oxygen, 132, 133–4, 185–6
Skin (*see also* dermatotoxicity, toxic effects)
  absorption of chemicals, 13–4, 16, 172–4, 188
  biotransformations in, 14, *14*
  exposure to chemicals, 15, 151–65, *152*, *155*, *161*, *163*
  irritation, 16, 19, 85
  keratinocytes, 13, 183
  Langerhans cells, 13, 181, 182, *182*, 183
  permeability, 173–4
  sebum, 12, 173
  structure, **12–5**, *12*, 13, 173
Smith, Captain John. *See* Captain John Smith
Smoke, 18, 152, 159, *164*, 170, 178
Solubility, 8, 10, 11, *11*, 13, 14, 16, 98, *98*, 149, 173
Spices, 59, 60, 77–8, *78*, 84, *109*, 157, 162, *163*
Stinging emergence, 48 (*see also* trichomes)
Sunlight, 5, 19, 66, 67, 186 (*see also* phototoxicity)
Swimmer's itch, 84–5, 148

T cells. *See* lymphocytes
Tea tree oil, 60, 121, 163, *166*
Tequila, 85
Thiophenes, phototoxic, 72–3, 134
Toxicity (intoxication) (*see also* dermatotoxicity)
  definition, 16
  LD_{50}, 175, *175*
  process, 172
  types, 16
Transport (conveyance), 8, 164, *164*, 172–3, *173*
Trichomes, 8, **47**, 53, **82**, 148, 152
Tumorigenesis, 186–7
Turpentine, 62, 123

Ultraviolet (uv) radiation, 19, 66, 128, 132, 180, 185, 187 (*see also* sunlight)
Urticaria. *See* Contact urticaria
Urushioids (except urushiols or laccols), 8, 39, *40*, 45, **89–90**, 103–6, 159
  definition, **10**, 106, 166
  effects, 16, 47, 51, 87, 101, 178, 187, 189
  degradation, 95, 99–100, *100*
  synthesis, 102–4, *103*, *104*
  unusual, 93
Urushiols, 10, *51*, 87, *88*, 96, *175*, *188*
  history, **88–92**
  physical properties and spectra, 11, *11*, 97, *209*
  reactions, 93–6, *94*, 95, 99–100, *100*, 101
  sources, *88*, 207
  structures, *207*
  synthesis, 102, 103, *103*, *104*

Vapors, allergenic, 9, 10, 69, 98, 160–1, 162
Vapor pressure, 11, *11*, 98, *98*, 120, 160
Vitiligo, 70, 71, 73, 180
Volatility, 11, 98, *98*, 123, 144, 145, 146, 160–1

Weed dermatitis, **55**, 155, 156, 159, 180